W9-AHB-482

Surgery

PreTest™ Self-Assessment and Review

Notice

Medicine is an ever-changing science. As new research and clinical experience broaden our knowledge, changes in treatment and drug therapy are required. The authors and the publisher of this work have checked with sources believed to be reliable in their efforts to provide information that is complete and generally in accord with the standards accepted at the time of publication. However, in view of the possibility of human error or changes in medical sciences, neither the authors nor the publisher nor any other party who has been involved in the preparation or publication of this work warrants that the information contained herein is in every respect accurate or complete, and they disclaim all responsibility for any errors or omissions or for the results obtained from use of the information contained in this work. Readers are encouraged to confirm the information contained herein with other sources. For example and in particular, readers are advised to check the product information sheet included in the package of each drug they plan to administer to be certain that the information contained in this work is accurate and that changes have not been made in the recommended dose or in the contraindications for administration. This recommendation is of particular importance in connection with new or infrequently used drugs.

Surgery
PreTest™ Self-Assessment and Review
Eleventh Edition

Lillian S. Kao, M.D.
Assistant Professor and Co-Director, Surgery Clerkship
University of Texas—Houston Medical School
Houston, Texas

McGraw-Hill
Medical Publishing Division

New York   Chicago   San Francisco   Lisbon   London   Madrid   Mexico City
Milan   New Delhi   San Juan   Seoul   Singapore   Sydney   Toronto

Surgery: PreTest™ Self-Assessment and Review, Eleventh Edition

Copyright © 2006 by The McGraw-Hill Companies, Inc. All rights reserved. Printed in the United States of America. Except as permitted under the United States Copyright Act of 1976, no part of this publication may be reproduced or distributed in any form or by any means, or stored in a data base or retrieval system, without the prior written permission of the publisher.

PreTest is a trademark of The McGraw-Hill Companies, Inc.

2 3 4 5 6 7 8 9 0   DOC/DOC   0 9 8 7 6

ISBN 0-07-145770-4

This book was set in Berkeley by North Market Street Graphics.
The editor was Catherine A. Johnson.
The production supervisor was Sherri Souffrance.
Project management was provided by North Market Street Graphics.
The cover designer was Mary McKeon / Pinpoint.
RR Donnelley was printer and binder.

This book is printed on acid-free paper.

Library of Congress Cataloging-in-Publication Data

Surgery : PreTest self-assessment and review.—11th ed. / [edited by] Lilian S. Kao.
    p. ; cm.
  Includes bibliographical references and index.
  ISBN 0-07-145770-4
    1. Surgery—Examinations, questions, etc.   I. Kao, Lilian S.
  [DNLM: 1. Surgical Procedures, Operative—Examination Questions. WO 18.2 S961 2006]
  RD37.2.S97 2006
  617.0076—dc22   2006041908

Student Reviewers

Daniel Krochmal
University of Michigan Medical School
Class of 2006

Alvin Kwok
University of Utah School of Medicine
Class of 2006

Kevin L. Olson
VCU/Medical College of Virginia
Class of 2005

Stacy Ugras
Weill Medical College of Cornell University
Class of 2006

Contents

Introduction

Each question in *Surgery: PreTest™ Self-Assessment and Review,* Eleventh Edition, is accompanied by an answer, a paragraph explanation, and a specific page reference to either a current journal article, a textbook, or both. A bibliography, which lists all the sources used in the book, follows the last chapter.

Perhaps the most effective way to use this book is to allow yourself one minute to answer each question in a given chapter; as you proceed, indicate your answer beside each question. By following this suggestion, you will be approximating the time limits imposed by the board examinations.

When you have finished answering the questions in a chapter, you should then spend as much time as you need verifying your answers and carefully reading the explanations. Although you should pay special attention to the explanations for the questions you answered incorrectly, you should read every explanation. The authors of this book have designed the explanations to reinforce and supplement the information tested by the questions. If, after reading the explanations for a given chapter, you feel you need still more information about the material covered, you should consult and study the references indicated.

Pre- and Postoperative Care

Questions

DIRECTIONS: Each item below contains a question followed by suggested responses. Select the **one best** response to each question.

1. A 48-year-old woman develops constipation postoperatively and self-medicates with milk of magnesium. She presents to clinic, at which time her serum electrolytes are checked, and she is noted to have an elevated serum magnesium level. Which of the following represents the earliest clinical indication of hypermagnesemia?

a. Loss of deep tendon reflexes
b. Flaccid paralysis
c. Respiratory arrest
d. Hypotension
e. Stupor

2. Five days after an uneventful cholecystectomy, an asymptomatic middle-aged woman is found to have a serum sodium level of 125 meq/L. Which of the following is the most appropriate management strategy for this patient?

a. Administration of hypertonic saline solution
b. Restriction of free water
c. Plasma ultrafiltration
d. Hemodialysis
e. Aggressive diuresis with furosemide

3. A 50-year-old patient presents with symptomatic nephrolithiasis. He reports that he underwent a jejunoileal bypass for morbid obesity when he was 39. Which of the following is a complication of jejunoileal bypass?

a. Pseudohyperparathyroidism
b. Hyperuric aciduria
c. Hungry bone syndrome
d. Hyperoxaluria
e. Sporadic unicameral bone cysts

4. Following surgery, a patient develops oliguria. You believe the patient is hypovolemic, but you seek corroborative data before increasing intravenous fluids. Which of the following values supports the diagnosis of hypovolemia?

a. Urine sodium of 28 meq/L
b. Urine chloride of 15 meq/L
c. Fractional excretion of sodium less than 1
d. Urine/serum creatinine ratio of 20
e. Urine osmolality of 350 mOsm/kg

5. A 45-year-old woman with Crohn's disease and a small intestinal fistula develops tetany during the second week of parenteral nutrition. The laboratory findings include Na 135 meq/L, K 3.2 meq/L, Cl 103 meq/L, HCO_3^- 25 meq/L, Ca 8.2 meq/L, Mg 1.2 meq/L, PO4 2.4 meq/L, and albumin 2.4. An arterial blood gas reveals a pH of 7.42, pCO_2 of 38 mmHg, and PO_2 of 84 mmHg. Which of the following is the most likely cause of the patient's tetany?

a. Hyperventilation
b. Hypocalcemia
c. Hypomagnesemia
d. Essential fatty acid deficiency
e. Focal seizure

6. A patient with a nonobstructing carcinoma of the sigmoid colon is being prepared for elective resection. Which of the following reduces the risk of postoperative infectious complications?

a. A single preoperative parenteral dose of antibiotic effective against aerobes and anaerobes
b. Avoidance of oral antibiotics to prevent emergence of *Clostridium difficile*
c. Postoperative administration for 48 h of parenteral antibiotics effective against aerobes and anaerobes
d. Postoperative administration of parenteral antibiotics effective against aerobes and anaerobes until the patient's intravenous lines and all other drains are removed
e. Redosing of antibiotics in the operating room if the case lasts for more than 2 h

7. A 75-year-old man with a history of myocardial infarction two years ago, peripheral vascular disease with symptoms of claudication after ½ block, hypertension, and diabetes presents with a large ventral hernia. He wishes to have the hernia repaired. Which of the following is the most appropriate next step in his preoperative workup?

a. A normal EKG precludes the need for further cardiac testing
b. He should undergo an exercise stress test
c. He should undergo coronary artery bypass prior to operative repair of his ventral hernia
d. He should undergo a persantine thallium stress test and echocardiography
e. His history of a myocardial infarction within three years is prohibitive for elective surgery. No further testing is necessary.

8. A previously healthy 55-year-old man undergoes elective right hemicolectomy for a Stage I ($T_2N_0M_0$) cancer of the cecum. His postoperative ileus is somewhat prolonged, and on the fifth postoperative day his nasogastric tube is still in place. Physical examination reveals diminished skin turgor, dry mucous membranes, and orthostatic hypotension. Pertinent laboratory values are as follows: arterial blood gases: pH 7.56, P_{CO_2} 50 mmHg, P_{O_2} 85 mmHg. Serum electrolytes (meq/L): Na^+ 132, K^+ 3.1, Cl^- 80; HCO_3^- 42. Urine electrolytes (meq/L): Na^+ 2, K^+ 5, Cl^- 6. What is the patient's acid-base abnormality?

a. Uncompensated metabolic alkalosis
b. Respiratory acidosis with metabolic compensation
c. Combined metabolic and respiratory alkalosis
d. Metabolic alkalosis with respiratory compensation
e. Mixed respiratory acidosis and respiratory alkalosis

9. A 52-year-old man with gastric outlet obstruction secondary to a duodenal ulcer presents with hypochloremic, hypokalemic metabolic alkalosis. Which of the following is the most appropriate therapy for this patient?

a. Infusion of 0.9% NaCl with supplemental KCl until clinical signs of volume depletion are eliminated
b. Infusion of isotonic (0.15 N) HCl via a central venous catheter
c. Clamping the nasogastric tube to prevent further acid losses
d. Administration of acetazolamide to promote renal excretion of bicarbonate
e. Intubation and controlled hypoventilation on a volume-cycled ventilator to further increase P_{CO_2}

10. A 23-year-old woman is brought to the emergency room from a halfway house, where she apparently swallowed a handful of pills. The patient complains of shortness of breath and tinnitus, but refuses to identify the pills she ingested. Pertinent laboratory values are as follows: arterial blood gases: pH 7.45, P_{CO_2} 12 mmHg, P_{O_2} 126 mmHg. Serum electrolytes (meq/L): Na^+ 138, K^+ 4.8, Cl^- 102, HCO_3^- 8. An overdose of which of the following drugs would be most likely to cause the acid-base disturbance in this patient?

a. Phenformin
b. Aspirin
c. Barbiturates
d. Methanol
e. Diazepam (Valium)

11. An 18-year-old previously healthy male is placed on intravenous heparin after having a pulmonary embolism after exploratory laparotomy for a small bowel injury following a motor vehicle collision. Five days later, his platelet count is 90,000/µL and continues to fall over the next several days. The patient's serum is positive for antibodies to the heparin-platelet factor complexes. Which of the following is the most appropriate next management step?

a. Cessation of all anticoagulation therapy
b. Cessation of heparin and immediate institution of high-dose warfarin therapy
c. Cessation of heparin and institution of low-molecular-weight heparin
d. Cessation of heparin and institution of lepirudin
e. Cessation of heparin and transfusion with platelets

12. A 65-year-old man undergoes a technically difficult abdominal-perineal resection for a rectal cancer during which he receives three units of packed red blood cells. Four hours later, in the intensive care unit, he is bleeding heavily from his perineal wound. Emergency coagulation studies reveal normal prothrombin, partial thromboplastin, and bleeding times. The fibrin degradation products are not elevated, but the serum fibrinogen content is depressed and the platelet count is 70,000/µL. Which of the following is the most likely cause of his bleeding?

a. Delayed blood transfusion reaction
b. Autoimmune fibrinolysis
c. A bleeding blood vessel in the surgical field
d. Factor VIII deficiency
e. Hypothermic coagulopathy

13. A 78-year-old man with a history of coronary artery disease and an asymptomatic reducible inguinal hernia requests an elective hernia repair. Which of the following would be a valid reason for delaying the proposed surgery?

a. Coronary artery bypass surgery three months earlier
b. A history of cigarette smoking
c. Jugular venous distension
d. Hypertension
e. Hyperlipidemia

14. A 68-year-old man is admitted to the coronary care unit with an acute myocardial infarction. His postinfarction course is marked by congestive heart failure and intermittent hypotension. On the fourth hospital day, he develops severe midabdominal pain. On physical examination, blood pressure is 90/60 mmHg and pulse is 110 beats per minute and regular; the abdomen is soft with mild generalized tenderness and distention. Bowel sounds are hypoactive; stool hematest is positive. Which of the following is the most appropriate next step in this patient's management?

a. Barium enema
b. Upper gastrointestinal series
c. Angiography
d. Ultrasonography
e. Celiotomy

15. A 30-year-old woman in the last trimester of pregnancy suddenly develops massive swelling of the left lower extremity. Which of the following would be the most appropriate workup and treatment?

a. Venography and heparin
b. Duplex ultrasonography and heparin
c. Duplex ultrasonography, heparin, and vena caval filter
d. Duplex ultrasonography, heparin, warfarin (Coumadin)
e. Impedance plethysmography, warfarin

16. A 20-year-old woman is found to have an activated partial thrombo-plastin time (APTT) of 78/32 on routine testing prior to cholecystectomy. Further investigation reveals a prothrombin time (PT) of 13/12 (patient/control), a template bleeding time of 13 min, and a platelet count of 350,000/mm^3. Which of the following characteristics of this woman's coagulopathy is true?

a. Infusion of purified factor VIII is usually required to normalize its concentration prior to surgery
b. Infusion of cryoprecipitate will not be followed by an improvement in coagulation
c. Most of these patients are, or become, seropositive for HIV
d. Epistaxis or menorrhagia is uncommon
e. Lack of platelet aggregation in response to ristocetin is a common feature of this disease

17. A 45-year-old man has been diagnosed with polycythemia vera. He has chronic cholelithiasis and repeated episodes of cholecystitis. A cholecystectomy is planned. Which of the following is not true?

a. The most frequent complication is likely to be intraoperative and postoperative hemorrhage
b. Fresh-frozen plasma should be infused before surgery
c. Phlebotomy should be performed to a hematocrit of 48% or less
d. Platelets should be brought to a level of less than 400,000
e. Emergency surgery should be preceded by dilution with Ringer's lactate to normal hematocrit and platelet levels

18. A victim of blunt abdominal trauma requires a partial hepatectomy. He is rapidly transfused with eight units of appropriately cross-matched packed red blood cells from the blood bank. He is noted in the recovery room to be bleeding from intravenous puncture sites and the surgical incision. His coagulopathy is likely due to thrombocytopenia and deficiencies of which clotting factors?

a. II only
b. II and VII
c. V and VIII
d. IX and X
e. XI and XII

19. A 62-year-old woman undergoes a lysis of adhesions and bowel resection for small-bowel obstruction secondary to radiation enteritis after treatment for ovarian cancer. A jejunostomy is placed to facilitate nutritional repletion. Which of the following statements is true regarding postoperative nutrition?

a. Enteral nutrition has no advantages over parenteral nutrition in postoperative patients
b. Institution of enteral feeding within 24 h postoperatively is safe
c. Institution of enteral feeding should be delayed until bowel function returns as evidenced by passage of flatus or a bowel movement
d. Parenteral nutrition should be instituted immediately postoperatively and continued until enteral feeds have been initiated
e. Return of gastric motility postoperatively occurs before return of small-bowel motility

20. A 65-year-old woman has a life-threatening pulmonary embolus five days following removal of a uterine malignancy. She is immediately heparinized and maintained in good therapeutic range for the next three days, then passes gross blood from her vagina and develops tachycardia, hypotension, and oliguria. Following resuscitation, an abdominal CT scan reveals a major retroperitoneal hematoma. Which of the following is the best next management step?

a. Immediately reverse heparin by a calculated dose of protamine and place a vena caval filter (e.g., a Greenfield filter)
b. Reverse heparin with protamine, explore and evacuate the hematoma, and ligate the vena cava below the renal veins
c. Switch to low-dose heparin
d. Stop heparin and observe closely
e. Stop heparin, give fresh-frozen plasma (FFP), and begin warfarin therapy

21. A 71-year-old man develops dysphagia for both solids and liquids and weight loss of 60 lb over the past six months. He undergoes endoscopy, demonstrating a distal esophageal lesion, and biopsies are consistent with squamous cell carcinoma. He is scheduled for neoadjuvant chemoradiation followed by an esophagectomy and preoperatively is started on total parenteral nutrition, given his severe malnutrition reflected by an albumin of <1. Which of the following is most likely to be a concern initially in starting total parenteral nutrition in this patient?

a. Hyperkalemia
b. Hypermagesemia
c. Hypoglycemia
d. Hypophosphatemia
e. Hypochloremia

22. An elderly diabetic woman with chronic steroid-dependent bronchospasm has an ileocolectomy for a perforated cecum. She is taken to the ICU intubated and is maintained on broad-spectrum antibiotics, renal dose dopamine, and a rapid steroid taper. On postoperative day 2, she develops a fever of 39.2°C (102.5°F), hypotension, lethargy, and laboratory values remarkable for hypoglycemia and hyperkalemia. Which of the following is the most likely explanation for her deterioration?

a. Sepsis
b. Hypovolemia
c. Adrenal insufficiency
d. Acute tubular necrosis
e. Diabetic ketoacidosis

23. A cirrhotic patient with abnormal coagulation studies due to hepatic synthetic dysfunction requires an urgent cholecystectomy. A transfusion of fresh-frozen plasma is planned to minimize the risk of bleeding due to surgery. What is the optimal timing of this transfusion?

a. The day before surgery
b. The night before surgery
c. On call to surgery
d. Intraoperatively
e. In the recovery room

24. On postoperative day 5, an otherwise healthy 55-year-old man recovering from a partial hepatectomy is noted to have a fever to 38.6°C (101.5°F). Which of the following is the most common nosocomial infection postoperatively?

a. Wound infection
b. Pneumonia
c. Urinary tract infection
d. Intraabdominal abscess
e. Intravenous catheter-related infection

25. Ten days after an exploratory laparotomy and lysis of adhesions in a patient who previously underwent a low anterior resection for rectal cancer followed by postoperative chemoradiation, a patient is noted to have succus draining from the wound. She appears to have adequate source control—she is afebrile with a normal white blood count. The output from the fistula is approximately 150 cc per day. Which of the following factors is most likely to result in failure of the enterocutaneous fistula to close?

a. Previous radiation
b. Previous chemotherapy
c. Recent surgery
d. History of malignancy
e. More than 100 cc output per day

26. A 26-year-old trauma victim is being resuscitated with packed red blood cells following an auto accident complicated by hypotension from a fractured pelvis and resultant hemorrhage. The patient becomes hypotensive with a normal central venous pressure (CVP), oliguric, and febrile and complains of flank pain. Which of the following is the most likely diagnosis?

a. Hypovolemic shock
b. Acute adrenal insufficiency
c. Gram-negative bacteremia
d. Transfusion reaction
e. Ureteral obstruction

27. A 16-year-old male with a history of severe hemophilia A is undergoing an elective inguinal hernia repair. Which of the following is the best option for preventing or treating a bleeding complication in the setting of this disease?

a. Fresh-frozen plasma
b. Combination of desmopressin and fresh-frozen plasma
c. Desmopressin (DDAVP)
d. Combination of ε-aminocaprioic acid and desmopressin
e. Factor IX concentrate

28. A patient who is a candidate for a coronary artery bypass has osteoarthritis and consumes nonsteroidal anti-inflammatory agents for the pain. Prior to surgery, which one of the following tests should be ordered?

a. APTT
b. PT
c. Reptilase time
d. Bleeding time
e. Thrombin time

29. A 63-year-old man undergoes a partial gastrectomy with Billroth II reconstruction for intractable peptic ulcer disease. Which of the following metabolic disturbances is not a potential consequence of this procedure?

a. Megaloblastic anemia
b. Iron-deficiency anemia
c. Osteoporosis
d. Osteitis fibrosa cystica
e. Steatorrhea

30. A 52-year-old woman undergoes a sigmoid resection with primary anastomosis for recurrent diverticulitis. She returns to the emergency room 10 days later with left flank pain and decreased urine output; laboratory examination is significant for a white blood cell (WBC) count of 20,000/mm³. She undergoes a CT scan that demonstrates new left hydronephrosis, but no evidence of an intraabdominal abscess. Which of the following is the most appropriate next step in management?

a. Intravenous pyelogram
b. Intravenous antibiotics and repeat CT in one week
c. Administration of intravenous methylene blue
d. No further management if urinalysis is negative for hematuria
e. Immediate reexploration

31. A 23-year-old woman undergoes total thyroidectomy for carcinoma of the thyroid gland. On the second postoperative day, she begins to complain of a tingling sensation in her hands. She appears quite anxious and later complains of muscle cramps. Which of the following is the most appropriate initial management strategy?

a. 10 mL 10% magnesium sulfate intravenously
b. Oral vitamin D
c. 100 μg oral Synthroid
d. Continuous infusion of calcium gluconate
e. Oral calcium gluconate

32. A 42-year-old man sustains a gunshot wound to the abdomen and is in shock. Multiple units of packed red blood cells are transfused in an effort to resuscitate him. He complains of numbness around his mouth and displays carpopedal spasm and a positive Chvostek's sign. An electrocardiogram demonstrates a prolonged QT interval. Which of the following is the most appropriate treatment?

a. Intravenous bicarbonate
b. Intravenous potassium
c. Intravenous calcium
d. Intravenous digoxin
e. Intravenous parathyroid hormone

33. A 65-year-old man has an enterocutaneous fistula originating in the jejunum secondary to inflammatory bowel disease. Which of the following would be the most appropriate fluid for replacement of his enteric losses?

a. D5W
b. 3% normal saline
c. Ringer's lactate solution
d. 0.9% sodium chloride
e. 6% sodium bicarbonate solution

34. A 62-year-old man is suffering from arrhythmias on the night of his triple coronary bypass. Potassium has been administered. His urine output is 20 to 30 mL/h. Serum potassium level is 6.2. Which of the following medications counteracts the effects of potassium without reducing the serum potassium level?

a. Sodium polystyrene sulfonate (Kayexalate)
b. Sodium bicarbonate
c. 50% dextrose
d. Calcium gluconate
e. Insulin

35. An in-hospital workup of a 78-year-old hypertensive, mildly asthmatic man who is receiving chemotherapy for colon cancer reveals symptomatic gallstones. Preoperative laboratory results are notable for a hematocrit of 24% and a urinalysis with 18 to 25 WBCs and gram-negative bacteria. On call to the operating room, the patient receives intravenous penicillin. His abdomen is shaved in the operating room. An open cholecystectomy is performed and, despite a lack of indications, the common bile duct is explored. The wound is closed primarily with a Penrose drain exiting a separate stab wound. On postoperative day 3, the patient develops a wound infection. Which of the following changes in the care of this patient could have decreased the chance of a postoperative wound infection?

a. Increasing the length of the preoperative hospital stay to prophylactically treat the asthma with steroids
b. Treating the urinary infection prior to surgery
c. Shaving the abdomen the night prior to surgery
d. Continuing the prophylactic antibiotics for three postoperative days
e. Using a closed drainage system brought out through the operative incision

36. A 72-year-old man undergoes a subtotal colectomy for a cecal perforation due to a sigmoid colon obstruction. He has had a prolonged recovery and has been on total parenteral nutrition (TPN) for two weeks postoperatively. After regaining bowel function, he experienced significant diarrhea. Examination of his abdominal wound demonstrates minimal granulation tissue. He complains that he has lost his taste for food. He also has increased hair loss and a new perioral pustular rash. Which of the following deficiencies does he most likely have?

a. Zinc
b. Selenium
c. Molybdenum
d. Chromium
e. Thiamine

37. A 12-year-old boy with a femur fracture after a motor vehicle collision undergoes operative repair. After induction of anesthesia, he develops a fever to 40°C (104°F), shaking rigors, and blood-tinged urine. Which of the following is the best treatment option?

a. Alkalinization of the urine, administration of mannitol, and continuation with the procedure
b. Administration of dantrolene sodium and continuation with the procedure
c. Administration of dantrolene sodium and termination of the procedure
d. Administration of intravenous steroids and an antihistamine agent with continuation of the procedure
e. Administration of intravenous steroids and an antihistamine agent with termination of the procedure

38. A 24-year-old Jehovah's Witness who was in a high-speed motorcycle collision undergoes emergent splenectomy. His estimated blood loss was 1500 mL. Which of the following is most accurate regarding his resuscitation?

a. Vasopressors should be primarily utilized for maintenance of his blood pressure
b. Synthetic colloids should be administered as the primary resuscitation fluid in a 3:1 ratio to replace the volume of blood lost
c. Crystalloid solutions should be administered in a 1:1 ratio to replace the volume of blood lost
d. 0.45% normal saline should be administered in a 3:1 ratio to replace the volume of blood lost
e. A non-anion-gap acidosis may result from large-volume resuscitation with 0.9% normal saline

39. A 53-year-old man with no significant medical problems undergoes lysis of adhesions for a small-bowel obstruction. Postoperatively, he is placed on lactated Ringer's solution for the first 24 h. Which of the following is true regarding lactated Ringer's?

a. It contains a higher concentration of sodium ions than does plasma
b. It is most appropriate for replacement of nasogastric tube losses
c. It is isosmotic with plasma
d. It has a pH of less than 7.0
e. It may induce a significant metabolic acidosis

40. Four days after surgical evacuation of an acute subdural hematoma, a 44-year-old man becomes mildly lethargic and develops asterixis. He has received 2400 mL of 5% dextrose in water intravenously each day since surgery, and he appears well hydrated. Pertinent laboratory values are as follows: serum electrolytes (meq/L): Na$^+$ 118, K$^+$ 3.4, Cl$^-$ 82, HCO$_3^-$ 24, serum osmolality 242 mOsm/L, and urine sodium 47 meq/L. Urine osmolality: 486 mOsm/L. A correct statement about this patient's fluid and electrolyte status is which of the following?

a. His low serum sodium indicates sodium deficiency, which should be treated with 3% saline infusion
b. He probably has the syndrome of inappropriate secretion of antidiuretic hormone
c. His blood glucose level should be checked because the hyponatremia may be artifactual
d. Water restriction is rarely effective in severe cases of hyponatremia
e. The underlying problem is the inappropriate excretion of sodium (renal sodium wasting)

41. A 43-year-old woman develops acute renal failure following an emergency resection of a leaking abdominal aortic aneurysm. One week after surgery, the following laboratory values are obtained: serum electrolytes (meq/L): Na^+ 127, K^+ 5.9, Cl^- 92, HCO_3^- 15, blood urea nitrogen 82 mg/dL, and serum creatinine 6.7 mg/dL. The patient has gained 4 kg since surgery and is mildly dyspneic at rest. Eight hours after these values are reported, the following electrocardiogram is obtained. Which of the following is the most appropriate initial treatment for this patient?

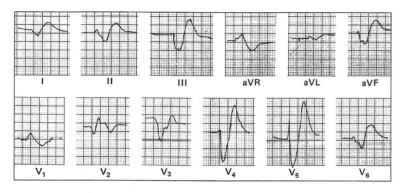

a. 10% calcium gluconate, 10 mL
b. 0.25 mg digoxin every 3 h for three doses
c. Oral Kayexalate
d. 100 mg lidocaine
e. Emergent hemodialysis

42. A 66-year-old obese woman has a prolonged length of stay in an intensive care unit after sustaining multiple injuries, including a severe head injury, in a motor vehicle collision. After one week in the hospital, she undergoes lower extremity duplex scanning and is found to have a left common femoral deep-venous thrombosis. Which of the following would not be an indication for the placement of a vena caval filter in this patient?

a. Recent intracranial hemorrhage
b. Presence of a complete venous occlusion of the common femoral vein
c. History of chronic pulmonary embolisms with pulmonary hypertension
d. Planned surgical procedure with contraindications for anticoagulation
e. Free-floating venous clot

43. A 63-year-old man with a 40-pack per year smoking history undergoes a low anterior resection for rectal cancer and on postoperative day 5 develops a fever, new infiltrate on chest x-ray, and leukocytosis. He is transferred to the intensive care unit for treatment of his pneumonia because of clinical deterioration. Which of the following is a sign of early sepsis?

a. Respiratory acidosis
b. Decreased cardiac output
c. Hypoglycemia
d. Increased arteriovenous oxygen difference
e. Peripheral vasodilation

44. A 60-year-old woman with no previous medical problems undergoes a total colectomy with diverting ileostomy for a cecal perforation secondary to a sigmoid stricture. Postoperatively, she has 2 L of ileostomy output per day. Her heart rate is 110 beats per minute, her respiratory rate is 16 breaths per minute, and her oxygen saturation is 98% on 2 L NC. Her laboratory values on postoperative day 6 are as follows: Na^+ 128, K^+ 3.0, Cl^- 102, and HCO_3^- 20. Which of the following statements is true?

a. Her laboratory abnormalities are most likely secondary to a Type IV renal tubular acidosis
b. Her laboratory abnormalities are most likely compensatory for a primary respiratory problem
c. She should be treated with fluid replacement and empiric treatment with oral Vancomycin
d. She should be treated with fluid replacement and stool-bulking agents
e. She should undergo immediate dialysis

45. A 39-year-old man is suspected of having had a transfusion reaction during resuscitation for an upper gastrointestinal (GI) bleed. Which of the following is appropriate in the management of this patient?

a. Removal of nonessential foreign body irritants, e.g., Foley catheter
b. Fluid restriction
c. 0.1 M HCl infusion
d. Steroids
e. Fluids and mannitol

46. A 45-year-old woman undergoes an uneventful laparoscopic cholecystectomy for which she receives one dose of cephalosporin. One week later, she returns to the emergency room with fever, nausea, and copious diarrhea and is subsequently diagnosed with pseudomembranous colitis. With respect to this disease, which one of the following statements is correct?

a. Surgical intervention is frequently required
b. After appropriate antibiotic therapy, the relapse rate is less than 5%
c. Tissue culture assay for *C. difficile* toxin B is neither sensitive nor specific; therefore, diagnosis should be based on clinical findings
d. If surgery is performed, a left hemicolectomy is usually adequate to treat pseudomembranous colitis
e. Indications for surgical treatment include intractable disease, failure of medical therapy, toxic megacolon, and colonic perforation

DIRECTIONS: The group of questions below consists of lettered options followed by a set of numbered items. For each numbered item, select the **one** lettered option with which it is **most** closely associated. Each lettered option may be used once, more than once, or not at all.

Questions 47–50

An average 70-kg man has a calculated basal energy expenditure of 1450 kcal/d. Match the following clinical situations with the appropriate daily energy requirement.

a. 1500 kcal/d
b. 2000 kcal/d
c. 2500 kcal/d
d. 3000 kcal/d
e. 4000 kcal/d

47. Sepsis

48. Multiple trauma, on a ventilator

49. Third-degree burns of 60% of body surface area (BSA)

50. Postoperative

Pre- and Postoperative Care

Answers

1. The answer is a. *(Brunicardi, p 49.)* The earliest clinical indication of hypermagnesemia is loss of deep tendon reflexes. States of magnesium excess are characterized by generalized neuromuscular depression. Clinically, severe hypermagnesemia is rarely seen except in those patients with advanced renal failure treated with magnesium-containing antacids. However, hypermagnesemia is produced intentionally by obstetricians who use parenteral magnesium sulfate ($MgSO_4$) to treat preeclampsia. $MgSO_4$ is administered until depression of the deep tendon reflexes is observed, a deficit that occurs with modest hypermagnesemia (over 4 meq/L). Greater elevations of magnesium produce progressive weakness, which culminates in flaccid quadriplegia and in some cases respiratory arrest due to paralysis of the chest bellows mechanism. Hypotension may occur because of the direct arteriolar relaxing effect of magnesium. Changes in mental status occur in the late stages of the syndrome and are characterized by somnolence that progresses to coma.

2. The answer is b. *(Brunicardi, pp 46, 52–54.)* The initial, and often definitive, management of hyponatremia is free-water restriction. Symptomatic hyponatremia, which occurs at serum sodium levels less than or equal to 120 meq/L, can result in headache, seizures, coma, and signs of increased intracranial pressure and may require infusion of hypertonic saline. Rapid correction should be avoided so as not to cause central pontine myelinolysis, manifested by neurologic symptoms ranging from seizures to brain damage and death. Additionally, a search for the underlying etiology of the hyponatremia should be undertaken. Acute severe hyponatremia sometimes occurs following elective surgical procedures due to a combination of appropriate stimulation of antidiuretic hormone and injudicious administration of excess free water in the first few postoperative days. Other potential etiologies include hyperosmolarity with free-water shifts from the intra- to the extracellular compartment (e.g., hyperglycemia), sodium depletion (e.g., gastrointestinal or renal losses, insufficient intake), dilution (e.g., drug-induced), and the syndrome of inappropriate secretion of anti-diuretic hormone (SIADH).

3. The answer is d. (*Greenfield, pp 769–770.*) Any patient who has lost much of the ileum (whether from injury, disease, or elective surgery) is at high risk of developing enteric hyperoxaluria if the colon remains intact. Calcium oxalate stones can subsequently develop due to excessive absorption of oxalate from the colon. Normally, fatty acids are absorbed by the terminal ileum, and calcium and oxalate combine to form an insoluble compound that is not absorbed. In the absence of the terminal ileum, unabsorbed fatty acids reach the colon, where they combine with calcium, leaving free oxalate to be absorbed. Unabsorbed fatty acids and bile acids in the colon also promote oxalate uptake by the colon. Subsequently, the excess oxalate is excreted by the kidneys, promoting calcium oxalate stone formation.

Hungry bone syndrome refers to rapid remineralization of bone leading to hypocalcemia and can be seen postoperatively in patients with secondary or tertiary hyperparathyroidism. Pseudohyperparathyroidism refers to hypercalcemia associated with the production of parathyroid-related peptide. A unicameral bone cyst is a benign lesion found in children.

4. The answer is c. (*Townsend, pp 314–316.*) A fractional excretion of sodium (FENa) of less than 1, which is calculated as (urine Na × serum creatinine) ÷ (serum sodium × urinary creatinine), supports a prerenal etiology for the patient's oliguria. When oliguria occurs postoperatively, it is important to differentiate between low output caused by the physiologic response to intravascular hypovolemia and that caused by acute tubular necrosis. A FENa of less than 1% in an oliguric setting indicates aggressive sodium reclamation in the tubules; values above this suggest tubular injury. In the setting of postoperative hypovolemia, all findings would reflect the kidney's efforts to retain volume: the urine sodium would be below 20 meq/L, the urine chloride would not be helpful except in the metabolically alkalotic patient, the urine osmolality would be over 500 mOsm/kg, the urine/serum creatinine ratio would be above 20, and the BUN-to-creatinine ratio would be above 20.

5. The answer is c. (*Brunicardi, pp 49, 55.*) Magnesium deficiency is common in malnourished patients and patients with large gastrointestinal fluid losses. The neuromuscular effects resemble those of calcium deficiency—namely, paresthesia, hyperreflexia, muscle spasm, and, ultimately, tetany. The cardiac effects are more like those of hypercalcemia. An electrocardiogram therefore provides a rapid means of differentiating between hypocalcemia (prolonged QT interval, T-wave inversion, heart blocks) and hypomagnesemia (prolonged QT and PR intervals, ST segment depression, flattening or inversion of p waves, torsade de pointes). Hypomagnesemia also causes potassium wasting by the kidney. Many hospital patients with refractory hypocalcemia will be found to be magnesium deficient. Often this deficiency becomes manifest during the response to parenteral nutrition when normal cellular ionic gradients are restored. A normal blood pH and arterial P_{CO_2} rule out hyperventilation. The serum calcium in this patient is normal when adjusted for the low albumin (add 0.8 mg/dL per 1 g/dL decrease in albumin). Hypomagnesemia causes functional hypoparathyroidism, which can lower serum calcium and thus result in a combined defect.

6. The answer is a. (*Townsend, pp 261–262.*) The appropriate dosing and timing of antibiotic prophylaxis to prevent surgical site infections in an elective procedure is a single dose, no greater than 1 h prior to the incision. Additionally, most textbooks recommend use of an oral, nonabsorbable antibiotic regimen effective against aerobes and anaerobes in combination with a mechanical bowel preparation before elective colon resections. There is no evidence to support the continuation of antibiotics for more than 12 h after an elective operation has been completed, and this practice should be avoided to prevent increasing microbial drug resistance. For complex, prolonged procedures, redosing of antibiotics may be appropriate during the procedure based on the drug's half-life. Broad-spectrum antibiotic coverage, including against anaerobic organisms, is required only in cases where such flora are anticipated, such as during colon resections; otherwise, cefazolin is the antibiotic of choice for cases requiring antibiotic prophylaxis.

7. The answer is d. (*Townsend, pp 222–223.*) The patient should undergo persantine thallium stress testing followed by echocardiography to assess his need for coronary angiogram with possible need for angioplasty, stenting, or surgical revascularization prior to repair of his hernia. Although exercise stress testing is an appropriate method for evaluating a patient's cardiac function preoperatively, this patient's functional status is limited by his peripheral vascular disease and therefore a pharmacologic stress test would be the preferred method of cardiac evaluation. An EKG should be performed in this patient with a history of cardiovascular disease, hypertension, and diabetes, but a normal EKG would not preclude further workup. While myocardial infarction (MI) within six months of surgery is considered to increase a patient's risk for a cardiac complication after surgery using Goldman's criteria, a remote history of MI is not prohibitive for surgery in and of itself.

8. The answer is d. (*Greenfield, pp 367–368.*) The patient has a metabolic alkalosis secondary to gastric losses of HCl, with compensatory hypoventilation as reflected by the elevated arterial pH and P_{CO_2} and supported by the absence of clinical lung disease. The P_{CO_2} would be normal if the metabolic akalosis was uncompensated. A respiratory acidosis with metabolic compensation would be characterized by decreased pH, increased P_{CO_2} levels, and increased bicarbonate levels. Mixed acid-base abnormalities should be suspected when the pH is normal but the P_{CO_2} and bicarbonate levels are abnormal or if the compensatory responses appear to be excessive or inadequate. The combination of respiratory acidosis and respiratory alkalosis is impossible.

9. The answer is a. (*Greenfield, pp 267–268.*) Infusion of 0.9% normal saline (sodium chloride) will correct his hypovolemia and his metabolic alkalosis. The development of a clinically significant metabolic alkalosis is secondary not only to the loss of acid or addition of alkali, but to renal responses that maintain the alkalosis. The normal kidney can tremendously augment its excretion of acid or alkali in response to changes in ingested load. However, in the presence of significant volume depletion and consequent excessive salt and water retention, the tubular maximum for bicarbonate reabsorption is increased. Correction of volume depletion alone is usually sufficient to correct the alkalosis, since the kidney will then excrete the excess bicarbonate. HCl infusion is usually unnecessary. Acetazolamide can be utilized to increase renal excretion of bicarbonate but should be avoided in volume-depleted individuals. Moreover, to the extent that acetazolamide causes natriuresis, it will exacerbate the volume depletion.

10. The answer is b. (*Brunicardi, p 52.*) This patient's history of tinnitus in conjunction with her mixed metabolic acidosis–respiratory alkalosis is pathognomonic of salicylate intoxication. Salicylates directly stimulate the respiratory center and produce respiratory alkalosis. By building up an accumulation of organic acids, salicylates also produce a concomitant metabolic acidosis. The patient is in a state of metabolic acidosis as shown by a markedly increased anion gap of 28 meq unmeasured anions per liter of plasma. However, the respiratory response is greater than can be explained by a compensatory response, since the patient is mildly alkalemic. The disturbance cannot be pure respiratory alkalosis, since the serum bicarbonate does not drop below 15 meq/L as a result of renal compensation and the anion gap does not vary by more than 1 to 2 meq/L from its normal value of 12 in response to a respiratory disturbance. The renal response to hyperventilation involves wasting of bicarbonate and compensatory retention of chloride; it does not involve a change in the concentration of unmeasured anions, such as albumin and organic acids.

Phenformin and methanol overdoses also produce high-anion-gap metabolic acidosis, but without the simultaneous respiratory disturbance. Sedatives, such as barbiturates or diazepam, would result in hypoventilation with respiratory acidosis.

11. The answer is d. (*Brunicardi, p 69.*) The patient has heparin-induced thrombocytopenia (HIT), which is a complication of heparin therapy, at both prophylactic and therapeutic doses. HIT is mediated by antibodies to the complexes formed by binding of heparin to platelet factor 4. In a previously unexposed patient, HIT typically manifests after five days as a decrease in platelet counts by 50% of the highest preceding value or to a level less than 100,000/mm^3. Complications of HIT are related to venous and/or arterial thromboembolic phenomena. Treatment of HIT consists of cessation of heparin (including low-molecular-weight heparins), institution of a nonheparin anticoagulant such as lepirudin, and conversion to oral warfarin when appropriate. Cessation of heparin alone is inadequate to prevent thromboembolic complications, and warfarin should not be started until the platelet count is above 100,000/mm^3. Platelet transfusion is not indicated, as HIT results in thrombotic rather than hemorrhagic complications.

12. The answer is c. (*Townsend, pp 118–120, 130, 298.*) Whenever significant bleeding is noted in the early postoperative period, the presumption should always be that it is due to an error in surgical control of blood vessels in the operative field. Hematologic disorders that are not apparent during the long operation are most unlikely to surface as problems postoperatively. Blood transfusion reactions can cause diffuse loss of clot integrity; the sudden appearance of diffuse bleeding during an operation may be the only evidence of an intraoperative transfusion reaction. In the postoperative period, transfusion reactions usually present as unexplained fever, apprehension, and headache—all symptoms difficult to interpret in the early postoperative period. Factor VIII deficiency (hemophilia) would almost certainly be known by history in a 65-year-old man, but if not, intraoperative bleeding would have been a problem earlier in this long operation. Moreover, factor VIII deficiency causes prolongation of the partial thromboplastin (PTT), which is normal in this patient. Severely hypothermic patients will not be able to form clots effectively, but clot dissolution does not occur. Care should be taken to prevent the development of hypothermia during long operations through the use of warmed intravenous fluid, gas humidifiers, and insulated skin barriers.

13. The answer is c. (*Townsend, pp 222–223.*) The work of Goldman and others has served to identify risk factors for perioperative myocardial infarction. The highest likelihood is associated with recent myocardial infarction: the more recent the event, the higher the risk up to six months. It should be noted, however, that the risk never returns to normal. A non-Q-wave infarction may not have destroyed much myocardium, but it leaves the surrounding area with borderline perfusion, thus the particularly high risk of subsequent perioperative infarction. Evidence of congestive heart failure, such as jugular venous distention, or S_3 gallop also carries a high risk, as does the frequent occurrence of ectopic beats. Old age (age > 70 years) and emergency surgery are risk factors independent of these others. Coronary revascularization by coronary artery bypass graft (CABG) tends to protect against myocardial infarction. Smoking, diabetes, hypertension, and hyperlipidemia (all of which predispose to coronary artery disease) are surprisingly not independent risk factors, although they may increase the death rate should an infarct occur. The value of this information and data derived from further testing is that it identifies the patient who needs to be monitored invasively with a systemic arterial catheter and pulmonary arterial catheter. Most perioperative infarcts occur postoperatively when the third-space fluids return to the circulation, which increases the preload and the myocardial oxygen consumption. This generally occurs around the third postoperative day.

14. The answer is c. *(Brunicardi, pp 1047–1049.)* In the absence of peritoneal signs, angiography is the diagnostic test of choice for acute mesenteric ischemia. Patients with peritoneal signs should undergo emergent laparotomy. Acute mesenteric ischemia may be difficult to diagnose. The condition should be suspected in patients with either systemic manifestations of arteriosclerotic vascular disease or low cardiac output states associated with a sudden development of abdominal pain that is out of proportion to the physical findings. Because of the risk of progression to small-bowel infarction, acute mesenteric ischemia is an emergency, and timely diagnosis is essential. Although patients may have lactic acidosis or leukocytosis, these are late findings. Abdominal films are generally unhelpful and may show a nonspecific ileus pattern. Since the pathology involves the small bowel, a barium enema is not indicated. Upper gastrointestinal series and ultrasonography are also of limited value. CT scanning has a sensitivity of 64 to 82% and is a good initial test, but should still be followed by angiography in a patient with clinically suspected acute mesenteric ischemia, even in the absence of findings on the CT scan. In addition to establishing the diagnosis in this stable patient, angiography may also assist with operative planning and elucidation of the etiology of the acute mesenteric ischemia. The cause may be embolic occlusion or thrombosis of the superior mesenteric artery, primary mesenteric venous occlusion, or nonocclusive mesenteric ischemia secondary to low cardiac output states. A mortality of 65 to 100% is reported. The majority of affected patients are at high operative risk, but since early diagnosis followed by revascularization or resectional surgery or both is the only hope for survival, celiotomy must be performed once the diagnosis of arterial occlusion or bowel infarction has been made. Initial treatment of nonocclusive mesenteric ischemia includes measures to increase cardiac output and blood pressure. Laparotomy should be performed if peritoneal signs develop.

15. The answer is b. *(Brunicardi, pp 811–821.)* Duplex ultrasound is the diagnostic modality of choice for detection of infrainguinal deep-venous thrombosis (DVT). Although venography is the gold standard, it is no longer routinely used, given the risks of local (thrombosis, pain) and contrast-related (allergic reaction, renal failure) complications. Impedance plethysmography, which measures changes in volume in the lower extremity as related to blood flow, is also used infrequently due to the superiority of duplex scanning in detecting DVTs. In pregnant women, anticoagulation for treatment of DVT is achieved with heparin, which does not cross the placenta, rather than warfarin, which is associated with the risk of spontaneous abortion and birth defects. The vena caval filter is not indicated because there is no contraindication to heparin therapy and no evidence of failure of anticoagulation therapy (pulmonary embolus in the face of adequate anticoagulation).

16. The answer is e. (*Greenfield, p 96.*) The patient has von Willebrand's disease (vWD), an autosomal dominant disorder that is manifested by a prolonged activated prothrombin time (aPTT) and, in 70% of patients, a failure to aggregate in response to the diagnostic reagent ristocetin. The deficiency of factor VIII activity (due to lack of von Willebrand factor which serves as a carrier for factor VIII) is generally less severe than in classic hemophilia and tends to fluctuate even in an untreated patient. However, the bleeding tendency is compounded by abnormal platelet function. This is responsible for the common occurrence of epistaxis and menorrhagia. Transfusion of cryoprecipitate provides vWF, whereas infusions of high-purity concentrates of factor VIII:C are not effective. These patients do not generally require treatment unless they need surgery or are severely injured. Because they do not receive frequent transfusions, patients with vWD are not at increased risk for HIV seropositivity.

17. The answer is b. (*Brunicardi, p 1304.*) Intraoperative and postoperative hemorrhage is a significant problem in the patient with polycythemia vera. Despite thrombocytosis, these patients have a hemorrhagic tendency generally ascribed to a qualitative deficiency of platelets. Elective surgery should be postponed until the hematocrit and platelet count reach normal levels. Alkylating agents, such as busulfan or chlorambucil, are effective in this regard. In the emergency situation, phlebectomy should be performed prior to operation and also an especially careful hemostatic technique should be employed. Infection is also a problem in patients with polycythemia vera, but hemorrhagic problems are the more frequently encountered complications.

18. The answer is c. (*Brunicardi, pp 77–79.*) When large amounts of banked blood are transfused, the recipient becomes deficient in factors V and VIII (the labile factors) and an acquired coagulopathy ensues. Since banked blood is also deficient in platelets, thrombocytopenia may also develop. Restoration of clotting factors can be achieved by transfusion of the patient with fresh-frozen plasma, which replaces vitamin K–dependent factors and is the only source of factor V. Platelets should also be transfused in thrombocytopenic patients.

19. The answer is b. (*Brunicardi, pp 31–32.*) The misconception that the entire bowel does not function in the early postoperative period is still widely held. Intestinal motility and absorption studies have clarified the patterns by which bowel activity resumes. The stomach remains uncoordinated in its muscular activity and does not empty efficiently for about 24 h after abdominal procedures. The small bowel functions normally within hours of surgery and is able to accept nutrients promptly, either by nasoduodenal or percutaneous jejunal feeding catheters or, after 24 h, by gastric emptying. The colon is stimulated in large measure by the gastrocolic reflex but ordinarily is relatively inactive for 3 to 4 days. Well-nourished patients who undergo uncomplicated surgical procedures can tolerate up to 10 days without full nutritional support before significant problems with protein breakdown begin to occur. Enteral nutrition is preferred over parenteral nutrition because of decreased risks of nosocomial infections and catheter-related complications.

20. The answer is a. (*Greenfield, p 100.*) In a heparinized patient with significant life-threatening hemorrhage, immediate reversal of heparin anticoagulation is indicated. Protamine sulfate is a specific antidote to heparin and should be given at 1 mg for each 100 U heparin if hemorrhage begins shortly after a bolus of heparin. For a patient in whom heparin therapy is ongoing, the dose should be based on the half-life of heparin (90 min). Since protamine is also an anticoagulant, only half the calculated circulating heparin should be reversed. The protaminization should be followed by placement of a percutaneous vena caval filter (Greenfield filter). In this critically ill patient, exploration of the retroperitoneal space would be surgically challenging and meddlesome.

21. The answer is d. (*Townsend, p 155.*) Hypophosphatemia is a complication of refeeding syndrome, which occurs in malnourished patients administered intravenous glucose. During periods of starvation, electrolytes are shifted to the extracellular space, and with refeeding, insulin levels rise and electrolytes are shifted back intracellularly, resulting in potential hypokalemia, hypomagnesemia, and hypophosphatemia. Early complications of TPN also include hyperglycemia, hyperchloremic acidosis, and volume overload with resultant heart failure. TPN, particularly in the extremely malnourished patient, should be started slowly; magnesium, potassium, and phosphate levels should be repleted; and dextrose infusions should be limited to prevent complications of refeeding.

22. The answer is c. (*Brunicardi, pp 1463–1465.*) Acute adrenal insufficiency can occur in patients with severe stress, infection, or trauma or as a result of abrupt cessation or too rapid tapering of chronic glucocorticoid therapy, and is classically manifested as changing mental status, increased temperature, cardiovascular collapse, hypoglycemia, and hyperkalemia. The diagnosis can be difficult to make and requires a high index of suspicion. Its clinical presentation is similar to that of sepsis; however, sepsis is generally associated with hyperglycemia and no significant change in potassium. The treatment for adrenal crisis is intravenous steroids, volume resuscitation, and other supportive measures to treat any new or ongoing stress. Dexamethasone is the steroid replacement of choice when empirically treating adrenal insufficiency since hydrocortisone can interfere with confirmatory testing (ACTH stimulation test). Steroid treatment can be subsequently converted to oral medication and tapered after treatment of the adrenal crisis.

23. The answer is c. (*Brunicardi, p 78.*) Transfusions with fresh-frozen plasma (FFP) to replenish vitamin K–dependent clotting factors should be administered on call to the operating room. The timing of transfusion is dependent on the quantity of each factor delivered and its half-life. The half-life of the most stable clotting factor, factor VII, is 4 to 6 h. Thus, transfusion of FFP on call to the operating room ensures that the transfusion is complete prior to the incision, with circulating factors to cover the operative and immediate postoperative period.

24. The answer is c. (*Brunicardi, p 353.*) The most common nosocomial infection is a urinary tract infection. Treatment consists of removal of an indwelling catheter as soon as possible and antibiotic therapy for cultures with greater than 100,000 CFU/mL. Pneumonias, wound infections, intraabdominal abscesses, and catheter-related bloodstream infections are also all causes of nosocomial infections, and a workup of a postoperative fever should also include careful examination of the patient and other diagnostic tests as appropriate (chest x-ray, blood cultures, abdominal/pelvic CT scan).

25. The answer is a. *(Brunicardi, p 347.)* Factors that predispose to fistula formation and may prevent closure include foreign body, radiation, inflammation, epithelialization of the tract, neoplasm, distal obstruction, and steroids. Treatment consists of source control, nutritional supplementation, wound care, and delayed surgical intervention if the fistula fails to close.

26. The answer is d. *(Townsend, p 130.)* Allergic and febrile reactions occur in about 1% of all transfusions. Hemolytic transfusion reactions are much less common (0.2%), with fatal reactions in 1 of 100,000 transfusions. Hemolytic transfusion reactions are due to the reaction of recipient antibodies against transfused antigens. These reactions can be both immediate and delayed. Symptoms of a hemolytic transfusion reaction include fever, chills, and pain and heat at the infusion site, as well as respiratory distress, anxiety, hypotension, and oliguria. During surgery, a hemolytic transfusion reaction can manifest as abnormal bleeding.

27. The answer is d. *(Townsend, pp 118–120.)* Hemophilia A is a disorder of or a deficiency of factor VIII, and for severe hemophilia, a combination of ε-aminocaproic acid (AMICAR), which is an inhibitor of fibrinolysis, and desmopressin (DDAVP), which is a synthetic analogue of antidiuretic hormone that increases levels of factor VIII and von Willebrand factor, can be used. DDAVP alone can be used for mild hemophilia A. Although fresh-frozen plasma (FFP) contains factor VIII, the levels are insufficient to prevent bleeding in hemophiliacs. However, cryoprecipitate or recombinant factor VIII can be used.

28. The answer is d. *(Townsend, p 122.)* Platelet dysfunction, measured by bleeding time, has been associated with a long list of drugs. Nonsteroidal anti-inflammatory agents, sulfa-based antibiotics, alcohol, thiazide diuretics, quinidine and quinine, and other drugs have been associated with thrombasthenia. Anytime platelet abnormalities are suspected, a careful review of the drugs the patient is receiving should be undertaken, and a measurement should be made of the platelet count and bleeding time. Platelet dysfunction does not affect APTT, PT, reptilase, or thrombin times.

29. The answer is d. *(Townsend, pp 1296–1297.)* Osteitis cystica fibrosa is a finding in patients with primary hyperparathyroidism and represents subperiosteal resorption, characteristically on the radial aspect of the middle phalanx. This is not a reported complication after partial gastrectomy. Patients who have undergone partial gastrectomy may, however, have osteoporosis secondary to impaired calcium absorption due to the Billroth II reconstruction (since calcium is normally absorbed in the proximal intestine—duodenum and jejunum). Fatty acids may also be malabsorbed due to inadequate mixing of bile salts and lipase with ingested fat, and therefore steatorrhea may result. Either megaloblastic anemia due to vitamin B_{12} deficiency (due to lack of intrinsic factor, which is necessary for B_{12} absorption and is normally produced by the parietal cells of the stomach) or microcytic anemia due to iron deficiency (due to decreased iron intake and impaired absorption in the duodenum) can result after partial gastrectomy.

30. The answer is a. *(Brunicardi, pp 175, 1606.)* The patient should undergo an intravenous pyelogram for a suspected ureteral injury. After gynecologic surgeries, colorectal surgery is the most common cause of iatrogenic ureteral injuries. Intraoperatively, intravenous administration of methylene blue or indigocyanine green may facilitate identification of an injury. However, delay in diagnosis is common, and patients may present with flank pain, fevers, and signs of sepsis, ileus, or decreased urine output. CT scan may demonstrate hydronephrosis or a fluid collection (urinoma). Initial diagnosis and management should include urinalysis, although hematuria may not always be present; percutaneous nephrostomy tube or retrograde ureteral catheterization; percutaneous drainage of fluid collections; and identification of the location of ureteral injury. Surgical management should be delayed if diagnosis is late (10 to 14 days), and operative strategy is dependent on the location of the injury. Diagnostic imaging such as a pyelogram or nuclear medicine scan may be helpful to identify the site of the injury.

31. The answer is d. *(Brunicardi, p 1448.)* Intravenous calcium infusion is the treatment for severe, symptomatic hypocalcemia, although, typically, oral calcium supplementation (up to 1 to 2 g every 4 h) is sufficient in patients with mild symptoms. Since post-thyroidectomy hypocalcemia is usually due to transient ischemia of the parathyroid glands and is self-limited, in most cases the problem is resolved in several days. In cases of persistent hypocalcemia, Vitamin D preparations may be necessary. There is no role for thyroid hormone replacement or magnesium sulfate in the treatment of hypocalcemia.

32. The answer is c. *(Brunicardi, p 50.)* Hypocalcemia is associated with a prolonged QT interval and may be aggravated by both hypomagnesemia and alkalosis. Additionally, massive transfusion is associated with hypocalcemia secondary to chelation with citrate in banked blood. Severe, symptomatic hypocalcemia, encountered most frequently following parathyroid or thyroid surgery or in patients with acute pancreatitis, should be treated with intravenous calcium gluconate. The myocardium is very sensitive to calcium levels; therefore, calcium is considered a positive inotropic agent. Calcium increases the contractile strength of cardiac muscle as well as the velocity of shortening. In its absence, the efficiency of the myocardium decreases. Hypocalcemia often occurs with hypoproteinemia, even though the ionized serum calcium fraction remains normal.

33. The answer is c. *(Brunicardi, pp 46, 52–53.)* Bile and the fluids found in the duodenum, jejunum, and ileum all have an electrolyte content similar to that of Ringer's lactate. Saliva, gastric juice, and right colon fluids have high K^+ and low Na^+ content. Pancreatic secretions are high in bicarbonate. It is important to consider these variations in electrolyte patterns when calculating replacement requirements following gastrointestinal losses.

34. The answer is d. *(Brunicardi, pp 47–48.)* Calcium gluconate does not affect the serum potassium level but rather counteracts the myocardial effects of hyperkalemia. Reduction of an elevated serum potassium level, however, is important to avoid the cardiovascular complications that ultimately culminate in cardiac arrest. Kayexalate is a cation exchange resin that is instilled into the gastrointestinal tract and exchanges sodium for potassium ions. Its use is limited to semiacute and chronic potassium elevations. Sodium bicarbonate causes a rise in serum pH and shifts potassium intracellularly. Administration of glucose initiates glycogen synthesis and uptake of potassium. Insulin can be used in conjunction with this to aid in the shift of potassium intracellularly.

35. The answer is b. *(Brunicardi, pp 118–120.)* The determinants of a postoperative wound infection include those related to the bacteria, the environment (i.e., the wound), and the host's defense mechanisms. Within this triad there are factors predetermined by the status of the patient [e.g., age, obesity, steroid dependence, multiple diagnoses (more than three), immunosuppression] and by the type of procedure (e.g., contaminated versus clean, emergent versus elective). However, there are several factors that can be optimized by the surgeon. Decreasing the bacterial inoculum and virulence by limiting the patient's prehospital stay, clipping the operative site in the operating room, administering perioperative antibiotics (within a 24-h period surrounding operation) with an appropriate antimicrobial spectrum, treating remote infections, avoiding breaks in technique, using closed drainage systems (if needed at all) that exit the skin away from the surgical incision, and minimizing the duration of the operation have all been shown to decrease postoperative infection. Making a wound less favorable to infection requires attention to basic Halstedian principles of hemostasis, anatomic dissection, and gentle handling of tissues as well as limiting the amount of foreign body and necrotic tissue in the wound. Although they are the most difficult factors to influence, host defense mechanisms can be improved by optimizing nutritional status, tissue perfusion, and oxygen delivery.

36. The answer is a. (*Townsend, p 156.*) The patient has a zinc deficiency. Alopecia, poor wound healing, night blindness or photophobia, anosmia, neuritis, and skin rashes are all characteristic of patients with zinc deficiency, which often results in the setting of excessive diarrhea. Selenium deficiency is characterized by the development of a cardiomyopathy. Molybdenum deficiency is manifested by encephalopathy due to toxic accumulation of sulfur-containing amino acids. Chromium deficiency can occur in patients on long-term TPN and is characterized by difficult-to-control hyperglycemia and peripheral neuropathy and encephalopathy. Thiamine deficiency results in beriberi, which includes symptoms of encephalopathy and peripheral neuropathy; patients with beriberi can also develop cardiovascular symptoms and cardiac failure.

37. The answer is c. (*Brunicardi, pp 356–357.*) The patient is manifesting symptoms of malignant hyperthermia (fevers, rigors, and myoglobinuria), which is treated by administration of dantrolene, immediate discontinuation of offending medication (which can include succinylcholine or halothane-based inhalational anesthetics), and supportive cooling measures. While urine alkalinization, loop diuretics, and mannitol are appropriate treatment measures for rhabdomyolysis, the underlying problem in this patient is malignant hyperthermia, which, because of its associated mortality of 30% in severe cases should be treated first and foremost. Malignant hyperthermia is not a manifestation of anaphylactic shock, and, therefore, steroids and antihistamines have no role in its treatment.

38. The answer is e. (*Townsend, p 98; Brunicardi, p 53.*) Following administration of large volumes of normal saline, a non-anion-gap metabolic acidosis can result from increased choloride concentrations. Normal saline and lactated Ringer's solution are examples of isotonic saline solutions, both of which can be used to replace the volume of blood lost in a ratio of 3:1. Hypotonic saline solutions such as 0.45% normal saline should not be used for acute resuscitation in hemorrhagic shock but are appropriate for postoperative fluid maintenance in the hemodynamically stable patient. The use of colloids in resuscitation of patients in hemorrhagic shock is controversial; in general, however, colloids can be used to replace blood volume lost in a ratio of 1:1. The definitive treatment of hypovolemic shock is fluid resuscitation, not initiation of vasopressors.

39. The answer is d. (*Townsend, p 98; Brunicardi, p 53.*) Isotonic saline solutions contain 154 meq/L of both sodium and chloride ions. Each ion is in a substantially higher concentration than is found in the normal serum (Na = 142 meq/L; Cl = 103 meq/L). When isotonic solutions are given in large quantities, they overload the kidney's ability to excrete chloride ion, which results in a dilutional acidosis. They also may intensify preexisting acidosis by reducing the base bicarbonate–carbonic acid ratio in the body. Isotonic saline solutions are particularly useful in hyponatremic or hypochloremic states and whenever a tendency to metabolic alkalosis is present, as occurs with significant nasogastric suction losses or vomiting. Administration of lactated Ringer's solution is appropriate for replacing gastrointestinal losses and correcting extracellular fluid deficits. Containing 130 meq/L sodium, lactated Ringer's is hyposmolar with respect to sodium and provides approximately 150 mL of free water with each liter given. Although this is ordinarily not a significant load, in some clinical situations it can be. Lactated Ringer's is sufficiently physiological to enable administration of large amounts without significantly affecting the body's acid-base balance. It is worth noting that both isotonic saline and lactated Ringer's are acidic with respect to the plasma: 0.9% NaCl/5% dextrose has a pH of 4.5, while lactated Ringer's has a pH of 6.5.

40. The answer is b. (*Brunicardi, pp 56–57.*) The patient presented has the syndrome of inappropriate antidiuretic hormone secretion (SIADH). Although this syndrome is associated primarily with diseases of the central nervous system or of the chest (e.g., oat cell carcinoma of the lung), excessive amounts of antidiuretic hormone are also present in most postoperative patients. The pathophysiology of SIADH involves an inability to dilute the urine; administered water is therefore retained, which produces dilutional hyponatremia. Body sodium stores and fluid balance are normal, as evidenced by the absence of the clinical findings suggestive of abnormalities of extracellular fluid volume. While hypertonic saline infusions can transiently improve hyponatremia, the appropriate therapy is to restrict water ingestion to a level below the patient's ability to excrete water. Hypertonic saline may be dangerous, since it can shift accumulated water into the extracellular fluid and precipitate pulmonary edema in the patient who suffers from low cardiac reserves. Hyperglycemia cannot account for the hyponatremia seen in this patient because the serum osmolality, as well as the serum sodium, is depressed. Hyponatremia resulting from hyperglycemia would be associated with an elevated serum osmolality.

41. The answer is a. (*Brunicardi, pp 47–48, 54.*) The electrocardiogram demonstrates changes that are essentially diagnostic of severe hyperkalemia. Correct treatment for the affected patient includes discontinuation of exogenous sources of potassium, administration of a source of calcium ions (which will immediately oppose the myocardial effects of potassium), and administration of sodium bicarbonate (which, by producing a mild alkalosis, will shift potassium into cells); each will temporarily reduce serum potassium concentration. Infusion of glucose and insulin would also effect a temporary transcellular shift of potassium. However, these maneuvers are only temporarily effective; definitive treatment calls for removal of potassium from the body. The sodium-potassium exchange resin sodium polystyrene sulfonate (Kayexalate) would accomplish this removal, but over a period of hours and at the price of adding a sodium ion for each potassium ion that is removed. Hemodialysis or peritoneal dialysis is probably required for this patient, since these procedures also rectify the other consequences of acute renal failure, but they would not be the first line of therapy, given the acute need to reduce the potassium level. Both lidocaine and digoxin would be not only ineffective but contraindicated, since they would further depress the myocardial conduction system.

42. The answer is b. (*Brunicardi, p 346; Greenfield, pp 1884–1885.*) The presence of a complete venous occlusion of the femoral vein is *not* an indication for caval interruption. Placement of a vena caval filter (Greenfield filter) is indicated in patients for whom anticoagulation is contraindicated (such as those who have had a recent intracranial or gastrointestinal bleed), for whom anticoagulation has failed (development of a DVT or pulmonary embolus on therapeutic doses of anticoagulants), who have a free-floating ileofemoral or vena caval venous clot, or who have chronic PE complicated by pulmonary hypertension.

43. The answer is e. (*Brunicardi, pp 98–99.*) It is important to identify and treat occult or early sepsis before it progresses to septic shock and the associated complications of multiple organ failure. An immunocompromised host may not manifest some of the more typical signs and symptoms of infection, such as elevated temperature and white cell count; this forces the clinician to focus on more subtle signs and symptoms. Early sepsis is a physiologically hyperdynamic, hypermetabolic state representing a surge of catecholamines, cortisol, and other stress-related hormones. Changing mental status, tachypnea that leads to respiratory alkalosis, and flushed skin are often the earliest manifestations of sepsis. Intermittent hypotension requiring increased fluid resuscitation to maintain adequate urine output is characteristic of occult sepsis. Hyperglycemia and insulin resistance during sepsis are typical in diabetic as well as nondiabetic patients. This relates to the gluconeogenic state of the stress response. The cardiovascular response to early sepsis is characterized by an increased cardiac output, decreased systemic vascular resistance, and decreased peripheral utilization of oxygen, which yields a decreased arteriovenous oxygen difference.

44. The answer is d. (*Brunicardi, pp 50–51.*) The patient has a non-gap metabolic acidosis, $[(Na^+) - (Cl^- + HCO_3^-) = (128) - (102 + 20) = 6]$, secondary to high output from her ileostomy with gastrointestinal losses of bicarbonate. This should be managed with fluid replacement and stool-bulking agents. The ionic composition of small-bowel fluid is Na^+ 140, K^+ 5, Cl^- 104, and HCO_3^- 30. Patients with large ileostomy outputs are at risk for dehydration with accompanying hyponatremia, hypokalemia, and non-anion-gap metabolic acidosis. While renal tubular acidosis (RTA) can be associated with a non-anion-gap metabolic acidosis, type IV RTAs are typically associated with hyperkalemia. Renal failure can result in an anion-gap, uremic acidosis and hyperkalemia, both of which may be indications for dialysis. Finally, while *C. difficile* colitis should be considered in postoperative patients with diarrhea, *C. difficile* enteritis is less common in a non-immunocompromised host, and Vancomycin is reserved for failures to metronidazole treatment.

45. The answer is e. *(Townsend, p 130.)* Hemolytic transfusion reactions lead to hypotension and oliguria. The increased hemoglobin in the plasma will be cleared via the kidneys, which leads to hemoglobinuria. Placement of an indwelling Foley catheter with subsequent demonstration of oliguria and hemoglobinuria not only confirms the diagnosis of a hemolytic transfusion reaction but is useful in monitoring corrective therapy. Treatment begins with discontinuation of the transfusion, followed by aggressive fluid resuscitation to support the hypotensive episode and increase urine output. Inducing diuresis through aggressive fluid resuscitation and osmotic diuretics is important to clear the hemolyzed red cell membranes, which can otherwise collect in glomeruli and cause renal damage. Alkalinization of the urine (pH > 7) helps prevent hemoglobin clumping and renal damage. Steroids do not have a role in the treatment of hemolytic transfusion reactions.

46. The answer is e. *(Brunicardi, p 1100.)* Indications for surgical treatment of *C. difficile* colitis are intractable disease, failure of medical therapy, toxic megacolon, and colonic perforation; surgical therapy consists of subtotal colectomy with end ileostomy. The diagnosis can be made by either detection of the characteristic appearance of pseudomembranes on endoscopy or detection of either toxin A or toxin B in the stool. Treatment is metronidazole for first-line therapy and oral vancomycine as a second-tier agent. Recurrence appears in up to 20% of patients.

47–50.   The answers are 47-b, 48-c, 49-d, 50-a. *(Greenfield, p 45.)* Resting energy expenditure (REE) can be calculated using indirect calorimetry and increases above basal levels depending on the disease process. The following table summarizes the REEs for various disease states:

Caloric Requirements for the Average Adult (70 kg) Man
(from Greenfield)

Disease process	Kcal/d
Basal	1450
Postoperative (uncomplicated)	1500–1700
Sepsis	2000–2400
Multiple trauma (ventilated)	2200–2600
Major burn	2500–3000

Critical Care: Anesthesiology, Blood Gases, and Respiratory Care

Questions

DIRECTIONS: Each item below contains a question followed by suggested responses. Select the **one best** response to each question.

51. A 75-year-old thin cachectic woman undergoes a tracheostomy for failure to wean from the ventilator. One week later, she develops significant bleeding from the tracheostomy. Which of the following would be an appropriate initial step in the management of this problem?

a. Remove the tracheostomy and place pressure over the wound
b. Deflate the balloon cuff on the tracheostomy
c. Attempt to reintubate the patient with an endotracheal tube
d. Upsize the tracheostomy
e. Perform fiberoptic evaluation immediately

52. A 53-year-old woman has been intubated for several days after sustaining a right pulmonary contusion after a motor vehicle collision as well as multiple rib fractures. Which of the following is a reasonable indication to attempt extubation?

a. Negative inspiratory force (NIF) of -15 cm H_2O
b. A PO_2 of 60 mmHg while breathing 30% inspired FiO_2 with a PEEP of 10 cm H_2O
c. Spontaneous respiratory rate of 35 breaths per minute
d. A rapid shallow breathing index of 80
e. Minute ventilation of 18 L/min

53. A 19-year-old male receives un-cross-matched blood during resuscitation after a gunshot wound to the abdomen. He develops fever, tachycardia, and oliguria during the transfusion and is diagnosed as having a hemolytic reaction. Which of the following treatments is most likely to be helpful?

a.   Administration of a loop diuretic such as furosemide
b.   Treating anuria with fluid and potassium replacement
c.   Acidifying the urine to prevent hemoglobin precipitation in the renal tubules
d.   Removing foreign bodies, such as Foley catheters, which may cause hemorrhagic complications
e.   Stopping transfusion immediately

54. A 74-year-old woman with a history of a previous total abdominal hysterectomy presents with abdominal pain and distention for three days. She is noted on plain films to have dilated small-bowel and air-fluid levels. She is taken to the operating room for a small-bowel obstruction. Which of the following inhalational anesthetics should be avoided because of accumulation in air-filled cavities during general anesthesia?

a.   Diethyl ether
b.   Nitrous oxide
c.   Halothane
d.   Methoxyflurane
e.   Trichloroethylene

55. A 61-year-old alcoholic man presents with severe epigastric pain radiating to his back. His amylase and lipase are elevated, and he is diagnosed with acute pancreatitis. Over the first 48 h, he is determined to have six Ranson's criteria, including a P_{O_2} less than 60 mmHg. His chest x-ray reveals bilateral pulmonary infiltrates, and his wedge pressure is low. Which of the following major alterations in pulmonary function is associated with adult respiratory distress syndrome (ARDS)?

a.   Hypoxemia
b.   Increased pulmonary compliance
c.   Increased resting lung volume
d.   Increased functional residual capacity
e.   Decreased dead-space ventilation

56. The curve depicted here plots the normal relationship of arterial P_{O_2} and percentage of hemoglobin saturation with other variables controlled at pH 7.4, P_aCO_2 40 mmHg, temperature 37°C (98.6°F), and hemoglobin 15 g/dL. Which of the following statements regarding this oxygen dissociation relationship is true?

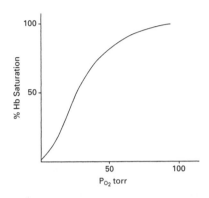

a. Modest decrements of arterial P_{O_2} have a major effect on alveolar oxygen uptake
b. Modest decrements of hemoglobin saturation have a major effect on tissue oxygen uptake
c. The curve shifts to the left with acidosis
d. The curve shifts to the left following banked blood transfusion
e. The curve is unaffected by chronic lung disease

57. A 64-year-old man afflicted with severe emphysema, who receives oxygen therapy at home, is admitted to the hospital because of upper gastrointestinal bleeding. The bleeding ceases soon after admission, and the patient becomes agitated and then disoriented; he is given 5 mg of intramuscular diazepam (Valium). Twenty minutes later he is unresponsive. Physical examination reveals a stuporous but arousable man who has papilledema and asterixis. Arterial blood gases are as follows: pH 7.17; P_{O_2} 42 mmHg; P_{CO_2} 95 mmHg. Which of the following is the best initial therapy for this patient?

a. Correct hypoxemia with high-flow nasal oxygen
b. Correct acidosis with sodium bicarbonate
c. Administer 10 mg intravenous dexamethasone
d. Intubate the patient
e. Call for neurosurgical consultation

58. A 62-year-old woman with a history of coronary artery disease presents with a pancreatic head tumor and undergoes a pancreaticoduodenectomy. Postoperatively, she develops a leak from the pancreaticojejunostomy anastomosis and becomes septic. A Swan-Ganz catheter is placed, which demonstrates an increased cardiac output and decreased systemic vascular resistance. She also develops acute renal failure and oliguria. Dopamine is started. Which of the following effects does dopamine have?

a. At high doses it increases splanchnic flow
b. At high doses it increases coronary flow
c. At low doses it decreases heart rate
d. At low doses it lowers peripheral resistance
e. It inhibits catecholamine release

59. A 29-year-old woman on oral contraceptives presents with abdominal pain. A CT scan of the abdomen demonstrates a large hematoma of the right liver with the suggestion of an underlying liver lesion. Her hemoglobin is 6, and she is symptomatic in terms of tachycardia and light-headedness. Because of her age, the patient wishes to know more about the risk of infection with blood transfusion. Which of the following statements regarding transmission of viral illness through homologous blood transfusion is true?

a. The most common viral agent transmitted via blood transfusion in the United States is human immunodeficiency virus (HIV)
b. Blood is routinely tested for cytomegalovirus (CMV) because CMV infection is often fatal
c. The most frequent infectious complication of blood transfusion continues to be viral meningitis
d. Up to 10% of those who develop posttransfusion hepatitis will develop cirrhosis or hepatoma or both
e. The etiologic agent in posttransfusion hepatitis remains undiscovered

60. A 68-year-old hypertensive man undergoes successful repair of a ruptured abdominal aortic aneurysm. He receives 9 L Ringer's lactate solution and four units of whole blood during the operation. Two hours after transfer to the surgical intensive care unit, the following hemodynamic parameters are obtained: systemic blood pressure (BP) 90/60 mmHg, pulse 110 beats per minute, central venous pressure (CVP) 7 mmHg, pulmonary artery pressure 28/10 mmHg, pulmonary capillary wedge pressure 8 mmHg, cardiac output 1.9 L/min, systemic vascular resistance 1400 (dyne·sec)/cm^5 (normal is 900 to 1300), PaO_2 140 mmHg (FiO_2: 0.45), urine output 15 mL/h (specific gravity: 1.029), and hematocrit 35%. Which of the following is the most appropriate management given this data?

a. Administration of a diuretic to increase urine output
b. Administration of a vasopressor agent to increase systemic blood pressure
c. Administration of a fluid challenge to increase urine output
d. Administration of a vasodilating agent to decrease elevated systemic vascular resistance
e. A period of observation to obtain more data

61. A 59-year-old man with a history of myocardial infarction two years ago undergoes an uneventful aortobifemoral bypass graft for aortoiliac occlusive disease. Six hours later he develops ST segment depression, and a 12-lead ECG shows anterolateral ischemia. His hemodynamic parameters are as follows: systemic BP 70/40 mmHg, pulse 100 beats per minute CVP 18 mmHg, pulmonary capillary wedge pressure (PCWP) 25 mmHg, cardiac output 1.5 L/min, and systemic vascular resistance 1000 (dyne·sec)/cm^5. Which of the following is the single best pharmacologic intervention for this patient?

a. Sublingual nitroglycerin
b. Intravenous nitroglycerin
c. A short-acting beta blocker
d. Sodium nitroprusside
e. Dobutamine

62. A 56-year-old man undergoes a left upper lobectomy. An epidural catheter is inserted for postoperative pain relief. Ninety minutes after the first dose of epidural morphine, the patient complains of itching and becomes increasingly somnolent. Blood-gas measurement reveals the following: pH 7.24, $PaCO_2$ 58, PaO_2 100, and HCO_3^- 28. Which of the following is the most appropriate initial therapy for this patient?

a. Endotracheal intubation
b. Intramuscular diphenhydramine (Benadryl)
c. Epidural naloxone
d. Intravenous naloxone
e. Alternative analgesia

63. A 71-year-old man returns from the OR after undergoing a triple coronary bypass. His initial cardiac index is 2.8 L/(min·m^2). Heart rate is then noted to be 55 beats per minute, BP is 110/80, wedge pressure is 15, and his cardiac index has dropped to 1.6 L/(min·m^2). He has a normal left ventricle. Which of the following maneuvers will increase his cardiac output?

a. Increase his peripheral vascular resistance
b. Increase his CVP
c. Increase his heart rate to 90 by electrical pacing
d. Increase his blood viscosity
e. Increase his inspired oxygen concentration

64. A 73-year-old woman with a long history of heavy smoking undergoes femoral artery–popliteal artery bypass for resting pain in her left leg. Because of serious underlying respiratory insufficiency, she continues to require ventilatory support for four days after her operation. As soon as her endotracheal tube is removed, she begins complaining of vague upper abdominal pain. She has daily fever spikes to 39°C (102.2°F) and a leukocyte count of 18,000/mL. An upper abdominal ultrasonogram reveals a dilated gallbladder, but no stones are seen. A presumptive diagnosis of acalculous cholecystitis is made. Which of the following is recommended regarding her treatment?

a. Nasogastric suction and broad-spectrum antibiotics
b. Immediate cholecystectomy with operative cholangiogram
c. Percutaneous drainage of the gallbladder
d. Endoscopic retrograde cholangiopancreatography (ERCP) to visualize and drain the common bile duct
e. Provocation of cholecystokinin release by cautious feeding of the patient

65. A 32-year-old man undergoes a distal pancreatectomy, splenectomy, and partial colectomy for a gunshot wound to the left upper quadrant of the abdomen. One week later he develops a shaking chill in conjunction with a temperature spike to 39.44°C (103°F). His blood pressure is 70/40 mmHg, pulse is 140 beats per minute, and respiratory rate is 45 breaths per minute. He is transferred to the ICU, where he is intubated and a Swan-Ganz catheter is placed. Which of the following is consistent with the expected initial Swan-Ganz catheter readings?

a. An increase in cardiac output
b. An increase in peripheral vascular resistance
c. An increase in pulmonary artery pressure
d. An increase in pulmonary capillary wedge pressure
e. An increase in central venous pressure

66. A 43-year-old trauma patient develops acute respiratory distress syndrome (ARDS) and has difficulty oxygenating despite increased concentrations of inspired oxygen. After the positive end-expiratory pressure (PEEP) is increased, the patient's oxygenation improves. What is the mechanism by which this occurs?

a. Decreasing dead-space ventilation
b. Decreasing the minute ventilation requirement
c. Increasing tidal volume
d. Increasing functional residual capacity
e. Resdistribution of lung water from the interstitial to the alveolar space

67. A 27-year-old man was assaulted and stabbed in the left chest between the areola and the sternum. He is hemodynamically unstable with jugular venous distention, distant heart sounds, and hypotension. Which of the following findings would be consistent with a diagnosis of hemodynamically significant cardiac tamponade?

a. More than a 10-mmHg decrease in systolic blood pressure at the end of the expiratory phase of respiration
b. Decreased right atrial pressures on Swan-Ganz monitoring
c. Equalization of pressures across the four chambers on Swan-Ganz monitoring
d. Compression of the left ventricle on echocardiography
e. Overfilling of the right atrium

68. A 55-year-old woman requires a laparotomy for ovarian cancer. She has a history of stable angina. Which of the following characteristics is most likely to predict perioperative ischemic events during her noncardiac surgery?

a. Angina
b. More than three premature ventricular contractions (PVCs) per minute
c. Dyspnea on exertion
d. Tricuspid regurgitation
e. Her age

69. A woman is to undergo local excision of a suspicious nevus on her back. The surgeon intends to perform this excision with a local anesthetic. Which of the following statements regarding the use of local anesthetic agents is true?

a. When used for infiltration anesthesia, the maximal safe total dose of lidocaine is 3.0 mg per kilogram of body weight
b. Addition of epinephrine (1:200,000) to the solution of lidocaine, procaine, or bupivacaine does not increase the maximal safe total dose but increases the duration of the block
c. Numerous individuals are hypersensitive to local anesthetics
d. A local anesthetic in contact with a nerve trunk will cause sensory loss but not motor paralysis in the area innervated
e. Rapid systemic administration of local anesthetics may produce death without signs of CNS stimulation

70. A 22-year-old man sustains severe blunt trauma to the back. He notes that he cannot move his lower extremities. He is hypotensive and brady-cardic. Which of the following is the best initial management of the patient?

a. Administration of phenylephrine
b. Administration of dopamine
c. Administration of epinephrine
d. Intravenous fluid bolus
e. Placement of a transcutaneous pacer

71. A 58-year-old woman with multiple comorbidities and previous cardiac surgery is in a high-speed motor vehicle collision. Because of hemodynamic instability, a Swan-Ganz catheter was placed. However, the pulmonary capillary wedge pressure (PCWP) and left ventricular end-diastolic pressure (LVEDP) do not appear to be correlating. Which of the following conditions may explain this lack of correlation?

a. Aortic stenosis
b. Aortic regurgitation
c. Coronary artery disease
d. Positive-pressure ventilation with positive end-expiratory pressure/continuous positive airway pressure (PEEP/CPAP)
e. Bronchospasm

72. A 70-year-old man with a history of two prior strokes requires a femoral-popliteal bypass for threatened leg ischemia. His family is concerned about the risk of another perioperative stroke. Which of the following statements concerning perioperative stroke is true?

a. The mortality after postoperative stroke is high
b. Most postoperative strokes occur directly after surgery and appear related to operative events
c. The risk of stroke correlates with the length of time since previous stroke
d. General state of health and severity of illness as measured by ASA classification are significant predictors of recurrent stroke
e. The risk of stroke correlates with a history of multiple strokes or poststroke transient ischemic attacks (TIAs)

73. An 18-year-old woman develops urticaria and wheezing after an injection of intravenous contrast for an abdominal CT scan. Her blood pressure is 120/60 mmHg, heart rate is 155 beats per minute, and respiratory rate is 30 breaths per minute. Which of the following is the most appropriate immediate therapy?

a. Intubation
b. Epinephrine
c. Beta blockers
d. Iodine
e. Fluid challenge

74. A patient develops a fever and tachycardia during a blood transfusion after a redo coronary artery bypass procedure. The nurse subsequently discovers that there was a mix-up in the cross-match due to a labeling error. Which of the following is diagnostic in a patient with an immediate hemolytic reaction secondary to a blood transfusion?

a. Serum haptoglobin above 50 mg/dL
b. Indirect bilirubin greater than 5 mg/dL
c. Direct bilirubin greater than 5 mg/dL
d. Positive Coombs test
e. Myoglobinuria

75. Your patient is receiving mechanical ventilation after surgery. A blood gas is sent to determine if weaning is possible. The P_{CO_2} is 40. Which of the following conclusions is appropriate?

a. There is probably a paradoxical aciduria
b. Alveolar ventilation is adequate
c. Arterial P_{O_2} will indicate the adequacy of alveolar ventilation
d. Arterial P_{O_2} will indicate the degree of ventilation-perfusion mismatch
e. Arterial P_{O_2} can be safely predicted to exceed 90 mmHg on room air

76. An obese 50-year-old woman undergoes a laparoscopic cholecystectomy. In the recovery room, she is found to be hypotensive and tachycardic. Her arterial blood gases reveal a pH of 7.29, Pa_{O_2} of 60 mmHg, and Pa_{CO_2} of 54 mmHg. Which of the following is the most likely cause of this patient's problem?

a. Acute pulmonary embolism
b. CO_2 absorption from induced pneumoperitoneum
c. Alveolar hypoventilation
d. Pulmonary edema
e. Atelectasis from high diaphragm

77. A 65-year-old man who had a 25-lb weight loss over the previous six months was diagnosed with adenocarcinoma of the distal esophagus. He undergoes a transhiatal esophagectomy complicated by a cervical leak. He is receiving enteral feeds through a jejunostomy tube. After a week, his physicians wish to assess his nutritional resuscitation. Which of the following is the best measure of adequacy of his nutritional support?

a. Urinary nitrogen excretion level
b. Total serum protein level
c. Serum albumin level
d. Serum transferrin level
e. Respiratory quotient

78. An elderly nursing home resident arrives at the emergency room moribund, with little helpful history. She is profoundly alkalotic by blood-gas measurement, and her urine shows an acid pH. Which of the following is a possible explanation for these findings?

a. Release of inappropriate antidiuretic hormone
b. Severe crush injury
c. Acute tubular necrosis
d. Gastric outlet obstruction
e. An eosinophilic pituitary adenoma

79. A 43-year-old man undergoes an extrapleural pneumonectomy for mesothelioma. During the procedure, dissection of the pulmonary artery is difficult and the surgeon is concerned for a pulmonary arterial air embolism. Which of the following observations by the anesthesiologist would support such a diagnosis?

a. Unexpected systemic hypertension
b. Rising right atrial filling pressures
c. Reduced systemic arterial oxygen saturation
d. Rising systemic CO_2 partial pressures
e. Falling end-tidal CO_2

80. A 72-year-old man undergoes resection of an abdominal aneurysm. He arrives in the ICU with a core temperature of 33°C (91.4°F) and shivering. Which of the following is a physiologic consequence of the shivering?

a. Rising mixed venous oxygen saturation
b. Increased production of carbon dioxide
c. Decreased consumption of oxygen
d. Rising base excess
e. Decreased minute ventilation

81. A 39-year-old woman with a known history of von Willebrand's disease has a ventral hernia after a previous Caesarean section and desires to undergo elective repair. Which of the following should be administered preoperatively?

a. High-purity factor VIII:C concentrates
b. Low-molecular-weight dextran
c. Fresh-frozen plasma (FFP)
d. Cryoprecipitate
e. Whole blood

82. You are the physician on call for the extracorporeal membrane oxygenation (ECMO) service. There are five calls today, but only one machine and one technologist available. Which of the following patients is the most appropriate recipient of this service?

a. A 1-day-old, full-term, anencephalic 4-kg boy suffering from meconium aspiration syndrome and hypoxia
b. A 75-year-old man with Alzheimer's disease, severe pneumonia, and elevated pulmonary arterial pressure
c. A neonate with a diagnosis of severe pulmonary hypoplasia who is in respiratory failure
d. A 5-year-old girl with rhabdomyosarcoma metastatic to the lungs
e. A 3-day-old boy preoperative for a congenital diaphragmatic hernia

83. A 72-year-old man has an altered sensorium after a high-speed motor vehicle collision and is placed in the intensive care unit for monitoring overnight. Which of the following strategies should be used in order to avoid the development of an aspiration pneumonia?

a. Nasogastric decompression
b. Steroids
c. Prophylactic antibiotics
d. Antacid administration
e. High positive end-expiratory pressure

84. A patient with severe neurological devastation after head trauma requires a secure long-term airway. Because of his body habitus, an open tracheostomy (as opposed to the percutaneous approach) is chosen. Which of the following is true regarding performance of the tracheostomy?

a. The strap muscles should be divided
b. The thyroid isthmus should be preserved
c. The trachea should be entered at the second or third cartilaginous ring
d. Only horizontal incisions should be used
e. Formal tracheostomy is preferable to cricothyroidotomy as an emergency procedure

85. Shortly after the administration of an inhalational anesthetic and succinylcholine for intubation prior to an elective inguinal hernia repair in a 10-year-old boy, he becomes markedly febrile and displays a tachycardia of 160, and his urine changes color to a dark red. Which of the following is the most appropriate treatment at this time?

a. Complete the procedure but pretreat with dantrolene prior to future elective surgery
b. Administer inhalational anesthetic agents
c. Administer succinylcholine
d. Hyperventilate with 100% oxygen
e. Acidify the urine to prevent myoglobin precipitation in the renal tubules

86. A 42-year-old man has had a rocky course for the three days following a bowel resection of intestinal perforation due to inflammatory bowel disease. His CVP had been 12 to 14 but is now 6, in the face of diminished blood pressure and oliguria. Which of the following is the most likely etiology of his hypotension?

a. Pulmonary embolism
b. Hypervolemia
c. Positive-pressure ventilation
d. Pneumothorax
e. Gram-negative sepsis

87. Acute renal failure occurs following aortic angiography in a 72-year-old man. His weight has been rising, his lungs show rales at both bases, and he is dyspneic. His fractional excretion of sodium is greater than 1. He has eosinophilia on his peripheral smear, an elevated erythrocyte sedimentation rate, and proteinuria with microscopic hematuria. Which of the following is the most likely cause of his renal failure?

a. Hypovolemia
b. Renal artery cholesterol embolism
c. Acute tubular necrosis
d. Cardiogenic shock
e. Aortic dissection

88. A 55-year-old woman has been hospitalized due to recurrent pancreatitis, ARDS, prolonged ileus, and need for parenteral nutrition. She demonstrates weakness, lassitude, orthostatic hypotension, nausea, and fever. Which of the following abnormalities is most likely to explain these symptoms?

a. Hypothermia
b. Hypokalemia
c. Hyperglycemia
d. Hyponatremia
e. Hypervolemia

89. A 19-year-old male sustains severe lower-extremity trauma including a femur fracture and a crush injury to his foot. He requires vascular reconstruction of the popliteal artery. On the day after surgery, he becomes dyspneic and hypoxemic and requires intubation and mechanical ventilation. Which of the following is the most likely etiology of his decompensation?

a. Aspiration
b. Atelectasis
c. Fat embolism syndrome
d. Fluid overload
e. Pneumonia

90. A 33-year-old woman is brought to the emergency room from the scene of a severe motor vehicle accident. She is combative and confused, uncooperative, and appears dusky and dyspneic. Which of the following is the most appropriate management of her airway?

a. Awake endotracheal intubation is indicated in patients with penetrating ocular injury
b. Steroids have been shown to be of value in the treatment of aspiration of acidic gastric secretions
c. The stomach may be assumed to be empty only if a history is obtained indicating no ingestion of food or liquid during the prior 8 h
d. Intubation should be performed as soon as possible (in the emergency room) if the patient is unstable
e. Cricothyroidotomy is contraindicated in the presence of maxillofacial injuries

91. Following a boating injury in an industrial-use river, a patient begins to display fever, tachycardia, and a rapidly expanding area of erythema, blistering, and drainage from a flank wound. An x-ray shows gas in the soft tissues. Which of the following measures is most appropriate?

a. Administration of an antifungal agent
b. Administration of antitoxin
c. Wide debridement
d. Administration of hyperbaric oxygen
e. Early closure of tissue defects

92. Following pelvic gynecologic surgery, a 34-year-old woman becomes dyspneic, her peripheral arterial oxygen saturation falls from 94% to 81%, and her measured PaO_2 is 52 on a 100% nonrebreathing mask. This is associated with which of the following?

a. Pulmonary thromboembolism
b. Lower abdominal surgery
c. Starvation
d. The upright position
e. Increased cardiac output

93. A 25-year-old trauma patient is brought to the emergency room and is noted to be hypothermic to 32°C (89.6°F). Which of the following is an inappropriate management strategy for this patient?

a. Heated and moisturized inhaled air
b. Initiation of continuous arteriovenous rewarming (CAVR)
c. Peritoneal lavage with heated solutions
d. Passive external rewarming
e. Use of heated intravenous fluids

94. A 72-year-old woman who is planning to undergo ventral hernia repair is on warfarin for atrial fibrillation. She is advised to cease her warfarin several days before her surgery and is hospitalized preoperatively for heparinization. During her hospital stay, she complains of severe abdominal and flank pain. Her prothrombin time (PT) is normal, but her aPTT (activated partial thromboplastin time) is elevated. An abdominal CT scan demonstrates a large retroperitoneal hematoma. Which of the following statements should be administered to reverse the effects of the heparin?

a. Thrombin
b. Vitamin K
c. Protamine sulfate
d. Aprotinin
e. Platelet transfusion

95. A 42-year-old refinery worker is transferred to your burn unit. He was dyspneic and in respiratory distress at the scene and was intubated by alert paramedics. Soot is suctioned from the tube. Which of the following is characteristic of this condition?

a. Smoke inhalation is a thermal rather than a chemical injury
b. Carbon monoxide levels are not likely to be elevated unless there is evidence of skin or oropharyngeal burns
c. Chest x-rays during the early postinhalation period show a characteristic ground-glass appearance
d. Damage to the upper respiratory tract is common and is usually found on laryngoscopy
e. The mortality associated with smoke inhalation is low in the absence of cutaneous burns

96. A young man was seen to swallow small packets containing an unknown substance during a drug bust. Which of the following would be an indication for laparotomy?

a. Refusal to take high doses of laxatives
b. Refusal to allow endoscopic retrieval
c. Refusal to allow digital rectal disimpaction
d. Intraintestinal drug packets evident on abdominal x-ray in an asymptomatic smuggler
e. Signs of toxicity from leaking drug packets

DIRECTIONS: Each group of questions below consists of lettered options followed by a set of numbered items. For each numbered item, select the **one** lettered option with which it is **most** closely associated. Each lettered option may be used once, more than once, or not at all.

Questions 97–99

Match the side effects with the appropriate anesthetic agent.

a. Nitrous oxide (N_2O)
b. Halothane
c. Methoxyflurane
d. Enflurane
e. Morphine

97. A 65-year-old man undergoing hip replacement experiences seizures after induction.

98. A patient's blood pressure falls from 124/68 to 88/56 shortly after induction.

99. A patient with bowel obstruction becomes increasingly distended after induction.

Questions 100–102

For each clinical problem, select the best method of physiologic monitoring necessary for the patient.

a. Central venous catheterization
b. Pulmonary artery catheterization
c. Blood-gas monitoring
d. Intracranial pressure monitoring
e. Arterial catheterization
f. Continuous ECG monitoring

100. A 74-year-old man has a 5-h elective operation for repair of an abdominal aortic aneurysm. He had a small myocardial infarction three years earlier. In the ICU on the first postoperative day, he is hypotensive and is receiving dobutamine by continuous infusion.

101. A 62-year-old woman underwent a right carotid endarterectomy for symptomatic high-grade carotid artery stenosis. Postoperatively, her blood pressure is 202/105, and she is started on a nitroprusside infusion.

102. A comatose 28-year-old woman sustained a depressed skull fracture in an automobile collision. She has been unconscious for six weeks. Her vital signs are stable and she breathes room air. Following her initial decompressive craniotomy, she has returned to the operating room twice due to intracranial bleeding.

Questions 103–105

For each test, select the coagulation factor(s) whose functions are measured.

a. Factor II
b. Factor V
c. Factor VIII
d. Platelets
e. Fibrinogen

103. A patient is receiving oral warfarin to effect anticoagulation because of an artificial heart valve. Prothrombin time is 21 (INR = 2.3).

104. A patient with heparin-induced thrombocytopenia is placed on hirudin and undergoes assessment of his clotting function. Thrombin time 30 s.

105. A patient is to undergo a coronary bypass. Bleeding time is 6 min.

Critical Care: Anesthesiology, Blood Gases, and Respiratory Care

Answers

51. The answer is c. (*Brunicardi, pp 338–339.*) The patient had a sentinel bleed from a tracheoinnominate artery fistula, which carries a greater than 50% mortality rate. If the bleeding has ceased, then immediate fiberoptic exploration in the operating room is indicated. If the bleeding is ongoing, several stopgap measures can be attempted while preparing for median sternotomy in the operating room, including inflation of the tracheostomy balloon to attempt compression of the innominate artery, reintubation of the patient with an endotracheal tube, and removal of the tracheostomy and placement of the finger through the site with anterior compression of the innominate artery.

52. The answer is d. (*Greenfield, pp 226–227; Brunicardi, pp 373–374.*) There are multiple predictors that have been used to assess readiness for extubation. No single parameter is 100% predictive; attempted extubation should be based on correction of the underlying pathology, clinical status and hemodynamic stability, and a combination of the following parameters. The rapid shallow breathing index is the ratio of the respiratory rate to tidal volume. There is evidence to suggest that an index between 60 and 105 predicts successful extubation. The negative inspiratory force should be at least greater than −20 cm H_2O. The patient should be weaned to 5 cm H_2O PEEP before attempting extubation. The minute ventilation, which is the product of the tidal volume and respiratory rate, should be less than 10 L/min. The spontaneous respiratory rate should also be below 20 breaths per minute.

53. The answer is e. (*Brunicardi, pp 79–80.*) Whenever a hemolytic reaction caused by an incompatible blood transfusion is suspected, transfusion should be stopped immediately. A Foley catheter should be inserted and hourly urine output should be monitored. Renal damage caused by precipitation of hemoglobin in the renal tubules is the major serious consequence of hemolysis. This precipitation is inhibited in an alkaline environment and is promoted in an acid environment. Stimulating diuresis with mannitol and alkalinizing the urine with sodium bicarbonate intravenously are indicated procedures. Fluid and potassium intake should be restricted in the presence of severe oliguria or anuria.

54. The answer is b. (*Greenfield, pp 450–451.*) Nitrous oxide has a low solubility compared with other inhalation anesthetics; nitrous oxide is more soluble in blood than nitrogen and is the only anesthetic gas less dense than air. As a result of these properties, nitrous oxide may cause progressive distension of air-filled spaces during prolonged anesthesia. Since nitrous oxide diffuses into gas-filled compartments faster than nitrogen can diffuse out, its use can lead to worsened distention, which may be undesirable (e.g., in an operation for intestinal obstruction).

55. The answer is a. (*Brunicardi, pp 344–345.*) Adult respiratory distress syndrome (ARDS) has been called "shock lung" or "traumatic wet lung" and occurs under a variety of circumstances. The diagnosis can be made based on bilateral pulmonary infiltrates on chest x-ray, a PaO_2 to FiO_2 ratio of less than 200, and pulmonary wedge pressures of less than 18 mmHg (low filling pressures exclude the diagnosis of pulmonary edema). Three major physiologic alterations include (1) hypoxemia usually unresponsive to elevations of inspired oxygen concentration; (2) decreased pulmonary compliance, as the lungs become progressively stiffer and harder to ventilate; and (3) decreased functional residual capacity. Progressive alveolar collapse occurs owing to leakage of protein-rich fluid into the interstitium and the alveolar spaces with the subsequent radiologic picture of diffuse fluffy infiltrates bilaterally. Ventilatory abnormalities develop that result in shunt formation, decreased resting lung volume, and increased dead-space ventilation.

56. The answer is d. (*Greenfield, pp 218–219.*) The shape of the oxygen dissociation curve translates into several physiologic advantages. The relatively flat slope above a PO_2 of 50 mmHg means that, in this region of the curve, hemoglobin saturation decreases slightly with decrements in PO_2; loading of oxygen at the alveolar level is therefore affected minimally, with mild to moderate degrees of hypoxemia. The steeper slope at the lower end of the curve means that as the hemoglobin becomes desaturated, arterial Po_2 drops only minimally and a gradient that favors oxygen diffusion into tissue cells is maintained. Acidosis, a rise in $Paco_2$, and elevation of temperature all shift the curve to the right, which enhances tissue oxygen uptake. Red blood cell organic phosphates, particularly 2,3-diphosphoglycerate (2,3-DPG), also affect the dissociation curve. Banked blood, being low in 2,3-DPG, shifts the curve to the left and therefore decreases tissue oxygen uptake. 2,3-DPG levels increase with chronic hypoxia. Chronic lung disease, therefore, results in a shift of the curve to the right, which enhances oxygen delivery to peripheral tissues.

57. The answer is d. (*Brunicardi, p 52.*) The patient presented in the question is suffering from acute, life-threatening respiratory acidosis that has been compounded, if not produced, by the injudicious administration of a central nervous system depressant. While hypoxemia must also be corrected, the immediate task is to correct the acidosis caused by carbon dioxide accumulation. Both disturbances can be resolved by skillful endotracheal intubation and ventilatory support. Both sodium bicarbonate and high-flow nasal oxygen would be inappropriate. Bicarbonate should not be administered because buffer reserves are already adequate (serum bicarbonate is still 34 meq/L based on the Henderson-Hasselbalch equation). Nasal oxygen administration is not warranted because both acidemia and hypoxemia are themselves potent stimulants to spontaneous ventilation. Headache, confusion, and papilledema are all signs of acute carbon dioxide retention and do not imply the presence of a structural intracranial lesion.

58. The answer is b. (*Greenfield, pp 212–213.*) Dopamine has a variety of pharmacologic characteristics that make it useful in critically ill patients. In low doses [1 to 5 mg/(kg·min)], dopamine affects primarily the dopaminergic receptors. Activation of these receptors causes vasodilation of the renal and mesenteric vasculature and mild vasoconstriction of the peripheral bed, which thereby redirects blood flow to kidneys and bowel. At these low doses, the net effect on the overall vascular resistance may be slight. As the dose rises [2 to 10 mg/(kg·min)], β_1-receptor activity predominates and the inotropic effect on the myocardium leads to increased cardiac output and blood pressure. Above 10 mg/(kg·min), α-receptor stimulation causes peripheral vasoconstriction, shifting of blood from extremities to organs, decreased kidney function, and hypertension. At all doses, the diastolic blood pressure can be expected to rise; since coronary perfusion is largely a result of the head of pressure at the coronary ostia, coronary blood flow should be increased.

59. The answer is d. (*Goodnough, pp 602–609.*) Cytomegalovirus (CMV) is harbored in blood leukocytes. CMV infection is endemic in the United States, and its prevalence increases steadily with age. While acute CMV infection may cause transient fever, jaundice, and hepatosplenomegaly in cases of large blood donor exposures, posttransfusion CMV infection (seroconversion) is not a significant clinical problem in immunocompetent recipients, and therefore blood is not routinely tested for the presence of CMV. Posttransfusion non-A, non-B hepatitis, however, not only represents the most frequent infectious complication of transfusion but also is associated with an incidence of chronic active hepatitis up to 16% and an 8 to 10% incidence of cirrhosis or hepatoma or both. The etiologic agent in over 90% of cases of posttransfusion hepatitis has been identified as hepatitis C.

60. The answer is c. (*Greenfield, pp 208–215.*) A ruptured abdominal aneurysm is a surgical emergency often accompanied by serious hypotension and vascular collapse before surgery and massive fluid shifts with renal failure after surgery. In this case, all the hemodynamic parameters indicate inadequate intravascular volume, and the patient is therefore suffering from hypovolemic shock. The low urine output indicates poor renal perfusion, while the high urine specific gravity indicates adequate renal function with compensatory free-water conservation. The administration of a vasopressor agent would certainly raise the blood pressure, but it would do so by increasing peripheral vascular resistance and thereby further decrease tissue perfusion. The deleterious effects of shock would be increased. A vasodilating agent to lower the systemic vascular resistance would lead to profound hypotension and possibly complete vascular collapse because of pooling of an already depleted vascular volume. This patient's blood pressure is critically dependent on an elevated systemic vascular resistance. To properly treat this patient, rapid fluid infusion and expansion of the intravascular volume must be undertaken. This can be easily done with lactated Ringer's solution or blood (or both) until improvements in such parameters as the pulmonary capillary wedge pressure, urine output, and blood pressure are noted.

61. The answer is e. (*Greenfield, pp 208–213.*) This patient has developed pump failure due to a combination of preexisting coronary artery occlusive disease and high preload following a fluid challenge; afterload remains moderately high as well because of systemic vasoconstriction in the presence of cardiogenic shock. Poor myocardial performance is reflected in the low cardiac output and high pulmonary capillary wedge pressure. Therapy must be directed at increasing cardiac output without creating too high a myocardial oxygen demand on the already failing heart. Administration of nitroglycerin could be expected to reduce both preload and afterload, but if given without an inotrope it would create unacceptable hypotension. Nitroprusside similarly would achieve afterload reduction but would result in hypotension if not accompanied by an inotropic agent. A beta blocker would act deleteriously by reducing cardiac contractility and slowing the heart rate in a setting in which cardiac output is likely to be rate-dependent. Dobutamine is a synthetic catecholamine that is becoming the inotropic agent of choice in cardiogenic shock. As a β_1-adrenergic agonist, it improves cardiac performance in pump failure both by positive inotropy and peripheral vasodilation. With minimal chronotropic effect, dobutamine only marginally increases myocardial oxygen demand.

62. The answer is d. (*Thoren, pp 687–694.*) Thoracic epidural narcotics have become an increasingly popular means of postoperative pain relief in thoracic and upper abdominal surgery. Local action on γ opiate receptors ensures pain relief and consequent improvement in respiration without vasodilation or paralysis. The less lipid-soluble opiates are effective for long periods. Their slow absorption into the circulation also ensures a low incidence of centrally mediated side effects, such as respiratory depression or generalized itching. When these do occur, the intravenous injection of an opiate antagonist is an effective antidote. The locally mediated analgesia is not affected. One poorly understood side effect, which is apparently unrelated to systemic levels, is a profound reduction in gastric activity. This may be an important consideration after thoracic surgery when an early resumption of oral intake is anticipated.

63. The answer is c. (*Brunicardi, pp 364–366.*) The cardiac index is computed by dividing the cardiac output by the body surface area; the cardiac output is the product of the stroke volume and the heart rate [CI = CO/BSA; CO = SV × HR; therefore, CI = (SV × HR)/BSA]. An increased heart rate will directly increase the cardiac output and cardiac index. The remaining choices will either decrease or not affect the stroke volume and consequently will not increase the cardiac index.

64. The answer is c. *(Brunicardi, p 1208.)* The development of acute postoperative cholecystitis is an increasingly recognized complication of the severe illnesses that precipitate admissions to the intensive care unit. The causes are obscure but probably lead to a common final pathway of gallbladder ischemia. The diagnosis is often extremely difficult because the signs and symptoms may be those of occult sepsis. Moreover, the patients are often intubated, sedated, or confused as a consequence of the other therapeutic or medical factors. Biochemical tests, though frequently revealing abnormal liver function, are nonspecific and nondiagnostic. Bedside ultrasonography is usually strongly suggestive of the diagnosis when a thickened gallbladder wall or pericholecystic fluid is present; nonvisualization of the gallbladder on a nuclear medicine (HIDA) scan can also be diagnostic. If diagnosis is delayed, mortality and morbidity are very high. Percutaneous drainage of the gallbladder is usually curative of acalculous cholecystitis and affords stabilizing palliation if calculous cholecystitis is present. Antibiotics without drainage are too cautious a choice for a patient with a potentially fatal complication. Operative intervention is indicated only if less invasive methods of treatment (percutaneous cholecystostomy tube) have failed, and ERCP is not indicated in the absence of ductal obstruction.

65. The answer is a. *(Greenfield, pp 208–213.)* The case presented is most consistent with septic shock from a postoperative intraabdominal abscess. In the early phase of septic shock, the respiratory profile is characterized by mild hypoxia with a compensatory hyperventilation and respiratory alkalosis. Hemodynamically, a hyperdynamic state is seen with an increase in cardiac output and a decrease in peripheral vascular resistance in the face of relatively normal central pressures. Initial therapy is aimed at resuscitation and stabilization. This includes fluid replacement and vasopressors as well as antibiotic therapy aimed particularly at gram-negative rods and anaerobes for patients with presumed intraabdominal collections, especially after bowel surgery. Laparotomy and drainage of a collection is the definitive therapy but should await stabilization of the patient and confirmation of the presence and location of such a collection.

66. The answer is d. *(Moore, pp 1306–1307.)* Positive end-expiratory pressure (PEEP) improves oxygenation by increasing functional residual capacity by keeping the alveoli open at the end of expiration. Extravascular lung water is shifted from the alveolar to the interstitial space. The overall result is to increase surface area for diffusive exchange of gases. Potential negative effects of increased PEEP include alveolar overdistention resulting in barotraumas (pneumothoraxes), decreased venous return and decreased cardiac output, and increased minute ventilation requirements due to increased dead-space ventilation.

67. The answer is c. *(Moore, pp 107–108.)* On physical exam, cardiac tamponade may manifest with Beck's triad (systemic hypotension, jugular venous distention, and distant heart sounds). Also, the patient may have pulsus paradoxus, which is manifested by a decrease in systolic blood pressure by more than 10 mmHg at the end of the inspiratory phase of respiration. On echocardiogram, there will be pericardial fluid and right atrial collapse. On Swan-Ganz monitoring, there will be equalization of pressures across the four chambers. The right atrial pressures and central venous pressure are increased and cardiac output is decreased.

68. The answer is c. *(Charlson, pp 637–648.)* The landmark study by Goldman in 1978 identified cardiac risk factors in noncardiac surgical patients that included previous infarction (particularly infarction within six months, but with increased risk continuing for life), functional impairment such as dyspnea on exertion, age over 70 years, mitral regurgitation, more than five premature ventricular contractions (PVCs) per minute, and a tortuous or calcified aorta. Angina alone was not a risk factor. Subsequent studies by others have differed regarding the importance of several of these factors, which probably reflects different comorbid characteristics in the study populations (e.g., diabetes and hypertension). Additional predictors of perioperative cardiac risk that achieved significance in some studies but not in others include cardiomegaly, upper abdominal or intrathoracic surgery, and intraoperative hypotension.

69. The answer is e. *(Greenfield, pp 453–454.)* The maximal safe total dose of lidocaine administered to a 70-kg man is 4.5 mg/kg, or approximately 30 to 35 mL of a 1% solution. The addition of epinephrine to lidocaine, procaine, or bupivacaine not only doubles the duration of infiltration anesthesia, but increases the maximal safe total dose by one-third by decreasing the rate of absorption of drug into the bloodstream. However, epinephrine-containing solutions should not be injected into tissues supplied by end arteries (e.g., fingers, toes, ears, nose, penis). Hypersensitivity to local anesthetics is uncommon and occurs most prominently with anesthetics of the ester type (procaine, tetracaine). While small nerve fibers seem to be most susceptible to the action of local anesthetics, these agents act on any part of the nervous system and on every type of nerve fiber. CNS toxicity usually appears as stimulation followed by depression, probably because of an early selective depression of inhibitory neurons; with a massive overdose, all neurons may be depressed simultaneously.

70. The answer is d. *(Brunicardi, p 100.)* The patient is in neurogenic shock as a result of a spinal cord injury. Neurogenic shock is characterized by loss of sympathetic tone peripherally as well as bradycardia due to loss of the reflexive increase in heart rate in response to hypotension. Initial treatment is with fluid resuscitation followed by initiation of vasoconstrictors such as dopamine or phenylephrine. Hypovolemia due to hemorrhage should also be ruled out in trauma patients.

71. The answer is d. *(Brunicardi, pp 364–368.)* When a Swan-Ganz pulmonary artery catheter is in the wedge position, that is, isolating the pulmonary arterial system from the pulmonary capillaries, the measured pulmonary capillary wedge pressure (PCWP) is usually equivalent to both the left atrial pressure (LAP) and the left ventricular end-diastolic pressure (LVEDP). However, pathologic processes in the pulmonary vasculature and heart valves may alter this relationship. Pulmonary vasoocclusive disease may elevate the PCWP independently of the LAP or LVEDP. Bronchospasm affecting the airway but not the pulmonary vasculature should not affect the validity of Swan-Ganz catheter readings. Mitral stenosis and regurgitation cause increased LAP and PCWP, which result in an overestimated LVEDP. However, aortic stenosis and regurgitation elevate the PCWP, LAP, and LVEDP equally. Accurate measurement of PCWP by a Swan-Ganz catheter may not be possible in the presence of positive airway pressure with PEEP/CPAP; transmission of the positive airway pressure to the pulmonary microvasculature via the alveoli, especially in the upper lung zones, results in measurement of alveolar pressure rather than LAP or LVEDP. Coronary artery disease does not affect the relationship between PCWP, LAP, and LVEDP.

72. The answer is a. (*Landercasper, pp 986–989.*) In an eight-year retrospective study of 173 consecutive patients with a documented medical history of stroke who underwent subsequent general anesthesia and surgery (excluding cardiac, cerebrovascular, and neurological surgery), five patients (2.9%) had documented postoperative strokes from 3 to 21 days (mean 12.2 days) after surgery. The risk of stroke did not correlate with age, sex, history of multiple strokes or poststroke transient ischemic attacks (TIAs), ASA classification, aspirin use, coronary artery disease, peripheral vascular disease, intraoperative blood pressure, time since previous stroke, or cause of previous stroke. The risk of recurrent stroke appears to be comparable with that for surgical patients who do not have a history of prior stroke and are undergoing cardiac and peripheral vascular surgery. Most recurrent strokes occur many hours to days following surgery and do not appear to be directly related to operative events. The mortality after postoperative stroke is high.

73. The answer is b. (*Greenfield, p 1661.*) This patient is having an anaphylactoid reaction with destabilization of the cardiovascular and respiratory systems. Anaphylactoid reactions are most commonly caused by iodinated contrast media, β-lactam antibiotics (e.g., penicillin), and *Hymenoptera* stings. Manifestations of anaphylactoid reactions include both lethal (bronchospasm, laryngospasm, hypotension, dysrhythmia) and nonlethal (pruritus, urticaria, syncope, weakness, seizure) phenomena. Epinephrine is the initial treatment for laryngeal obstruction and bronchospasm, followed by histamine antagonists (H_1 and H_2 blockers), aminophylline, and hydrocortisone. Vasopressors and fluid challenges may be given for shock. Conscious patients are usually stabilized with injected or inhaled epinephrine, while unconscious patients and those with refractory hypotension or hypoxia should be intubated.

74. The answer is d. (*Brunicardi, pp 78–79.*) Most transfusion reactions are hemolytic and are due to clerical errors that result in administration of blood with major (ABO) and minor antigen incompatibility. Intravascular hemolysis results in hemoglobinemia. Because haptoglobin binds hemoglobin via a receptor located on macrophages, serum haptoglobin levels are decreased; haptoglobin level less than 50 mg/dL is one criterion for a transfusion reaction. Additionally, hemoglobinuria with a free hemoglobin level greater than 5 mg/dL is another criterion. A positive Coombs test is diagnostic. Indirect hyperbilirubinemia and anemia may be seen in delayed transfusion reactions, which occur between 2 and 10 days after a transfusion. Delayed transfusion reactions can occur due to antibodies to Rh antigens and are characterized by extravascular hemolysis.

75. The answer is b. *(Brunicardi, pp 50–52.)* Because of the highly efficient diffusion characteristics of carbon dioxide, $PaCO_2$ levels are reliable indicators of adequacy of alveolar ventilation. A $PaCO_2$ of 40 mmHg is the normal value. Paradoxical aciduria occurs when hypokalemic metabolic alkalosis is present, as the kidney excretes hydrogen ion in an effort to conserve potassium ion. Though a $PaCO_2$ of 40 mmHg is not incompatible with metabolic alkalosis, it would ordinarily be higher, as the patient tries to conserve carbolic acid by hypoventilating to compensate. PaO_2 levels are influenced by so many other variables (e.g., age, concentration of inspired O_2, altitude) that no inferences can be made about adequacy of alveolar ventilation from PaO_2 alone, nor can PaO_2 be safely predicted by the presence of normocarbia. The ventilation-perfusion mismatch is a reflection of the gradient between alveolar and arterial oxygen tension in relationship to percentage of inspired O_2.

76. The answer is c. *(Brunicardi, p 52.)* Because of the ease with which carbon dioxide diffuses across the alveolar membranes, $PaCO_2$ is a highly reliable indicator of alveolar ventilation. In this postoperative patient with respiratory acidosis and hypoxemia, the hypercarbia is diagnostic of alveolar hypoventilation. Acute hypoxemia can occur with pulmonary embolism, pulmonary edema, and significant atelectasis, but in all those situations the $PaCO_2$ should be normal or reduced, as the patient hyperventilates to improve oxygenation. The absorption of gas from the peritoneal cavity may transiently affect the $PaCO_2$, but should have no effect on oxygenation.

77. The answer is c. *(Greenfield, pp 937–939.)* The serum albumin level provides a rough estimate of protein nutritional adequacy. The accuracy of this estimate is affected by the long half-life of albumin (three weeks) and the vagaries of hemodilution. The acute-phase serum proteins have a very short half-life (hours) and may also provide good short-term indications of nutritional status. Transferrin is one of these acute-phase proteins, but unfortunately its levels, too, are influenced by changes in intravascular volume and, along with the other acute-phase reactants, rise nonspecifically during acute illness. All the listed responses provide some useful information about nutrition and adequacy of replacement.

78. The answer is d. *(Brunicardi, pp 50–52.)* The body has elaborate mechanisms to compensate for metabolic acidosis. Not only do most body functions work better in an acidotic state, but the patient is able to move toward correction of the pH by excreting acid urine and by hyperventilating to "blow off" carbonic acid. On the other hand, we are poorly equipped to deal with metabolic alkalosis. We cannot hold our breath to save acid because the respiratory center overrides our efforts as the $PaCO_2$ rises and the PaO_2 falls. The kidney cannot make urine under any circumstance that is very far above normal pH. In the subtraction alkalosis that accompanies gastric outlet obstruction with loss of gastric acid by vomiting or suction, the potassium depletion and volume deficits provoke exchange of sodium for hydrogen ion in the distal tubule, with resultant exacerbation of the metabolic alkalosis. All the other conditions listed would be expected to produce acidosis; consequently, acid urine would not be paradoxical.

79. The answer is e. *(Brunicardi, p 134.)* Air carried into the pulmonary arterial vasculature creates an abnormal blood-air interface that leads to denaturing of plasma proteins and creates amorphous proteinaceous and cellular debris and endothelial injury. The ensuing increased capillary permeability results in alveolar flooding. The occlusion of pulmonary vessels increases the proportion of ventilated but underperfused alveoli. The increment in dead space results in a drop in end-tidal carbon dioxide.

80. The answer is b. *(Brunicardi, p 356.)* Shivering is the physiologic effort of the body to generate heat to maintain the core temperature. In healthy persons, shivering increases the metabolic rate by three to five times and results in increased oxygen consumption and carbon dioxide production. In critically ill patients, these metabolic consequences are almost always counterproductive and should be prevented with other means employed to correct systemic hypothermia. In the presence of vigorous shivering, oxygen debt in the muscles and lactic acidemia develop.

81. The answer is d. *(Greenfield, p 96.)* Von Willebrand disease is similar to true hemophilia in frequency of occurrence. It is being diagnosed more commonly today because of more reliable assays for factor VIII. This autosomal dominant disorder (recessive transmission can occur) is characterized by a diminution in factor VIII:C (procoagulant) activity. The reduction in activity is not as great as in classic hemophilia, and the clinical manifestations are more subtle. These manifestations are often overlooked until an episode of trauma or surgery makes them apparent. Treatment requires correcting the bleeding time and providing factor VIII R:WF (the von Willebrand factor). Only cryoprecipitate is reliably effective. High purity factor VIII:C concentrates, effective in hemophilia, lack the von Willebrand factor and are consequently undependable.

82. The answer is e. *(Greenfield, pp 1506, 1921–1922.)* Extracorporeal membrane oxygenation (ECMO) is a form of cardiopulmonary support that is useful in the setting of potentially reversible pulmonary or cardiac disease. Treatment of meconium aspiration syndrome, sepsis, pneumonia, and congenital diaphragmatic hernia (pre- or postoperatively) are thus appropriate uses. The technique is also applicable in some circumstances as a bridge to cardiac or lung transplantation since the outlook for survival is quite good if the child can be maintained in a good physiological state until donor organs are available. Hypoplastic lungs do not have enough surface area to perform adequate gas exchange and are unlikely to mature to a point where they can sustain life. Babies with hypoplastic lungs will be bypass-dependent for life and consequently are not candidates for institution of ECMO therapy.

83. The answer is a. *(Moore, pp 367–368.)* Immediate emptying of the stomach after traumatic injury and nasogastric decompression are important for the prevention of aspiration of gastric contents. Elevation of the head of the bed is also recommended for ICU patients. Prophylactic antibiotics are not indicated in high-risk patients, even after gross aspiration. Although gross aspiration results in a chemical pneumonitis, antibiotics are indicated only if pneumonia develops. Antacids result in loss of the protective effect of acidification of gastric contents and subsequent colonization with gram-negative organisms, and therefore should be avoided. Sucralfate may be a better choice for stress ulcer prophylaxis. Steroids are not indicated. High positive end expiratory pressure is not required in patients unless respiratory failure develops.

84. The answer is c. *(Brunicardi, p 542.)* Although tracheostomy is occasionally an emergency procedure, it can be more effectively performed in an operating room, where hemostasis and antisepsis are readily achieved. Most authorities recommend a horizontal incision; however, limited direct midline incisions have the advantage of not opening any unnecessary tissue planes and perhaps reducing the incidence of bleeding complications. Both approaches have advocates. In either case, the skin incision is made just below the cricoid cartilage, the strap muscles are spared and retracted, the thyroid isthmus is divided if necessary, and the trachea is entered at the second tracheal ring. The second and third tracheal rings are incised vertically, allowing placement of the tracheostomy tube. The first tracheal ring and the cricoid cartilage must be left intact.

85. The answer is d. *(Brunicardi, pp 356–357.)* The cause of malignant hyperthermia is unknown, but it is associated with inhalational anesthetic agents and succinylcholine. It may develop in an otherwise healthy person who has tolerated previous surgery without incident. It should be suspected in the presence of a history of unexplained fever, muscle or connective tissue disorder, or a positive family history (evidence suggests an autosomal dominant inheritance pattern). In addition to fever during anesthesia, the syndrome includes tachycardia, increased O_2 consumption, increased CO_2 production, increased serum K^+, myoglobinuria, and acidosis. Rigidity rather than relaxation following succinylcholine injection may be the first clue to its presence. Treatment of malignant hyperthermia should include prompt conclusion of the operative procedure and cessation of anesthesia, hyperventilation with 100% oxygen, and administration of intravenous dantrolene. The urine should be alkalinized to protect the kidneys from myoglobin precipitation. If reoperation is necessary, the physician should premedicate heavily, alkalinize the urine, and avoid depolarizing agents such as succinylcholine. Pretreatment for 24 h with dantrolene is helpful; it is thought to act directly on muscle fiber to attenuate calcium release.

86. The answer is e. *(Greenfield, pp 229–230.)* Determination of CVP has been helpful in the overall hemodynamic assessment of the patient. This pressure can be affected by a variety of factors including those of cardiac, noncardiac, and artifactual origin. Venous tone, right ventricular compliance, intrathoracic pressure, and blood volume all influence CVP. Vasoconstrictor drugs, positive pressure ventilation (with and without PEEP), mediastinal compression, and hypervolemia all increase CVP. Acute pulmonary embolism, when clinically significant, elevates CVP by causing right ventricular overload and increased right atrial pressure. Sepsis, on the other hand, decreases CVP through both the release of vasodilatory mediators and the loss of intravascular plasma volume due to increased capillary permeability. Trends in CVP measurement are more reliable than isolated readings.

87. The answer is b. (*Greenfield, p 1581.*) Cholesterol atheroembolism is a known complication of angiography or aortic manipulation during surgery and can result in lower extremity ischemia, acute myocardial infarction, ischemic bowel, and acute or chronic renal failure. Eosinophilia is strongly suggestive of cholesterol atheroembolization, and other laboratory findings include microscopic hematuria or proteinuria and elevated inflammatory mediators such as erythrocyte sedimentation rate. A fractional excretion of sodium (FeNa) of greater than 1 suggests a renal cause of acute renal failure as opposed to prerenal causes such as hypovolemia or cardiogenic shock. Thoracic aortic dissections can result in acute renal failure if they involve the renal arteries and may present with hematuria and elevations in BUN and creatinine. However, aortic dissections are typically associated with significant chest pain.

88. The answer is d. (*Brunicardi, pp 1463–1465.*) Clinical manifestations of adrenocortical insufficiency include hyperkalemia, hyponatremia, hypoglycemia, fever, weight loss, and dehydration. There is excessive sodium loss in the urine, contraction of the plasma volume, and perhaps hypotension or shock. Classic hyperpigmentation is present in chronic Addison's disease only. Addison's disease may present in newborns as a congenital atrophy, as an insidious chronic state often due to tuberculosis, as an acute dysfunction secondary to trauma or adrenal hemorrhage, or as a semiacute adrenal insufficiency seen during stress or surgery. In this last instance, signs and symptoms include nausea, lassitude, vomiting, fever, progressive salt wasting, hyperkalemia, and hypoglycemia. It may be confirmed by measurements of urinary Na^+ loss and absence of response to ACTH.

89. The answer is c. (*Greenfield, p 375.*) Fat embolism syndrome is a relatively uncommon complication of long-bone fractures and is characterized by acute respiratory failure, altered mental status, and petechiae.

Unfortunately, there are no reliable diagnostic tests, and management is supportive only. Pulmonary edema is unlikely in an otherwise healthy 19-year-old male without chest trauma or evidence of a cardiac contusion. Aspiration is unlikely in an awake patient with normal mental status. Pneumonias typically present with fever and/or leukocytosis, productive cough, and a new infiltrate on chest x-ray. Atelectasis in and of itself is not a cause for respiratory failure.

90. The answer is d. (*Moore, pp 177–199.*) Securing a stable airway is one of the most fundamental and important aspects of the management of the severely injured patient. The level of control required will vary from a simple oropharyngeal airway to tracheostomy, depending on the clinical situation. Full control of the airway should be secured in the emergency room if the patient is unstable. Endotracheal intubation will usually be the method chosen, but the physician should be prepared to do a tracheotomy if attempts at peroral or pernasal intubation are failing or are impractical because of maxillofacial injuries. The most dangerous period is just prior to and during the initial attempts to get control of the airway. Manipulation of the oronasopharynx may provoke combative behavior or vomiting in a patient already confused by drugs, alcohol, hypoxia, or cerebral trauma. The risk of aspiration is high during these initial attempts, and the physician should make no assumptions about the state of the contents of the patient's stomach. Antacids are recommended just prior to the intubation attempt, if feasible. Although steroids have been recommended in the past, they are no longer considered of value in the management of aspiration of acidic gastric juice. The best management requires prevention of the complication of aspiration. In a reasonably cooperative patient, awake intubation with topical anesthesia may help to prevent some of the risks of hypotension, arrhythmia, and aspiration associated with the induction of anesthesia. If awake intubation is inappropriate, then an alternative is rapid-sequence induction with a thiobarbiturate followed by muscle paralysis with succinylcholine. If elevated intracranial pressure is suspected, or if a penetrating eye injury exists, awake intubation is contraindicated.

91. The answer is c. (*Brunicardi, p 434.*) Necrotizing skin and soft tissue infections may produce insoluble gases (hydrogen, nitrogen, methane) through anaerobic bacterial metabolism. While the term "gas gangrene" has come to imply clostridial infection, gas in tissues is more likely not to be due to *Clostridium* species but rather to other facultative and obligate anaerobes, particularly streptococci. Though fungi have also been implicated, they are less often associated with rapidly progressive infections. Treatment for necrotizing soft tissue infections includes repeated wide debridement, with wound reconstruction delayed until a stable, viable wound surface has been established. The use of hyperbaric oxygen in the treatment of gas gangrene remains controversial, due to lack of proven benefit, difficulty in transporting critically ill patients to hyperbaric facilities, and the risk of complications. Antitoxin has neither a prophylactic nor a therapeutic role in the treatment of necrotizing infections.

92. The answer is a. *(Greenfield, p 1918.)* Abnormalities of ventilation-perfusion ratio result from the shunting of blood to a hypoventilated lung or from the ventilation of hypoperfused regions of lung tissue. When this imbalance is extreme, as following massive pulmonary thromboembolism, the effect is life-threatening hypoxemia. Other common predisposing factors in the postoperative patient that contribute to this maldistribution include the assumption of a supine position, thoracic and upper abdominal incisions, obesity, atelectasis, and reduced cardiac output.

93. The answer is d. *(Greenfield, pp 414–416.)* Passive rewarming should be reserved for patients with only mild hypothermia, which is defined as between 34°C (93.2°F) and 36°C (96.8°F). Active core rewarming techniques are indicated in patients with severe hypothermia (less than 32°C or 89.6°F) and include infusion of heated intravenous fluids (or blood products if needed), inhalation of heated moisturized air, lavage of body cavities with heated solutions, and continuous arteriovenous rewarming (CAVR). Other less aggressive active external rewarming techniques include use of heated lights, warm blankets, heating pads, and immersion in warm water.

94. The answer is c. *(Greenfield, pp 98–102.)* Heparin is reversed by the administration of protamine sulfate. Spontaneous retroperitoneal hemorrhage is a rare but potentially fatal complication of anticoagulation. Heparin is much more frequently associated with spontaneous retroperitoneal hemorrhage than are oral agents. Advanced patient age and poor regulation of coagulation times also increase the likelihood of bleeding complications. Most cases of retroperitoneal hemorrhage present with flank pain and signs of peritoneal irritation suggestive of an acute intraabdominal process. CT scans are most useful in confirming the diagnosis and following the course of the bleeding. Successful management is usually nonoperative and consists of the discontinuation of anticoagulants, reversal of anticoagulation, possible transfusion of clotting factors, and repletion of intravascular volume with intravenous fluids. Warfarin inhibits synthesis of vitamin K–dependent clotting factors, whereas heparin potentiates antithrombin III activity. Aprotinin is a protease inhibitor that decreases the inflammatory and fibrinolytic response and is used in patients undergoing cardiopulmonary bypass surgery to reduce bleeding complications. Lepirudin is an anticoagulant that is used in patients who develop heparin-induced thrombocytopenia. Thrombin can be used topically as a hemostatic agent.

95. The answer is e. (*Brunicardi, pp 200–204.*) The mortality from isolated smoke inhalation injuries is low in the absence of cutaneous burns. Smoke inhalation injuries, as opposed to respiratory burns (which result from thermal injury), result from epithelial injury from chemical irritation of the tracheobronchial tree and alveoli. Most patients admitted for this injury have elevated carboxyhemoglobin levels from carbon monoxide poisoning, but a minority have physical evidence of skin burns or oropharyngeal burns. Chest films initially are often negative even in those patients who subsequently develop respiratory failure from pulmonary edema or pneumonitis. Patients with elevated carboxyhemoglobin levels or evidence of smoke inhalation should be observed regardless of normal arterial blood gases and chest x-ray; hyperbaric oxygen should be considered in patients with neurologic symptoms and carbon monoxide poisoning, as it reduces the half-life of carboxyhemoglobin. Visible damage to the respiratory tract is not a frequent finding.

96. The answer is e. (*Robinson, 709–711.*) Some drug smugglers, often called body packers or mules, ingest cocaine- or heroin-filled packets and retrieve them at a later date from their stools. The drugs are usually contained in latex or plastic packets. Rupture or leakage of even one bag carries the risk of severe toxicity and death. Although conservative medical management with moderate doses of laxatives is usually safe in stable body packers, close physiologic monitoring is necessary until all packets are passed. High doses of laxatives, digital rectal disimpaction, or endoscopic removal create a high risk of rupture of the bags and therefore are generally discouraged. Emergency surgery is indicated when complications develop.

97–99. The answers are 97-d, 98-e, 99-a. *(Greenfield, pp 450–451.)* Nitrous oxide (N_2O) is a frequently used inhalation analgesic. However, because the minimum alveolar anesthetic concentration (MAC) is so high (over 100), true anesthesia at 1 atm cannot be obtained without compromising oxygen delivery to the patient. Since nitrous oxide is 30 times more soluble than nitrogen in blood, it enters a collection of trapped air at a rate faster than that at which nitrogen leaves the collection. Thus, the trapped air will increase in volume. If the trapped air is a result of bowel obstruction, intestinal distension will increase. Halothane is a very potent anesthetic with an MAC of 0.75. Cardiovascular depression results from a number of different mechanisms. Hypotension and decreased cardiac output have been associated with a direct depression of myocardial muscle fibers and peripheral vascular smooth muscle fibers. An effect on the medullary vasomotor centers as well as on sympathetic ganglionic transmissions to the heart has been reported. Enflurane is a halogenated inhalation anesthetic with an MAC of 1.2. It is similar to halothane in its anesthetic characteristics. However, in a small number of normal patients it may induce electroencephalographic changes similar to those seen in epilepsy. Methoxyflurane is the most potent and least volatile halogenated inhalation anesthetic, with an MAC of 0.16. Its clinical use has been curtailed because of the high risk of nephrotoxicity of the free fluoride ions released during its biodegradation. Morphine is a potent narcotic agent. Its use during general anesthesia can potentiate the analgesic effects of the inhalation agents. It causes histamine release with the risk of hypotension if given in a large bolus dose.

100–102. The answers are 100-b, 101-e, 102-d. *(Brunicardi, pp 364–375.)* This patient requires pulmonary artery catheter readings to allow his physicians to assess his volume status and need for ongoing inotropic support. Furthermore, the patient continues to be hypotensive and requires further investigation as to the etiology that would subsequently dictate treatment (volume, afterload reduction, etc). Central venous monitoring alone does not allow the physician to assess cardiac function.

A patient who is hypertensive after a carotid endarterectomy is at risk for hemorrhagic stroke and therefore requires aggressive blood pressure management, occasionally with a continuous infusion of nitroglycerin or nitroprusside. Beat-to-beat monitoring of the blood pressure is essential. A patient who has suffered blunt head trauma requiring repeated surgeries for intracranial bleeding will likely be monitored with an intracranial pressure device. Other indications for intracranial pressure monitoring include subarachnoid hemorrhage, hydrocephalus, postcraniotomy status, and Reye's syndrome. Measurement of intracranial pressure (ICP) allows the physician to determine and optimize the cerebral perfusion pressure (which is the difference between the mean arterial pressure and the ICP).

103–105. The answers are 103-a, 104-e, 105-d. (*Brunicardi, pp 63–65; Greenfield, pp 106–107.*) Prothrombin time measures the speed of coagulation in the extrinsic pathway. A tissue source of procoagulant (thromboplastin) with calcium is added to plasma. The test will detect deficiencies in factors II, V, VII, X, and fibrinogen and is used to monitor patients receiving coumadin derivatives. However, even small amounts of heparin will artificially prolong the clotting time, so that accurate prothrombin times can be obtained only when the patient has not received heparin for at least 5 h.

The intrinsic pathway is measured by the partial thromboplastin time. This test is sensitive for defects in the contact and intrinsic phases of coagulation (II, V, VIII, IX, X, XI, XII, fibrinogen) and is used to monitor the status of patients on heparin.

The bleeding time assesses the interaction of platelets and the formation of the platelet plug. Therefore it will pick up deficiencies in both qualitative and quantitative platelet function. Ingestion of aspirin within one week of the test will alter the result.

The thrombin time assesses qualitative abnormalities in fibrinogen and the presence of inhibitors to fibrin polymerization. A standard amount of fibrin is added to a fixed volume of plasma and clotting time is measured.

Skin: Wounds, Infections, and Burns; Hands; Plastic Surgery

Questions

DIRECTIONS: Each item below contains a question followed by suggested responses. Select the **one best** response to each question.

106. A 45-year-old woman is seen with wasting of the intrinsic muscles of the hand, weakness, and pain in the wrist. Which of the following nerves has most likely been injured?

a. Ulnar nerve
b. Radial nerve
c. Brachial nerve
d. Axillary nerve
e. Thenar and hypothenar nerves

107. A 68-year-old woman is to have a suspected melanoma excised from her trunk. It appears to be a thin melanoma, less than 1 mm deep. Which of the following is the smallest margin recommended for excision?

a. 3 mm
b. 5 mm
c. 1 cm
d. 2 cm
e. 5 cm

108. A patient has a clean incision and then closure of the incision to excise an unwanted benign nevus. With regard to the healing process, which of the following statements is correct?

a. Collagen content reaches a maximum at approximately one week after injury
b. Monocytes are essential for normal wound healing
c. Fibroblasts appear in the wound within 24 to 36 h after the injury
d. The function of monocytes in wound healing is limited to phagocytosis of bacteria and debris
e. Early in wound healing, type I collagen is predominant

109. While you are on duty in the emergency room, a 12-year-old boy arrives with pain and inflammation over the ball of his left foot and red streaks extending up the inner aspect of his leg. He remembers removing a wood splinter from the sole of his foot on the previous day. Which of the following is the most likely infecting organism?

a. *Clostridium perfringens*
b. *Clostridium tetani*
c. *Staphylococcus*
d. *Escherichia coli*
e. *Streptococcus*

110. A 35-year-old man with new diagnosis of Crohn's disease presents with rapidly enlarging painful ulcerations on the lower extremities. Cultures of the lesion are negative, and skin biopsy reveals no evidence of malignancy. Which of the following is the most appropriate treatment option?

a. Surgical debridement of the wound with skin grafting
b. Local wound care with silver sulfadiazine
c. Topical corticosteroids
d. Systemic steroids and immunosuppressants
e. Saphenous vein stripping and compressive stockings

111. Following a weekend of snowmobiling, a 42-year-old man comes to the emergency department with pain, numbness, and discoloration of his right forefoot. You diagnose frostbite. Which of the following is the proper initial treatment?

a. Debridement of the affected part followed by silver sulfadiazine dressings
b. Administration of corticosteroids
c. Administration of vasodilators
d. Immersion of the affected part in water at 40 to 44°C (104 to 111.2°F)
e. Rewarming of the affected part at room temperature

112. A 54-year-old woman cuts her hand with a kitchen knife. There is evidence of tendon injury. Which of the following is true regarding the muscles of the hand?

a. The flexor digitorum superficialis inserts on the distal phalanx
b. The flexor digitorum profundus inserts on the middle phalanx
c. The tendons of the flexor digitorum superficialis arise from a common muscle belly
d. The best results for repair of a flexor tendon are obtained with injuries in the fibroosseous tunnel (zone 2)
e. The process of healing a tendon injury involves formation of a tenoma

113. Intraoperative record keeping is important. The OR staff cannot determine which cases were classified as clean versus contaminated. Which of the following is considered a clean-contaminated case?

a. Open cholecystectomy for cholelithiasis
b. Herniorrhaphy with mesh repair
c. Lumpectomy with axillary node dissection
d. Appendectomy with walled-off abscess
e. Gunshot wound to the abdomen with injuries to the small bowel and sigmoid colon

114. A 65-year-old woman presents with a 1-cm lesion with a pearly border on her nose, and punch biopsy is consistent with a basal cell carcinoma. She is scheduled to undergo Mohs surgery. Which of the following statements is true regarding this technique?

a. Mohs surgery results in a larger cosmetic defect because of the emphasis on obtaining negative margins circumferentially
b. The major benefit of Mohs surgery is a shorter operating time
c. Mohs surgery is indicated for all basal and squamous cell carcinomas
d. Frozen sections are not necessary if Mohs surgery is performed
e. There is no difference in cure rates between wide local excision and Mohs surgery

115. A 60-year-old woman presents with the skin lesion shown here, which has been present for 10 years. She reports a history of radiation treatments to that hand for eczema. Which of the following statements is true concerning this lesion?

a. It is more malignant than basal cell carcinoma
b. It occurs more frequently in brunettes
c. It rarely metastasizes to regional lymph nodes
d. It should be treated by radiation therapy
e. It is rarely associated with chronic sun exposure

116. A 25-year-old man is brought to the emergency room after sustaining burns during a fire in his apartment. He has blistering and erythema of his face, left upper extremity, and chest, with frank charring of his right upper extremity. He is agitated, hypotensive, and tachycardic. Which of the following statements concerning this patient's initial wound management is correct?

a. Topical antibiotics should not be used, as they will encourage growth of resistant organisms
b. Early excision of facial and hand burns is especially important
c. Escharotomy should be performed only if neurologic impairment is imminent
d. Excision of areas of third-degree or deep second-degree burns usually takes place three to seven days after injury
e. Split-thickness skin grafts over the eschar of third-degree burns should be performed immediately in order to prevent fluid loss

117. A 24-year-old firefighter sustains 30% TBSA burns to his torso, face, and extremities. His wounds are treated topically with silver nitrate. Which of the following complications is associated with use of this agent?

a. Hypernatremia
b. Metabolic acidosis
c. Hyperchloremia
d. Neutropenia
e. Methemoglobinemia

118. A 54-year-old man sees you because of a growth on his lip. He works in construction and is usually outdoors. The biopsy report confirms squamous cell carcinoma. Which of the following is true?

a. The lesion often arises in areas of persistent hyperkeratosis
b. More than 90% of cases occur on the upper lip
c. The lesion constitutes 30% of all cancers of the oral cavity
d. Radiotherapy is considered inappropriate treatment for these lesions
e. Initial metastases are to the ipsilateral posterior cervical lymph nodes

119. A 40-year-old woman complains of pain in her right wrist. There are also paresthesias in her hand. With regard to her diagnosis, which of the following statements is correct?

a. It is rarely secondary to trauma
b. It may be associated with pregnancy
c. It most often causes dysesthesia during waking hours
d. It is often associated with vascular compromise
e. Surgical treatment involves release of the extensor retinaculum

120. A 60-year-old diabetic man undergoes resection of an infected boil on his back. The wound is left open for packing and cleansing. Week by week, the wound grows smaller. Which of the following is true concerning wound contracture?

a. It is the primary process affecting closure of a sutured or stapled surgical wound
b. Bacterial colonization significantly slows the process of contraction
c. It may account for a maximum of 50% decrease in the size of a wound
d. It is based on specialized fibroblasts that contain actin myofilaments
e. The percentage reduction of wound size is increased with increased adherence of skin to underlying tissue

121. A 70-year-old man is concerned when his dentist finds a white patch on his oral mucosa during a routine exam. Proper management should include which of the following?

a. Excisional biopsy of all lesions
b. Application of topical antibiotics
c. Low-dose radiation therapy
d. Ascertaining that dentures fit properly
e. Application of topical chemotherapeutic agents

122. An 8-lb infant, born following uncomplicated labor and delivery, is noted to have a unilateral cleft lip and palate. Which of the following is true?

a. The child almost certainly has other congenital anomalies
b. Rehabilitation requires adjunctive speech therapy
c. Lip repair is indicated at one year of age
d. Palate repair is indicated prior to six months of age
e. Cosmetic revisions to the nose should be performed at the same time as cleft lip repair

123. A 40-year-old woman undergoes wide excision of a pigmented lesion of her thigh. Pathologic examination reveals malignant melanoma that is Clark's level IV. Findings on examination of the groin are normal. Which of the following is true regarding treatment of her melanoma?

a. Radiotherapy will be an important part of subsequent therapy
b. The likelihood of groin node metastases is remote
c. Immunotherapy is an effective form of adjunctive treatment for metastatic malignant melanoma
d. Groin dissection is not indicated unless and until groin nodes become palpable
e. Intralesional bacille Calmette-Guérin (BCG) administration has been found to aid in local control in the majority of patients

124. A 42-year-old woman has a childhood history of a third-degree scald burn to her right lower extremity that did not require skin grafting. She states that she experienced trauma to the wound one year ago and since then she has had persistent nonhealing of the area. A biopsy of the wound is performed. Which of the following is the most likely diagnosis?

a. Angiosarcoma
b. Malignant melanoma
c. Squamous cell carcinoma
d. Kaposi's sarcoma
e. Keloid

125. A 13-year-old male is in a motor vehicle collision in which the car caught fire. He sustained a circumferential burn but no fractures or other soft tissue trauma to his left lower extremity during extrication from the burning vehicle. Several hours after admission, he complains of numbness and severe pain in his left calf. On examination, he has a palpable, although weak, dorsalis pedis pulse. Which of the following is the most appropriate management?

a. Four-compartment fasciotomies
b. Medial and lateral escharatomies
c. CT scan of the left lower extremity
d. MRI of the left lower extremity
e. Left lower extremity angiogram

126. During a bar brawl, a 19-year-old male sustains a 4-inch laceration on his left arm from glass and presents to the emergency room the following morning, 10 h later. He is neurovascularly intact and the wound is deep, extending down to fascia. Which of the following is the most appropriate management of the wound?

a. Closure of the skin only and administration of oral antibiotics for one week
b. Closure of the skin and subcutaneous tissue and administration of oral antibiotics for one week
c. A single dose of intravenous antibiotics and closure of the skin only
d. A single dose of intravenous antibiotics and closure of the skin and subcutaneous tissue
e. Local wound care without wound closure or antibiotics

127. A 59-year-old woman undergoes an exploratory laparotomy for peritonitis and is found to have perforated diverticulitis. She undergoes a sigmoid resection with an end colostomy. She is administered a third-generation cephalosporin within 1 h prior to the incision and the antibiotic is continued postoperatively. One week later, she develops an intraabdominal abscess, which is percutaneously drained. *Bacteroides fragilis* is isolated from the cultures. Which of the following statements regarding her perioperative antibiotic regimen is most accurate?

a. The preoperative dose of antibiotics should have been given closer to the time of incision
b. The patient should have received several doses of antibiotics prior to laparotomy
c. The patient should have received a first-generation cephalosporin
d. The patient did not have adequate gram-negative coverage
e. The patient did not have adequate anaerobic coverage

128. A 30-year-old man with a history of Crohn's disease develops an enterocutaneous fistula and is placed on total parenteral nutrition through a right subclavian central venous catheter. After five days, the patient develops a fever and leukocytosis; CT scan of the abdomen reveals no intraabdominal abscess. The subclavian catheter insertion site is inspected and noted to be erythematous and painful. Blood cultures are positive. Which of the following organisms is the most likely cause of his fever?

a. Coagulase-positive staphylococci
b. Coagulase-negative staphylococci
c. Group A streptococcus
d. Enterococcus
e. *Escherichia coli*

DIRECTIONS: The group of questions below consists of lettered options followed by a set of numbered items. For each numbered item, select the **one** lettered option with which it is **most** closely associated. Each lettered option may be used once, more than once, or not at all.

Questions 129–131

Match each lower extremity lesion with its correct etiology.

a. Ischemic ulcer
b. Venous stasis ulcer
c. Diabetic ulcer
d. Pyoderma gangrenosum
e. Marjolin's ulcer

129. A 43-year-old man with a painless ulceration over the left medial malleolus with surrounding brany induration

130. A 69-year-old man with a history of diabetes mellitus with pain in the balls of his feet at night with an ulcer over the lateral aspect of his right fifth toe

131. A 52-year-old woman with a history of diabetes mellitus with an ulcer on the plantar surface of her right heel

Skin: Wounds, Infections, and Burns; Hands; Plastic Surgery

Answers

106. The answer is a. (*Townsend, pp 2208–2209.*) The ulnar nerve innervates 15 of the 20 intrinsic muscles of the hand. The musculocutaneous, radial, ulnar, and median nerves are all important to hand function. The musculocutaneous and radial nerves allow forearm supination; the radial nerve alone innervates the extensor muscles. The median nerve is the "eye of the hand" because of its extensive contribution to sensory perception; it also maintains most of the long flexors, the pronators of the forearm, and the thenar muscles.

107. The answer is c. (*Brunicardi, pp 442–445.*) The appropriate margin for wide excision of melanomas is dependent on the depth of the lesion. For thin lesions, less than or equal to 1 mm in depth, a 1-cm margin is adequate. For intermediate (1 to 4 mm) and thick (>4 mm) lesions, a 2-cm margin is recommended.

108. The answer is b. (*Brunicardi, pp 224–230.*) Wound healing is an overlapping sequence of inflammation, proliferation, and remodeling. The inflammatory phase is characterized by a rapid influx of neutrophils, followed in about two days by an influx of mononuclear cells. These monocytes act not only by phagocytosing debris and bacteria, but also by secreting numerous growth factors including tumor necrosis factor (TNF), transforming growth factor, platelet-derived growth factor (PDGF), and fibroblast growth factor, which are essential to normal wound healing. Angiogenesis and collagen formation take place during the proliferative phase of wound healing. Fibroblasts, which enter the wound at about day 3, continue to proliferate with increasing collagen deposition. Throughout the proliferative phase, type III collagen predominates. Collagen content is maximal at two to three weeks, at which time the remodeling phase begins. Type III collagen, which is elastic fibrils, is gradually replaced by rigid fibrils, or type I collagen, at this time. During remodeling, collagen deposition and degradation reach a steady state, which may continue for up to one year.

109. The answer is e. (*Greenfield, pp 192–193.*) The significant observation in this question is the description of lymphangitic inflammatory streaking up the inner aspect of the patient's leg. This is highly suggestive of a streptococcal infection, and the presumptive therapy should be high doses of a bactericidal antibiotic. Penicillin remains the mainstay of therapy against presumed streptococcal infections. Most streptococcal cellulitis is adequately treated by penicillin, elevation of the infected extremity, and attention to the local wound to ascertain adequate local drainage and absence of any persisting foreign body. However, the clinician must be alert to the possibility of a more fulminant and life- or limb-threatening infection by clostridia, microaerophilic streptococci, or other potentially synergistic organisms that can produce rapidly progressive deep infections in fascia of muscle. Close observation of the wound is essential, and aggressive debridement in the operating room is mandatory at the slightest suggestion that fasciitis or myonecrosis may be ensuing.

110. The answer is d. (*Brunicardi, p 436.*) The patient has pyoderma gangrenosum, which is a rare cause of cutaneous ulcerations that can be associated with inflammatory bowel disease as well as other immune disorders. The mainstay of treatment is systemic steroids and immunosuppressants such as cyclosporine. Surgical debridement without medical therapy is not recommended, and local wound care alone or topical steroids are not therapeutic. Saphenous vein ligation and compressive stockings would be more appropriate treatment options in patients with venous stasis ulcers.

111. The answer is d. (*Moore, pp 1104–1105.*) Many methods of treating frostbite have been tried throughout the years. These include massage, warm-water immersion, and covering the affected area. Rapid warming by immersion in water slightly above normal body temperature (40 to 44°C, or 104 to 111.2°F), is the most effective method; however, because the frostbitten region is numb and especially vulnerable, it should be protected from trauma or excessive heat during treatment. Further treatment may include elevation to minimize edema, administration of antibiotics and tetanus toxoid, and debridement of necrotic skin as needed.

112. The answer is e. *(Brunicardi, pp 2025–2056.)* Each digit has two long flexors, called "superficial" and "deep," according to the relative position of the muscle bellies. In the fingers, each superficial flexor tendon divides around the corresponding deep tendon to reach its insertion on the base of the middle phalanx. The deep flexor tendon continues to its insertion on the base of the distal phalanx. Only the deep flexors can flex the distal interphalangeal joint. Since the tendons of the deep flexors share a common muscle belly, only the superficial flexors can move a finger when the adjacent fingers are immobilized. These tendons are prevented from bowstringing across the joints by the flexor retinaculum of the wrists and the fibroosseous tunnels, which extend from the distal palmar crease to the middle phalanx. They run within synovial sheaths and are nourished by vincula tendinum (short mesenteries). The process of healing a tendon injury involves the formation of a tenoma, which tends to become adherent to the surrounding sheath. A difficult balance has to be struck between the desire to prevent adhesions by early mobilization and the risk of rupturing an unhealed tendon. Verdan has divided the hand into six regions according to the anatomy surrounding the tendons. Zone 2, sometimes referred to as no-man's land, refers to the fibroosseous tunnels. Repair in this region is fraught with difficulty.

113. The answer is a. *(Brunicardi, pp 118–120.)* Open cholecystectomy is a clean-contaminated case. Surgical wounds can be divided into three categories based on the amount of bacterial contamination. Clean wounds are those in which no part of the respiratory, gastrointestinal, or genitourinary tract is entered. Examples include herniorrhaphy and breast surgery. Clean-contaminated wounds encompass those cases in which these systems are entered, but without evidence of active infection or gross spillage. Examples include elective cholecystectomy or elective colon resection with adequate bowel preparation. Contaminated wounds are those in which there is active infection (perforated appendicitis with abscess) or gross spillage (gunshot wound with large- or small-bowel injuries). While contaminated and clean-contaminated wounds require perioperative antibiotics, clean wounds need not be treated with prophylactic antibiotics.

114. The answer is e. *(Brunicardi, p 440.)* There is no difference in cure rate between Mohs surgery and wide local excision of a basal cell carcinoma. Mohs surgery describes a technique for resecting either basal or squamous cell carcinomas on the face or near the nose or eye in order to achieve the optimal cosmetic result. Resection of the tumor is performed in small increments with immediate frozen section analysis in order to ensure negative margins. The disadvantage of the Mohs technique is the longer time required.

115. The answer is a. (*Brunicardi, p 440.*) Squamous cell carcinoma occurs in people who have had chronic sun exposure, chronic ulcers or sinus tracts (draining osteomyelitis), or a history of radiation or thermal injury (Marjolin's ulcer). It is more invasive, grows more rapidly, and metastasizes more frequently than basal cell carcinoma. It occurs more frequently in blondes and fair-skinned people. A radiation-induced carcinoma, or one arising in a burn scar, should not be treated with radiation therapy for fear of further damage.

116. The answer is d. (*Brunicardi, pp 204–209.*) Early wound management is characterized by early excision of areas of devitalized tissue, with the exception of deep wounds of the palms, soles, genitals, and face. Staged excision of deep partial-thickness or full-thickness burns occurs between three and seven days after the injury. There are several proven advantages to early excision, including decreased hospital stay and lower cost. This is especially true of burns encompassing more than 30 to 40% of the total body surface area. In conjunction with early excision, topical antimicrobials such as silver sulfadiazine are extremely important in delaying colonization of the newly excised or fresh burn wounds. Permanent coverage through split-thickness skin grafting usually occurs more than one week after injury. Skin autograft requires a vascular bed and therefore cannot be placed over eschar. Meticulous attention to deep circumferential burns is crucial in the management of burn patients. Progressive tissue edema may lead to progressive vascular and neurologic compromise. Because the blood supply is the initial system affected, frequent assessment of flow is vital, with longitudinal escharotomy performed at the first sign of vascular compromise. A low threshold should be maintained in performing an escharotomy in the setting of severely burned limbs.

117. The answer is e. (*Brunicardi, pp 212–213.*) One rare complication of silver nitrate is methemoglobinemia; the more common complication is hyponatremia and other electrolyte imbalances. Other topical agents used to treat burns include silver sulfadiazine and mafenide acetate. The main complications associated with them are neutropenia for silver sulfadiazine and metabolic acidosis secondary to inhibition of carbonic anhydrase for mafenide acetate.

118. The answer is a. *(Brunicardi, pp 518–519.)* Squamous cell carcinoma of the lip is the most common malignant tumor of the lip and constitutes 15% of all malignancies of the oral cavity. Basal cell carcinomas do occur on the lip, but much less frequently. There is a strong association between squamous cell tumors of the lip and sun exposure. Therefore, these lesions are more common in the southern United States and in occupational groups who work out of doors. Because of its greater sun exposure, the lower lip is the site of more than 90% of such lesions. Persistent hyperkeratosis precedes 35 to 40% of these lesions. The incidence of metastases increases with the size of the lesion, and spread is usually via lymphatics to the ipsilateral submental node. Contralateral nodal metastases are rare unless the lesion crosses the midline. Approximately 10 to 15% of all patients have metastases at the time of diagnosis. These lip tumors are very responsive to radiotherapy, which works well for small to medium-sized lesions. Large lesions treated with radiotherapy usually require surgical reconstruction. Radiotherapy should not be used in patients who will have ongoing sun exposure to the area because radiation therapy sensitizes the tissues to solar trauma.

119. The answer is b. *(Townsend, p 2221.)* Signs and symptoms of carpal tunnel syndrome are related to the distribution of the median nerve. This nerve, which passes through the carpal tunnel in the wrist with the finger flexor tendons, may suffer compression from fibrous scarring or malalignment following a fracture of the wrist. Nerve compression may also occur in patients with rheumatoid arthritis who develop flexor tenosynovitis. In women, the syndrome frequently first appears during pregnancy and recurs during the premenstrual phase of subsequent menstrual cycles. In these cases, symptoms are presumably the result of the effects of fluid retention and pressure on the median nerve owing to tissue swelling. In many instances, symptoms are limited to nocturnal pain and paresthesias. If conservative treatment of carpal tunnel syndrome is unsuccessful, surgical treatment may be required. Open and endoscopic techniques have been employed, both of which release adhesions of the median nerve and divide the transverse carpal ligament. The extensor retinaculum is located on the dorsal aspect of the wrist and contains the six compartments of extensor tendons.

120. The answer is d. *(Brunicardi, pp 224–230.)* While epithelialization is responsible for the healing of a closed incision, wound contraction is the primary method of closure in open wounds. During this process, the skin surrounding the wound is pulled over the wound surface and may account for up to a 90% reduction in the size of an open wound. In areas of greater adherence of skin to underlying tissue, the ability of contraction to close the wound is hindered due to the decreased mobility of the skin. Therefore, in areas of tight skin adherence such as the leg, contraction may only account for 30 to 40% reduction in wound size. Fibroblasts in the open wound, which predominate during the proliferative phase, contain increasing numbers of actin microfilaments, thereby becoming myofibroblasts. These specialized fibroblasts are thought to be responsible for wound contraction either through intrinsic cellular contraction or attachment to collagen strands. Bacterial colonization does not harm the process of wound contraction and surgical wound healing. While wound infection is often difficult to diagnose in open wounds, it is generally accepted that bacterial counts of 1 million bacteria per gram of tissue are deleterious to wound closure.

121. The answer is d. *(Townsend, pp 833–834.)* White patches in the oral cavity (leukoplakia) sometimes are incorrectly interpreted as a premalignant condition. Microscopic examination of leukoplakia may in fact reveal hyperplasia, keratosis, or dyskeratosis, of which the last finding is the most serious because of its association with malignancy. Only about 5% of patients with leukoplakia develop cancer. A suggested treatment protocol for patients with thin lesions advocates a program of strict oral hygiene and avoidance of alcohol and tobacco. Biopsy is reserved only for those with thick lesions (since carcinoma in situ may be present). Radiation therapy is contraindicated. Approximately 50% of all oral cancers occur in patients who have associated areas of hyperkeratosis and dyskeratosis. Chronic irritation, such as with poorly fitting dentures, may result in leukoplakia.

122. The answer is b. *(Townsend, pp 2187–2189.)* Clefts of the lip and palate occur relatively frequently (1 in 750 live births); they may be unilateral or bilateral and can vary from a small notch to a complete cleft of the lip and palate. Most clefts occur as isolated anomalies, but occasionally they are associated with neurologic, orthopedic, or cardiac anomalies. A frequently recommended protocol for management is lip repair in the first 3 months of life and palate repair at 12 to 18 months. Other cosmetic procedures can be performed late in childhood and adolescence. Palate repair after two years of age is associated with a high incidence of speech impairment, often requiring speech therapy; repair in the early months of life can lead to a hazardous loss of blood that is poorly tolerated by the infant. Repair of the lip usually should be accomplished as soon as the infant is sufficiently stabilized to tolerate anesthesia with reasonable safety. Ten to twelve weeks is often recommended as the time for lip repair. At this age, the affected baby usually can be converted to dropper or cup feedings in the postoperative period, which thereby facilitates healing of the lip by reducing the need for suckling with the freshly wounded tissues.

123. The answer is d. (*Townsend, pp 781–794.*) The survival of patients with malignant melanoma correlates with the depth of invasion (Clark) and the thickness of the lesion (Breslow). It is widely held that patients with thin lesions (<0.76 mm) and Clark level I and II lesions are adequately managed by wide local excision. The incidence of nodal metastases rises with increasing Clark level of invasion such that a level IV lesion has a 30 to 50% incidence of nodal metastases. Lymph node dissection for melanoma is generally reserved for patients with a positive sentinel lymph node or clinically positive lymph nodes. The sentinel lymph node is the first node that drains a particular nodal basin and can be identified with preoperative injection of ^{99m}Tc sulfur colloid around the lesion and detection with a gamma counter intraoperatively and/or intraoperative injection of blue dye. Sentinel lymph node biopsy is performed for lesions greater than 1 mm in size, and the topic is controversial for thinner lesions, given the low likelihood of metastasis. The sentinel lymph node is analyzed using histologic staining, immunostaining, and reverse transcription polymerase chain reaction testing. Immunotherapy has not been successful in controlling widespread metastatic melanoma even when added to chemotherapy. Intralesional administration of BCG has been demonstrated to control local skin lesions in only 20% of patients. Dinitrochlorobenzene (DNCB) can also be used.

124. The answer is c. (*Brunicardi, pp 216, 446.*) A Marjolin's ulcer refers to a squamous cell carcinoma that develops in a chronic wound such as a previous burn scar or a sinus tract secondary to osteomyelitis. Although basal cell carcinoma, melanoma, and other malignancies can develop in a chronic wound, squamous cell carcinoma is the most common. The mainstay of treatment is surgical excision or amputation. Kaposi's sarcoma usually presents as multifocal lesions on the extremities that may be associated with immunocompromised individuals, and the mainstay of therapy is radiation. Keloids can occur in areas of previous burn and represent an overexuberance of wound healing. Surgical excision alone is associated with a high recurrence rate, and other adjunctive modalities that have been utilized include injection of steroids, radiation, external compression, and topical retinoids.

125. The answer is b. (*Townsend, p 578.*) The patient should undergo medial and lateral escharotomies of his left lower extremity. Based on his clinical history of a circumferential, full-thickness burn and on his symptoms of numbness and pain, the patient has compartment syndrome. The presence of pedal pulses does not preclude the diagnosis of compartment syndrome. If the diagnosis is in question, compartment pressures can be measured, and a pressure of greater than 30 to 40 mmHg is diagnostic. Compartment syndromes secondary to burns are a result of increased pressure secondary to tissue edema and lack of elasticity of the burnt skin (eschar), causing compression of the blood vessels. Fasciotomies are rarely required.

126. The answer is e. (*Townsend, p 264.*) The wound should not be closed because the elapsed time to presentation was greater than 6 h. Wounds that are dirty or contaminated (e.g., animal bites), that are traumatically induced by a puncture, gunshot, or crush injury, or that are older than 6 h should be left open. Prophylactic antibiotics have not been demonstrated to prevent wound infections.

127. The answer is e. (*Townsend, pp 261–277.*) Third-generation cephalosporins provide good coverage against most gram-negative bacteria, but have poor activity against anaerobic bacteria (e.g., *B. fragilis*). Clindamycin or metronidazole can be used in addition to a third-generation cephalosporin to provide anaerobic coverage. Other alternatives include a combination of a penicillin/β-lactamase inhibitor or a cefoxitin or cefotetan, both of which are second-generation cephalosporins. Prophylactic antibiotics against anaerobic organisms are indicated only in cases where they are likely to be encountered (e.g., bowel cases). Prophylactic antibiotics should optimally be administered intravenously within 1 h prior to incision. Continuation of postoperative antibiotics for more than 24 h is indicated in patients with preexisting infection, for example, secondary to perforated viscera, but not after routine elective operations.

128. The answer is b. (*Townsend, p 269–270.*) The most common organism in patients with nosocomial bacteremia is coagulase-negative staphylococcus.

129–131. The answers are 129-b, 130-a, 131-c. (*Townsend, p 2197.*) Venous stasis ulcers are typically located over the medial malleolus, are painless, and may be associated with brawny induration. Treatment consists of leg elevation, compression stockings, local wound care, and occasionally surgical debridement. Ischemic ulcers are often associated with other symptoms of severe peripheral vascular disease such as rest pain, and are commonly located on the dorsum of the foot or the lateral first or fifth toes. Patients with ischemic ulcers should undergo urgent evaluation for lower extremity revascularization. Diabetic ulcers are often associated with trauma or pressure secondary to sensory neuropathy and typically occur on the plantar surface of the foot. Treatment should include optimization of the patient's blood sugars, protective shoewear, and debridement of necrotic tissue. Pyoderma gangrenosum can be associated with underlying disorders such as inflammatory bowel disease, rheumatic heart disease, or malignancy. The lesions are painful ulcerations surrounded by erythema. Treatment consists primarily of corticosteroids and immunosuppressants. A Marjolin's ulcer is a squamous cell carcinoma that arises in a chronic wound and is treated with surgical excision.

Trauma and Shock

Questions

DIRECTIONS: Each item below contains a question followed by suggested responses. Select the **one best** response to each question.

132. A teenage boy falls from his bicycle and is run over by a truck. On arrival in the emergency room, he is awake and alert and appears frightened but in no distress. The chest radiograph suggests an air-fluid level in the left lower lung field and the nasogastric tube seems to coil upward into the left chest. Which of the following is the next best step in his management?

a. Placement of a left chest tube
b. Thoracotomy
c. Laparotomy
d. Esophagogastroscopy
e. Diagnostic peritoneal lavage

133. A 10-year-old boy was the backseat belted passenger in a high-speed motor vehicle collision. On presentation to the emergency room, he is awake, alert, and hemodynamically stable. He is complaining of abdominal pain and he has an ecchymosis on his anterior abdominal wall where the seatbelt was located. Which of the following statements is true regarding need for additional workup?

a. The boy can be safely discharged home without any other workup, since his abdominal pain is probably secondary to his abdominal wall ecchymosis
b. The boy can be safely discharged home if his amylase level is normal
c. The boy can be safely discharged home if abdominal plain films are negative for the presence of free air
d. The boy can be safely discharged home if an abdominal CT scan is negative
e. The boy should be observed regardless of negative test results

134. A 65-year-old man who smokes cigarettes and has chronic obstructive pulmonary disease falls and fractures the third, fourth, and fifth ribs in the left anterolateral chest. Chest x-ray is otherwise normal. Which of the following would be the most appropriate next step in his management?

a. Strapping the chest with adhesive tape
b. Admission to the hospital and treatment with oral analgesia
c. Tube thoracostomy
d. Placement of an epidural for pain management
e. Surgical fixation of the fractured ribs

135. A 36-year-old man who was hit by a car presents to the emergency room with decreased mental status. On examination, his abdominal exam is mildly tender. An ultrasound examination is performed and reveals free fluid in the abdomen. What is the most likely organ to have been injured in this patient?

a. Liver
b. Kidney
c. Spleen
d. Intestine
e. Pancreas

136. A 52-year-old man is pinned against a loading dock, severely injuring the right lower extremity, which is pulseless, pallid, and insensate. Angiography discloses a popliteal artery injury with obstruction. At surgery, the popliteal vein is also transected. The patient also has a fractured femur, a pelvic fracture, and a tender abdomen. His blood pressure is 85/60. Which of the following is the best management strategy for his vascular injuries?

a. Repair of the popliteal vein with simple closure
b. Repair of the popliteal vein with saphenous vein patch
c. Repair of the popliteal vein with a synthetic interposition graft
d. Ligation of the popliteal vein
e. Amputation of the right lower extremity above the knee

137. A 27-year-old man sustains a single gunshot wound to the left thigh. In the emergency room, he is noted to have a large hematoma of his medial thigh. He complains of paresthesias in his foot. On examination, there are weak pulses palpable distal to the injury and the patient is unable to move his foot. Which of the following is the most appropriate initial management of this patient?

a. Angiography
b. Immediate exploration and repair in the operating room
c. Fasciotomy of the anterior compartment of the calf
d. Observation for resolution of spasm
e. Local wound exploration at the bedside

138. A 25-year-old woman arrives in the emergency room following an automobile accident. She is acutely dyspneic with a respiratory rate of 60 breaths per minute. Breath sounds are markedly diminished on the right side. Which of the following is the best first step in the management of this patient?

a. Take a chest x-ray
b. Draw arterial blood for blood-gas determination
c. Decompress the right pleural space
d. Perform pericardiocentesis
e. Administer intravenous fluids

139. A 17-year-old male is stabbed in the left seventh intercostal space, midaxillary line. He presents to the emergency room with a heart rate of 86, blood pressure of 125/74, and oxygen saturation of 98%. Breath sounds are equal bilaterally. Which of the following is the most appropriate next step in his workup?

a. Local exploration of the wound
b. Left tube thoracostomy
c. Diagnostic peritoneal lavage
d. CT scan of the abdomen
e. Echocardiography

140. Your hospital is conducting an ongoing research study involving the hormonal response to trauma. Blood is drawn regularly (with IRB approval) for various studies. Which of the following values are likely to be seen after a healthy 36-year-old man is hit by a bus and sustains a ruptured spleen and a lacerated small bowel?

a. Increased secretion of insulin
b. Increased secretion of thyroxine
c. Decreased secretion of vasopressin (ADH)
d. Decreased secretion of glucagon
e. Decreased secretion of aldosterone

141. A 29-year-old man sustained a gunshot wound to the right upper quadrant. He is taken to the operating room and, after management of a liver injury, is found to have a complete transection of the common bile duct with significant tissue loss. Which of the following is the optimal surgical management of this patient's injury?

a. Choledochoduodenostomy
b. Loop choledochojejunostomy
c. Primary end-to-end anastomosis of the transected bile duct
d. Roux-en-Y choledochojejunostomy
e. Bridging of the injury with a T tube

142. You evaluate an 18-year-old male who sustained a right-sided cervical laceration during a gang fight. Your intern suggests nonoperative management and observation. Which of the following is a relative rather than an absolute indication for neck exploration?

a. Expanding hematoma
b. Dysphagia
c. Dysphonia
d. Pneumothorax
e. Hemoptysis

143. Following blunt abdominal trauma, a 12-year-old girl develops upper abdominal pain, nausea, and vomiting. An upper gastrointestinal series reveals a total obstruction of the duodenum with a coiled spring appearance in the second and third portions. In the absence of other suspected injuries, which of the following is the most appropriate management of this patient?

a. Gastrojejunostomy
b. Nasogastric suction and observation
c. Duodenal resection
d. TPN to increase the size of the retroperitoneal fat pad
e. Duodenojejunostomy

144. A 29-year-old man sustains a closed humeral shaft fracture and on examination in the emergency room is noted to have a radial nerve injury. Which of the following statements is true regarding his treatment and prognosis?

a. Immediate exploration with primary repair of the radial nerve should be undertaken
b. Fracture reduction and observation is the initial management strategy of choice
c. Delayed exploration after six to eight weeks with sural nerve graft results in the best long-term function
d. The incidence of recovery from a closed radial nerve palsy is only 50% with nonoperative management
e. Nerve regeneration occurs at the rate of approximately 0.1 mm/d.

145. An 18-year-old male was assaulted and sustained significant head and facial trauma. Which of the following is the most common initial manifestation of increased intracranial pressure?

a. Change in level of consciousness
b. Ipsilateral (side of hemorrhage) pupillary dilation
c. Contralateral pupillary dilation
d. Hemiparesis
e. Hypertension

146. A 28-year-old man is brought to the emergency room for a severe head injury after a fall. He was intubated in the field for his decreased level of consciousness. He is tachycardic and hypotensive. On examination, he is noted to have an obvious skull fracture and his right pupil is dilated. Which of the following is the most appropriate method for initially reducing his intracranial pressure?

a. Elevation of the head of the bed
b. Saline-furosemide (Lasix) infusion
c. Mannitol infusion
d. Intravenous dexamethasone (Decadron)
e. Hyperventilation

147. A 45-year-old man was an unhelmeted motorcyclist involved in a high-speed collision. He was ejected from the motorcycle and was noted to be apneic at the scene. After being intubated, he was brought to the emergency room, where he is noted to have a left dilated pupil that responds only sluggishly. What is the pathophysiology of his dilated pupil?

a. Infection within the cavernous sinus
b. Herniation of the uncal process of the temporal lobe
c. Laceration of the corpus callosum by the falx cerebri
d. Occult damage to the superior cervical ganglion
e. Cerebellar hypoxia

148. A 31-year-old man is brought to the emergency room following an automobile accident in which his chest struck the steering wheel. Examination reveals stable vital signs and no evidence of respiratory distress, but the patient exhibits multiple palpable rib fractures and paradoxical movement of the right side of the chest. Chest x-ray shows no evidence of pneumothorax or hemothorax. Which of the following is the most appropriate initial management of this patient?

a. Intubation, mechanical ventilation, and positive end-expiratory pressure
b. Stabilization of the chest wall with sandbags
c. Stabilization with towel clips
d. Immediate operative stabilization
e. Pain control, chest physiotherapy, and close observation

149. A 30-year-old man is stabbed in the arm. There is no evidence of vascular injury, but he cannot flex his three radial digits. Which of the following structures has he most likely injured?

a. Flexor pollicis longus and flexor digitus medius tendons
b. Radial nerve
c. Median nerve
d. Thenar and digital nerves at the wrist
e. Ulnar nerve

150. Following a 2-h firefighting episode, a 36-year-old fireman begins complaining of a throbbing headache, nausea, dizziness, and visual disturbances. He is taken to the emergency room, where his carboxyhemoglobin (COHb) level is found to be 31%. Which of the following is the most appropriate next step in his treatment?

a. Begin an immediate exchange transfusion
b. Transfer the patient to a hyperbaric oxygen chamber
c. Begin bicarbonate infusion and give 250 mg acetazolamide (Diamox) intravenously
d. Administer 100% oxygen by mask
e. Perform flexible bronchoscopy with further therapy determined by findings

151. An elderly male pedestrian collides with a bicycle-riding pizza delivery man and suffers a unilateral fracture of his pelvis through the obturator foramen. Which of the following is the best management of this injury?

a. External pelvic fixation
b. Angiographic visualization of the obturator artery with surgical exploration if the artery is injured or constricted
c. Direct surgical approach with internal fixation of the ischial ramus
d. Short-term bed rest with gradual ambulation as pain allows after three days
e. Hip spica cast

152. An 18-year-old male climbs up a utility pole to retrieve his younger brother's kite. An electrical spark jumps from the wire to his metal belt buckle and burns his abdominal wall, knocking him to the ground. Which of the following guides his treatment plan?

a. Injuries are generally more superficial than those from thermal burns
b. Intravenous fluid replacement is based on the percentage of body surface area burned
c. Electric burns often result in a transient traumatic optic neuropathy
d. Evaluation for fracture of the other extremities and visceral injury is indicated
e. Cardiac conduction abnormalities are unlikely

153. A 22-year-old man is examined following a motor vehicle accident. His right leg is injured, as are his elbow and clavicle. Which of the following fractures or dislocations is most likely to result in an associated vascular injury?

a. Knee dislocation
b. Closed posterior elbow dislocation
c. Midclavicular fracture
d. Supracondylar femur fracture
e. Tibial plateau fracture

154. A 23-year-old previously healthy man presents to the emergency room after sustaining a single gunshot wound to the left chest. The entrance wound is 3 cm inferior to the nipple and the exit wound is just below the scapula. A chest tube is placed that drains 400 mL of blood and continues to drain 50 to 75 mL/h during the initial resuscitation. Initial blood pressure of 70/0 mmHg has responded to 2 L crystalloid and is now 100/70 mmHg. Abdominal examination is unremarkable. Chest x-ray reveals a reexpanded lung and no free air under the diaphragm. Which of the following is the best next step in his management?

a. Admission and observation
b. Peritoneal lavage
c. Exploratory thoracotomy
d. Exploratory celiotomy
e. Local wound exploration

155. A patient is brought to the emergency room after a motor vehicle accident. He is unconscious and has a deep scalp laceration and one dilated pupil. His heart rate is 120 beats per minute, blood pressure is 80/40 mmHg, and respiratory rate is 35 breaths per minute. Despite rapid administration of 2 L normal saline, the patient's vital signs do not change significantly. Which of the following is the most appropriate next step in the workup of his hypotension?

a. Neurosurgical consultation for emergent ventriculostomy to manage his intracranial pressure
b. Neurosurgical consultation for emergent craniotomy for suspected subdural hematoma
c. Emergent burr hole drainage at the bedside for suspected epidural hematoma
d. Administration of mannitol and hyperventilation to treat his elevated intracranial pressure
e. Abdominal ultrasound (Focused Assessment with Sonography in Trauma, or FAST)

156. A 25-year-old man is involved in a gang shoot-out and sustains an abdominal gunshot wound from a .22 pistol. At laparotomy, it is discovered that the left transverse colon has incurred a through-and-through injury with minimal fecal soilage of the peritoneum. Which of the following is the most appropriate management of this patient?

a. A colostomy should be performed regardless of the patient's hemodynamic status to decrease the risk of an intraabdominal infection
b. Primary repair should be performed but only in the absence of hemodynamic instability
c. Primary repair should be performed with placement of an intraabdominal drain next to the repair
d. Primary repair should be performed and intravenous antibiotics administered for 14 days
e. The patient should undergo a two-stage procedure with resection of the injured portion and reanastomosis 48 h later when clinically stabilized

157. A 34-year-old prostitute with a history of long-term intravenous drug use is admitted with a 48-h history of pain in her left arm. She is tachycardic to 130 and her systolic blood pressure is 80 mmHg. Physical examination is remarkable for crepitus surrounding needle track marks in the antecubital space with a serous exudate. The plain x-ray of the arm is shown here. Which of the following is the most appropriate next step in her management?

a. Treatment with penicillin G and close observation
b. MRI of the arm
c. CT scan of the arm
d. Surgical exploration and debridement
e. Hyperbaric oxygen therapy

158. A 47-year-old man is extracted from an automobile after a motor vehicle accident. The patient has a steering wheel bruise on the anterior chest. His ECG shows some premature ventricular complexes, and his cardiac isoenzymes are elevated. There is suspicion of a cardiac contusion. Which of the following is the best next step in this patient's workup?

a. Elevated cardiac isoenzyme levels sensitively identify patients at risk for life-threatening arrhythmias
b. The majority of patients have abnormalities on the initial ECG after injury
c. Cardiac imaging such as echocardiography is sensitive in detecting wall motion abnormalities or valvular dysfunction
d. Echocardiography is a good predictor of subsequent cardiac complications such as arrhythmias and pump failure
e. All patients diagnosed with myocardial contusion should be monitored in an intensive care unit setting for 72 h

159. A 70-year-old man sustained several fractures and a ruptured spleen after a fall from 20 ft. Which of the following best represents his body's response to the injury?

a. Decreased liver gluconeogenesis
b. Inhibition of skeletal muscle breakdown by interleukin 1 and tumor necrosis factor (TNF, cachectin)
c. Decreased urinary nitrogen loss
d. Hepatic synthesis of acute-phase reactants
e. Decreased glutamine consumption by fibroblasts, lymphocytes, and intestinal epithelial cells

160. A 36-year-old man sustains a gunshot wound to the left buttock. He is hemodynamically stable. There is no exit wound, and an x-ray of the abdomen shows the bullet to be located in the right lower quadrant. Which of the following is most appropriate in the management of his suspected rectal injury?

a. Barium studies of the colon and rectum
b. Barium studies of the bullet track
c. Endoscopy of the bullet track
d. Angiography
e. Sigmoidoscopy in the emergency room

161. An 18-year-old previously healthy male is dropped off in the emergency room by a friend after being shot in a gang-related shoot-out. He is taken emergently to the operating room, where he is noted to have a large liver laceration in the left lateral segment; bleeding is controlled with hepatorrhaphy and packing. He also undergoes repair of a stomach injury. Postoperatively he is noted to have an intraabdominal fluid collection, which is drained. The output from the drain is bilious and totals 150 cc per day. A HIDA scan demonstrates an active biliary leak from a tertiary radical. Which of the following is the best initial management option for this patient?

a. Relaparotomy for formal left lateral hepatectomy
b. Relaparotomy with placement of larger drains
c. Relaparotomy with Roux-en-Y hepatico-jejunostomy
d. Endoscopic retrograde cholangiopancreaticogram with stent placement
e. Bowel rest with total parenteral nutrition to decrease bile output

162. A 48-year-old man sustains a gunshot wound to the right upper thigh just distal to the inguinal crease. Peripheral pulses are palpable in the foot, but the foot is pale, cool, and hypesthetic. The patient is taken emergently to surgery. Which of the following is not reliably excluded by the presence of palpable distal pulses?

a. Significant arterial injury
b. Significant injury to adjacent motor nerve trunks
c. Significant injury to adjacent long bones
d. Significant injury to adjacent veins
e. Subsequent development of a compartment syndrome and the need for fasciotomy

163. A 62-year-old woman is seen after a three-day history of fever, abdominal pain, nausea, and anorexia. She has not urinated for 24 h. She has a history of previous abdominal surgery for inflammatory bowel disease. Her blood pressure is 85/64, and her pulse is 136. Her response to this physiologic state includes which of the following?

a. Increase in sodium and water excretion
b. Increase in renal perfusion
c. Decrease in cortisol levels
d. Hyperkalemia
e. Hypoglycemia

164. A 20-year-old man presents after being punched in the right eye and assaulted to the head. On a facial CT scan, she is noted to have a blowout fracture of the right orbital floor. Which of the following findings mandates immediate surgical intervention?

a. A fracture 25% of the orbital floor
b. 1 mm of enopthalmos
c. Periorbital ecchymosis
d. Inability to move the right eye upward
e. Traumatic optic neuropathy

165. A 33-year-old woman is seen in the ER with severe rectal bleeding. She has a history of ulcerative colitis. Her blood pressure is 78/56, her pulse is 144, and she is pale and clammy. Which of the following responses is likely to occur after administration of Ringer's lactate solution?

a. Increase in serum lactate concentration
b. Impairment of liver function
c. Improvement in hemodynamics by alleviating the deficit in the interstitial fluid compartment
d. Increase in metabolic acidosis
e. Increase in the need for blood transfusion

166. An 18-year-old high school football player is kicked in the left flank. Three hours later he develops hematuria. His vital signs are stable. An intravenous pyelogram demonstrates extravasation of contrast into the renal parenchyma. Which of the following is the most appropriate treatment for this patient?

a. Resumption of normal daily activity excluding sports
b. Exploration and suture of the laceration
c. Exploration and wedge resection of the left kidney
d. Nephrostomy
e. Antibiotics and serial monitoring of blood count and vital signs

167. A 32-year-old man is in a high-speed motorcycle collision and presents with an obvious pelvic fracture. On examination, he has a scrotal hematoma and blood at his urethral meatus. Which of the following is the most appropriate next step in his management?

a. Placement of a Foley catheter
b. Cystoscopy
c. CT of the pelvis
d. Retrograde urethrogram
e. Nephrostomy tube placement

168. A 17-year-old male sustains a small-caliber gunshot wound to the midepigastrium with no obvious exit wound. His abdomen is very tender; he is taken to the operating room and the bullet appears to have tracked through the midpancreas. Which of the following is correct regarding this type of injury?

a. Most injuries do not involve adjacent organs
b. Management of a ductal injury to the left of the mesenteric vessels is Roux-en-Y pancreaticojejunostomy
c. Management of a ductal injury in the head of the pancreas is pancreaticoduodenectomy
d. Small peripancreatic hematomas need not be explored to search for pancreatic injury
e. The major cause of death is exsanguination from associated vascular injuries

169. A 43-year-old man is examined in the trauma bay after being stabbed in the chest with a long kitchen knife. A chest tube is placed and 800 mL of blood is recovered, with subsequent drainage of approximately 50 mL/h. Resuscitation is best facilitated by which of the following?

a. Placement of long 18-gauge subclavian vein catheters
b. Placement of percutaneous femoral vein catheters
c. Bilateral saphenous vein cutdowns
d. Placement of short, large-bore percutaneous peripheral intravenous catheters
e. Infusion of cold whole blood

170. The victim of a motor vehicle accident who was in shock is delivered to your trauma center by a rural ambulance service with the pneumatic antishock garment (PASG) in place and inflated. Blood pressure is 110/86. X-rays reveal a pelvic fracture. Which of the following statements is true regarding the use of this garment?

a. Elevates blood pressure by an autotransfusion effect, with augmentation of venous return and cardiac output
b. Is not recommended for control of persistent bleeding in the setting of severe pelvic fracture
c. Increases peripheral vascular resistance
d. Expedites assessment of lower-body injuries in the trauma patient
e. Should be terminated by means of prompt deflation as soon as the trauma patient reaches the emergency department

171. A radio transmission is received in your trauma unit stating that a victim of a motor vehicle collision is en route to your ER with no vital signs. The ambulance is 3 min away. As you formulate your plan, which of the following situations would constitute an indication for emergency room thoracotomy?

a. Massive hemothorax following blunt trauma to the chest
b. Blunt trauma to multiple organ systems with obtainable vital signs in the field but none on arrival in the emergency room
c. Rapidly deteriorating patient with cardiac tamponade from penetrating thoracic trauma
d. Penetrating thoracic trauma and no signs of life in the field
e. Penetrating abdominal trauma and no signs of life in the field

172. A 22-year-old man sustains a gunshot wound to the abdomen. At exploration, an apparently solitary distal small-bowel injury is treated with resection and primary anastomosis. On postoperative day 7, small-bowel fluid drains through the operative incision. The fascia remains intact. The fistula output is 300 mL/d and there is no evidence of intraabdominal sepsis. Which of the following is the most appropriate treatment strategy?

a. Early reoperation to close the fistula tract
b. Broad-spectrum antibiotics
c. Total parenteral nutrition
d. Somatostatin to lower fistula output
e. Loperamide to inhibit gut motility

173. A 26-year-old man sustains a gunshot wound to the left thigh. Exploration reveals that a 5-cm portion of superficial femoral artery is destroyed. Which of the following is the most appropriate regarding his management?

a. Debridement and end-to-end anastomosis
b. Debridement and repair with an interposition prosthetic graft
c. Debridement and repair with an interposition arterial graft
d. Debridement and repair with an interposition vein graft
e. Ligation and observation

174. The patient shown in this chest x-ray film and contrast study was hospitalized after a car collision in which he suffered blunt trauma to the abdomen. He sustained several left rib fractures, but was hemodynamically stable. Which of the following statements is true regarding the injury demonstrated in the films?

a. The injury depicted is the most frequent organ injury in the setting of blunt trauma to the abdomen
b. Delayed operative repair is indicated after the patient's rib fractures are allowed to stabilize
c. Surgical treatment of this injury is indicated during this hospitalization
d. Early repair of this injury is preferably accomplished through a left posterolateral thoracotomy
e. If this injury is incidentally discovered during a surgical exploration, it should not be repaired

175. A 56-year-old woman sustains blunt abdominal trauma from an assault. Her blood pressure is 107/56 and her pulse is 92. She complains of abdominal pain. She undergoes CT scanning of the abdomen and pelvis, which demonstrates a splenic injury. Which of the following would preclude an attempt at nonoperative management of the patient?

a. Presence of a subcapsular hematoma involving more than 25% of the surface area of the spleen
b. Presence of a subcapsular hematoma involving more than 50% of the surface area of the spleen
c. Evidence of a blush on CT scan
d. An RBC count of 120,000/μL on diagnostic peritoneal lavage
e. Peritoneal signs on abdominal exam

176. A 49-year-old man was the restrained driver in a motor vehicle collision. He decelerated rapidly in order to avoid hitting another car and swerved into a ditch. He complains of chest pain. Which of the following findings on chest x-ray would be most suspicious for an aortic injury?

a. Multiple right-sided rib fractures
b. A left pulmonary contusion
c. A left pneumothorax
d. Widening of the mediastinum greater than 8 cm
e. Pneumomediastinum

177. A 29-year-old woman was hit by a car while crossing the street. She is hemodynamically unstable with a heart rate of 124 beats per minute and a systolic blood pressure of 82/45. The ultrasound machine is broken, and therefore a diagnostic peritoneal lavage is performed. Which of the following findings on DPL is an indication for exploratory laparotomy in this patient?

a. Aspiration of 5 cc of gross blood initially
b. Greater than 50,000/μL red blood cells
c. Greater than 100,000/μL red blood cells
d. Greater than 100/μL white blood cells
e. Greater than 250/μL white blood cells

178. A 27-year-old construction worker falls about 30 ft from a scaffold. At the scene, he complains of inability to move his lower extremities. On arrival in the emergency room, he has a heart rate of 45 beats per minute and a blood pressure of 78/39. His extremities are warm and pink. His blood pressure improves with 1 L of crystalloid. A central venous catheter is placed for further resuscitation and his central venous pressure is 2 mmHg. Which of the following is the best initial treatment strategy for improving his blood pressure?

a. Immediate celiotomy
b. Fluid resuscitation with crystalloids
c. Administration of O-negative blood
d. Administration of a peripheral vasoconstrictor
e. Administration of intravenous corticosteroids

179. A 22-year-old man undergoes an exploratory laparotomy after a gunshot wound to the abdomen. The patient has multiple injuries including a significant liver laceration, multiple small bowel and colon injuries, and an injury to the infrahepatic vena cava. The patient receives 35 units of packed red blood cells, 15 L of crystalloid, 12 units of FFP, and a 12-pack of platelets. The patient's abdomen is packed closed and he is taken to the intensive care unit for further resuscitation. Which of the following is a sequela of intraabdominal hypertension (abdominal compartment syndrome)?

a. Decreased peak airway pressure
b. Increased cardiac output
c. Decreased systemic vascular resistance
d. Decreased plasma renin and aldosterone
e. Increased intracranial pressure

180. A 10-year-old girl is the unrestrained backseat passenger in a high-speed motor vehicle collision. She is intubated in the field for unresponsiveness and on presentation to the emergency room, her heart rate is 160 beats per minute and her blood pressure is 60/35. She weighs 40 kg. Which of the following is the most appropriate recommendation for her fluid resuscitation?

a. Bolus 1 L of normal saline initially
b. Bolus 1 L of 5% albumin initially
c. Bolus 400 cc of packed RBCs initially
d. Blood transfusion should be initiated if there is only a transient response to the first bolus
e. Blood transfusion should be initiated after one repeat bolus if there is no response to the first bolus

DIRECTIONS: The group of questions below consists of lettered options followed by a set of numbered items. For each numbered item, select the **one** lettered option with which it is **most** closely associated. Each lettered option may be used once, more than once, or not at all.

Questions 181–185

An 18-year-old female is transported to your trauma unit after sustaining a side-impact collision on her side of the car. She is hypotensive and in respiratory distress, and has distended neck veins. For each immediately life-threatening injury of the chest, select the proper intervention.

a. Endotracheal intubation
b. Cricothyroidotomy
c. Subxiphoid window
d. Tube thoracostomy
e. Occlusive dressing

181. Laryngeal obstruction

182. Open pneumothorax

183. Flail chest

184. Tension pneumothorax

185. Pericardial tamponade

Trauma and Shock

Answers

132. The answer is c. (*Greenfield, p 340.*) The patient has an acute diaphragmatic rupture, which occurs in about 4% of patients who sustain either blunt abdominal or chest trauma, and should be treated with immediate laparotomy, which allows both for examination of the intraabdominal solid and hollow viscera for associated injuries and for adequate exposure of the diaphragm to allow secure repair. Because of the risk of vascular compromise of the contents of the hernia, exacerbated by the negative thoracic pressure, acute diaphragmatic rupture should be repaired immediately. Diagnosis may be difficult. The finding of an air-fluid level in the left lower chest with a nasogastric tube entering it after blunt trauma to the abdomen is diagnostic of diaphragmatic rupture with gastric herniation into the chest. Esophagogastroscopy is of limited value. CT scanning and MRI may be useful adjuncts, but neither can definitively rule out diaphragmatic rupture. Diagnostic peritoneal lavage is neither sensitive nor specific for diaphragmatic injuries, particularly in the absence of significant hemorrhage. Diaphragmatic repair can be accomplished via the left chest, but laparotomy is the procedure of choice for acute traumatic rupture for the stated reasons.

133. The answer is e. (*Townsend, pp 513, 518.*) The presence of an abdominal wall ecchymosis from a seatbelt, or a "seatbelt sign," should raise suspicion for an enteric or mesenteric injury. Therefore, these patients should be observed closely for worsening abdominal pain, fevers, or signs of sepsis, even in the face of negative diagnostic tests. Serum amylase levels, plain films of the abdomen, abdominal CT scans, and diagnostic peritoneal lavage (DPL) all have low sensitivity for small-bowel injuries. CT scan findings of free air, or thickening of the small-bowel wall or mesentery, or free fluid in the absence of solid organ injury should raise suspicion of a hollow viscus injury. DPL findings of a WBC count greater than 500/μL, an elevated amylase value, or detection of bile, bacteria, or food fibers should prompt exploratory laparotomy to rule out a bowel injury.

134. The answer is d. (*Greenfield, pp 323–324.*) Patients with lower rib fractures may have associated abdominal injuries and should undergo appropriate evaluation (e.g., ultrasound examination, CT scanning, or peritoneal lavage). Epidural catheters, continuous narcotic infusions, and patient-controlled analgesia are the most effective methods for ensuring pain control in hospitalized patients with rib fractures. Patients who are elderly, have multiple rib fractures, demonstrate ventilatory compromise, or have underlying respiratory problems (such as chronic obstructive pulmonary disease or smoking) are at increased risk for pulmonary complications (atelectasis, pneumonia, respiratory failure) and should be hospitalized. Patients with minor fracture injuries and no significant comorbidities may be managed at home with oral analgesics and appropriate instructions for coughing and deep breathing. Attempts to relieve pain by immobilization or splinting, such as strapping the chest, merely compound the problem of inadequate ventilation. Tube thoracostomy is indicated only if pneumothorax is diagnosed. Intercostal nerve blocks often provide prolonged periods of pain relief, but have been largely replaced by epidural catheters and intravenous narcotic administration. Rib fractures heal spontaneously, without need for surgical fixation.

135. The answer is c. *(Greenfield, pp 340–341.)* The spleen is the organ most likely to be damaged in blunt abdominal trauma, and splenic and liver injuries combined account for 75% of all blunt intraabdominal injuries. The diagnosis of injuries resulting from blunt abdominal trauma is difficult; injuries are often masked by associated injuries. Thus, trauma to the head or chest, together with fractures, frequently conceals intraabdominal injury. Apparently trivial injuries may rupture abdominal viscera in spite of the protection offered by the rib cage. Abdominal ultrasound (Focused Assessment with Sonography in Trauma, or FAST) is a rapid diagnostic test used to evaluate for free intraperitoneal fluid and has largely replaced diagnostic peritoneal lavage (DPL) as the test of choice for evaluation for abdominal injury after blunt trauma. Abdominal CT scans are more specific than either ultrasound or DPL for hepatic, splenic, and renal injuries and can be performed in hemodynamically stable patients who are candidates for nonoperative therapy.

136. The answer is d. *(Greenfield, pp 365–366.)* Ligation rather than venous repair is the treatment of choice in hemodynamically unstable patients. However, the role of venous repair in hemodynamically stable patients with combined arterial and venous extremity injuries is controversial. Proximal veins should be repaired to avoid the sequelae of chronic venous insufficiency. Repairs can be performed primarily with suture closure, using saphenous vein patches, or using synthetic interposition grafts. Amputation may be necessary in the setting of extensive soft tissue and skeletal injuries in conjunction with the vascular injury.

137. The answer is b. (*Greenfield, pp 365–366.*) Immediate exploration and repair is mandated for acute arterial insufficiency in the presence of neurologic symptoms. The five P's of arterial injury include pain, paresthesias, pallor, pulselessness, and paralysis. In the extremities, the tissues most sensitive to anoxia are the peripheral nerves and striated muscle. The early developments of paresthesias and paralysis are signals that there is significant ischemia present, and immediate exploration and repair are warranted. The presence of palpable pulses does not exclude an arterial injury because this presence may represent a transmitted pulsation through a blood clot. When severe ischemia is present, the repair must be completed within 6 to 8 h to prevent irreversible muscle ischemia and loss of limb function. Delay to obtain an angiogram or to observe for change needlessly prolongs the ischemic time. Fasciotomy may be required but should be done in conjunction with and after reestablishment of arterial flow. Local wound exploration at the bedside is not recommended because brisk hemorrhage may be encountered without the securing of prior proximal and distal vascular control.

138. The answer is c. (*Greenfield, pp 326–327.*) Tension pneumothorax is a life-threatening problem requiring immediate treatment. A lung wound that behaves as a ball or flap valve allows escaped air to build up pressure in the intrapleural space. This causes collapse of the ipsilateral lung and shifting of the mediastinum and trachea to the contralateral side, in addition to compression of the vena cava and contralateral lung. Sudden death may ensue because of a decrease in cardiac output; hypoxemia; and ventricular arrhythmias. To accomplish rapid decompression of the pleural space, a large-gauge needle should be passed into the intrapleural cavity through the second intercostal space at the midclavicular line. This may be attached temporarily to an underwater seal with subsequent insertion of a chest tube after the life-threatening urgency has been relieved. Tension pneumothorax produces characteristic x-ray findings of ipsilateral lung collapse, mediastinal and tracheal shift, and compression of the contralateral lung. Occasionally, adhesions prevent complete lung collapse, but the tension pneumothorax is evident because of the mediastinal displacement.

139. The answer is c. (*Greenfield, pp 320, 338.*) Diaphragmatic or abdominal injuries should be suspected in patients with a penetrating injury below the nipples; diagnostic peritoneal lavage (DPL) is an appropriate test to evaluate for an abdominal injury in penetrating abdominal trauma. CT scan has a low sensitivity for diagnosing abdominal injuries in the setting of penetrating trauma. Local wound exploration is contraindicated in penetrating trauma to the chest, given the risk of creating a pneumothorax. An immediate tube thoracostomy is indicated in patients with a suspected tension pneumothorax or in the hemodynamically unstable patient with a suspected pneumo- or hemothorax (e.g., decreased breath sounds). In hemodynamically stable patients without clinical evidence of a pneumothorax, a chest x-ray should be obtained prior to tube thoracostomy. Echocardiography is appropriate for the evaluation for a pericardial effusion in the setting of a penetrating cardiac injury and should be performed for penetrating wounds between the clavicle and costal margin and medial to the midclavicular line.

140. The answer is a. (*Brunicardi, pp 5–9.*) Though the immediate release of catecholamines causes a transient drop in insulin levels, shortly thereafter there is a significant rise in plasma insulin levels in injured humans. Because of increased peripheral insulin resistance in conjunction with increased insulin production, the overall net effect after severe injury is that of hyperglycemia. Since injured patients are highly hypermetabolic, it might be expected that the activity of the thyroid hormones would be increased following injury. This is not the case, however, and increased levels of the thyroid hormones are not seen. Vasopressin (ADH) is regulated by serum osmolality. In the postinjury period, many factors are at play that provoke the excretion of vasopressin. Glucagon secretion is normal or increased after injury; not only are aldosterone levels elevated, but the diurnal fluctuations ordinarily seen are lost.

141. The answer is d. (*Moore, pp 656–657.*) Traumatic injury to the common bile duct must be considered in two separate categories. Complete transection of the common bile duct can be handled in many ways. If the patient is unstable and time is limited, simply placing a T tube in either end of the open common bile duct and staging the repair is the treatment of choice. In a stable patient with a transected bile duct and a loss of tissue, a biliary enteric bypass is preferred. This can be accomplished by Roux-en-Y choledochojejunostomy or cholecystojejunostomy. The jejunum is favored over the duodenum because a lateral duodenal fistula is avoided if the anastomosis leaks. For similar reasons, the defunctionalizing of the jejunal limb is also preferable. This can be accomplished by creating a Roux-en-Y limb of jejunum. Primary end-to-end repair of a completely transected common bile duct can be performed if there is no significant tissue loss and an anastomosis can be performed without significant tension. Primary repair under tension is associated with an increased likelihood of a subsequent stricture. Primary repair is the procedure of choice if the common bile duct is lacerated or only partially transected.

142. The answer is d. (*Greenfield, pp 314–315.*) All hemodynamically unstable patients with a penetrating neck wound should be explored, while management of asymptomatic, stable patients with neck injuries that penetrate the platysma is more controversial. In the past, treatment of asymptomatic, stable patients with zone II (between the lower border of the cricoid cartilage to the angle of the mandible) injuries was mandatory operative exploration. However, proponents for selective management of these patients argue that there is a high rate of negative explorations of the neck (40 to 60%) and that serious injuries can be overlooked despite operative exploration. Furthermore, studies have demonstrated similar incidences of overall mortality with either selective or mandatory exploration. Stable patients with zone III (between the angle of the mandible and the skull), zone I (between the sternal notch and the lower border of the cricoid cartilage), or multiple neck wounds, should undergo initial angiography irrespective of the ultimate treatment plan. For zone II injuries, algorithms exist for nonoperative management of asymptomatic patients that employ observation alone or combinations of vascular and aerodigestive contrast studies and endoscopy. Nevertheless, recognition of acute signs of airway distress (stridor, hoarseness, dysphonia), visceral injury (subcutaneous air, hemoptysis, dysphagia), hemorrhage (expanding hematoma, unchecked external bleeding), or neurologic symptoms referable to carotid injury (stroke or altered mental status) or lower cranial nerve or brachial plexus injury requires formal neck exploration. Pneumothorax would mandate a chest tube; the necessity for exploration would depend on clinical judgment and institutional policy.

143. The answer is b. (*Greenfield, p 348.*) Duodenal hematomas result from blunt abdominal trauma, and they should be managed initially with observation in patients not undergoing laparotomy to rule out other associated injuries. They present as a proximal bowel obstruction with abdominal pain and occasionally a palpable right upper quadrant mass. An upper gastrointestinal series is almost always diagnostic, with the classic coiled spring appearance of the second and third portions of the duodenum secondary to the crowding of the valvulae conniventes (circular folds) by the hematoma. Observation is the initial management strategy in patients with no other injuries, since the vast majority of duodenal hematomas resolve spontaneously. However, in patients undergoing immediate laparotomy for other associated injuries, duodenal exploration with drainage of the hematoma is indicated. Also, patients whose obstructive symptoms do not resolve after two weeks should undergo exploration and evacuation of the hematoma in order to rule out a perforation or injury to the head of the pancreas. Surgical bypass and duodenal resection are not indicated in the initial management of a duodenal hematoma.

144. The answer is b. (*Greenfield, p 2121.*) The initial management of choice for closed radial nerve palsies is fracture reduction and observation, since the prognosis is excellent—the incidence of recovery is close to 90%. Operative intervention may be indicated after several months if function does not appear to be returning; either primary repair or reconstruction with sural nerve graft can be employed at that time.

Transection of a peripheral nerve results in hemorrhage and in retraction of the severed nerve ends. Almost immediately, degeneration of the axon distal to the injury begins. Degeneration also occurs in the proximal fragment back to the first node of Ranvier. Phagocytosis of the degenerated axonal fragments leaves a neurilemmal sheath with empty cylindrical spaces where the axons were. Several days following the injury, axons from the proximal fragment begin to regrow. If they make contact with the distal neurilemmal sheath, regrowth occurs at about the rate of 1 mm/d. However, if associated trauma, fracture, infection, or separation of neurilemmal sheath ends precludes contact between axons, growth is haphazard and a traumatic neuroma is formed.

145. The answer is a. (*Greenfield, pp 295–297.*) Closed head injuries may result in cerebral concussion owing to depression of the reticular formation of the brainstem. This type of injury is usually reversible. Local bleeding and swelling (intracranial or extracranial) produce an increase in intracranial pressure. A characteristic symptom pattern occurs, initiated by progressive depression of mental status.

146. The answer is e. (*Greenfield, p 299.*) Emergency measures to reduce intracranial pressure include hyperventilation, mannitol infusion, and elevation of the head of the bed (reverse Trendelenburg position). However, in the face of inadequate volume resuscitation, osmotic diuresis with mannitol and placement of the patient in reverse Trendelenburg may exacerbate the patient's hypotension. CT scanning should be performed as soon as possible along with neurosurgical evaluation in order to determine the need for operative drainage or decompression.

147. The answer is b. (*Greenfield, pp 295–297.*) Increasing intracranial pressure tends to displace brain tissue away from the source of the pressure; if the pressure is sufficient, herniation of the uncal process through the tentorium cerebri occurs. Pupillary dilation is caused by compression of the ipsilateral oculomotor nerve and its parasympathetic fibers. If the pressure is not relieved, the brainstem will herniate through the foramen magnum and cause death. Hypertension and bradycardia are preterminal events.

148. The answer is e. (*Greenfield, pp 324–325, 328–329.*) Management of flail chest consists of adequate analgesia, chest physiotherapy, and mechanical ventilation if respiratory compromise develops. Flail chest is diagnosed in the presence of paradoxical respiratory movement in a portion of the chest wall. At least two fractures in each of three adjacent rib or costal cartilages are required to produce this condition. The complications of flail chest are no longer believed to arise from this paradoxical motion, but rather that the underlying pulmonary parenchymal injury with resultant hypoventilation can lead to atelectasis, pneumonia, and respiratory failure. Indications for mechanical ventilation include significant impedance to ventilation by the flail segment, large pulmonary contusion, an uncooperative patient (e.g., owing to head injury), general anesthesia for another indication, and the development of respiratory failure. Chest stabilization with sandbags or towel clips is no longer used. Surgical stabilization is performed only if thoracotomy is to be performed for another indication.

149. The answer is c. *(Brunicardi, pp 1764–1770.)* The motor components of the median nerve maintain the muscular function of most of the long flexors of the hand as well as the pronators of the forearm and the thenar muscles. The median nerve is also an extremely important sensory innervator of the hand and is commonly described as the "eye of the hand" because the palm, the thumb, and the index and middle fingers all receive their sensation via the median nerve.

150. The answer is d. *(Greenfield, p 444.)* Carbon monoxide (CO) is the leading cause of toxin-related death in the United States. It is produced by the incomplete combustion of fossil fuels and is emitted by virtually all gas-powered engines and appliances that burn fossil fuel, such as home furnaces, water heaters, stoves, pool heaters, kerosene heaters, and charcoal fires. Tobacco smoke—particularly smoke released from the tip of the cigarette, which has 2.5 times more CO than inhaled smoke—produces a significant amount of the gas; nonsmokers working in closed quarters with smokers may have carboxyhemoglobin (COHb) levels as high as 15%, easily enough to cause headache and some impairment of judgment. Firefighters are at particularly high risk for CO intoxication. The pathophysiology of CO poisoning is unclear. It is known to cause an adverse shift in the oxygen-hemoglobin dissociation curve, to cause direct cardiovascular depression, and to inhibit cytochrome a_3. Tissue hypoxia is the result. Treatment is directed toward increasing the partial pressures of O_2 to which the transalveolar hemoglobin is exposed. In most cases, administering 100% oxygen through a tightly fitted face mask will result in a serum elimination half-life of COHb of 80 min (compared with 520 min when breathing room air). In severe cases, where coma, seizures, or respiratory failure are present, the partial pressure of O_2 is increased by administering it in a hyperbaric chamber with an atmospheric pressure of 2.8. In this situation the serum elimination half-life is reduced to 23 min. In any case, the oxygen therapy should continue until the COHb levels reach 10%.

151. The answer is d. *(Moore, pp 779–803.)* Most pelvic fractures are the result of automobile-pedestrian accidents, and these fractures are a frequent cause of death. The pelvis is extremely vascular with a diffuse blood supply that makes hemorrhage common and surgical control of bleeding difficult. This patient has a type II fracture (single break in pelvic ring) through a non-weight-bearing portion of the pelvis. These fractures are best treated by bed rest until hemodynamic stability is ensured and thereafter by gentle ambulation as pain permits. The clinician must watch carefully for associated injuries to the bladder, urethra, and colon and be alert to the many other possible concurrent injuries to an elderly patient who has suffered a collision, even a low-velocity attack from a pizza man.

152. The answer is d. (*Moore, pp 1086–1087.*) The treatment of electrical injury should be modified from that of thermal burns because tissue damage is much deeper than is apparent at first inspection. The heat generated is proportional to the resistance to the flow of current. Bone, fat, and tendons offer the greatest resistance. Therefore, the tissue deep within the center of an extremity may be injured while more superficial tissues are spared. For this reason, the quantification of fluid requirements cannot be based on the percentage of body surface area involved, as in the Parkland, Brooke, or Baxter formulas used to calculate fluid replacement after thermal burns. Massive fluid replacement is usually essential. A brisk urine output is desirable because of the likelihood of myonecrosis with consequent myoglobinuria and renal damage. As with deep thermal burns, debridement, skin grafting, and amputation of extremities may be required following electrical injury. However, fasciotomy is more frequently required than escharotomy with electrical injury because deep myonecrosis results in increased intracompartmental pressures and compromised limb perfusion. In addition, distant fractures may result, owing to vigorous muscle contraction during the accident or if subsequent falls occur. Cardiac or respiratory arrest may occur if the pathway of the current includes the heart or brain. An electrical current can also damage the pulmonary alveoli and capillaries and lead to respiratory infections, a major cause of death in these victims. Electrical burns can also result in cataract development even months after the injury, and therefore these patients require ophthalmologic follow-up.

153. The answer is a. (*Bunt, pp 226–228.*) In a four-year retrospective study of 569 at-risk parajoint fractures or dislocations resulting from blunt trauma, there was only a 1.5% incidence of associated vascular injury. Angiograms and vascular surgical consultations were obtained when vascular compromise was suspected owing to clinical examination or Doppler confirmation of flow abnormalities. While vascular injuries due to fractures on either side of a joint (e.g., supracondylar femur fracture or tibial plateau fracture) were uncommon, major joint dislocations were more commonly associated with vascular injury. An exception to this rule is the type III supracondylar humerus fracture, where displacement of bone may injure or entrap the tethered brachial artery. Clavicular fractures are rarely associated with significant vascular injury. The highest rate of vascular injury occurs with knee dislocations because of the extreme force required to dislocate the joint. In open elbow dislocations, the brachial artery is often disrupted by forcible hyperextension of the joint; closed elbow dislocations are rarely associated with vascular injury unless the dislocation is anterior.

154. The answer is d. (*Greenfield, pp 327, 334–335.*) Gunshot wounds to the lower chest are often associated with intraabdominal injuries. The diaphragm can rise to the level of T4 during maximal expiration. Therefore, any patient with a gunshot wound below the level of T4 should be subjected to abdominal exploration. Exploratory thoracotomy is not automatically indicated because most parenchymal lung injuries will stop bleeding and heal spontaneously with the use of tube thoracostomy alone. Indications for thoracic exploration for bleeding are 1500 mL of blood on initial chest tube placement or persistent bleeding at a rate of 200 mL/h for 4 h or 100 mL/h for 8 h. Peritoneal lavage is not indicated even when the abdominal examination is unremarkable. As many as 25% of patients with negative physical findings and negative peritoneal lavage will have significant intraabdominal injuries in this setting. These injuries include damage to the colon, kidney, pancreas, aorta, and diaphragm. Local wound exploration is not recommended because the determination of diaphragmatic injury with this technique is unreliable.

155. The answer is e. (*Greenfield, pp 297–299.*) Except in the rare circumstance, hypotension in a trauma patient should be presumed to be secondary to hypovolemia and not the head injury. When cardiovascular collapse occurs as a result of rising intracranial pressure, it is generally accompanied by hypertension, bradycardia, and respiratory depression. On the other hand, loss of consciousness following head trauma should be assumed to be due to intracranial hemorrhage until proved otherwise. A thorough evaluation of the head-injured patient includes assessment for other potentially life-threatening injuries including abdominal, thoracic, and pelvic hemorrhage. Appropriate workup should be initiated (chest and pelvic x-rays, abdominal evaluation with FAST exam or DPL). Rarely, a patient may have sufficient hemorrhage from a scalp laceration to cause hypotension, but caution should be used in attributing hypotension and tachycardia solely to such an injury.

156. The answer is b. (*Greenfield, pp 352–353.*) Primary repair of traumatic colon injuries can be safely performed in the absence of risk factors such as gross fecal contamination, shock on presentation, multiple other injuries, or delayed intervention. Alternatives to primary repair include end colostomy with mucous fistula or Hartmann's pouch and protection of a primary repair in the distal colon by formation of a proximal colostomy or ileostomy.

157. The answer is d. (*Greenfield, pp 193–194.*) In patients with suspected necrotizing fasciitis, an infection of the superficial and deep fascia that is associated with high rates of morbidity and mortality, prompt surgical exploration is mandatory. While CT and MRI may be useful adjuncts in the diagnosis of necrotizing fasciitis, they should not be performed in unstable patients or patients in whom the diagnosis is likely. Treatment consists of prompt surgical debridement and intravenous antibiotics. Most of these infections are polymicrobial, although monomicrobial necrotizing soft tissue infections can be caused by *Group A beta-hemolytic Streptococcus* or *Clostridium*. If the latter is suspected, high-dose penicillin G should be administered. Hyperbaric oxygen may be used as an adjunct; however, its efficacy has never been proven in clinical trials.

158. The answer is c. (*Greenfield, p 331.*) The spectrum of blunt cardiac injuries includes myocardial contusion, rupture, and internal (chamber and septal) disruptions such as traumatic septal defects, papillary muscle tears, and valvular tears. Myocardial contusions are by far the most common of these injuries. They usually occur in persons who sustain a direct blow to the sternum, as seen in a driver whose sternum is forcibly compressed by the steering column in a deceleration injury. They may have external signs of thoracic trauma, including sternal tenderness, abrasions, ecchymosis, palpable crepitus, rib fractures, or flail segments. Overall, fewer than 10% of patients have conduction abnormalities, dysrhythmias, or ischemic patterns on initial ECG. Elevated cardiac isoenzyme levels are specific for myocardial injury, but they lack clinical significance in patients without ECG abnormalities or hemodynamic instability. Echocardiography provides a sensitive assessment of ventricular wall motion and ejection fraction after blunt chest trauma, but is a poor predictor of the significant cardiac complications of pump failure and arrhythmia. Patients without evidence of ECG abnormalities on presentation and who are hemodynamically stable do not require extended ICU monitoring. Virtually all patients who develop cardiac complications display ECG abnormalities on arrival in the emergency room or within the first 24 h. Since an abnormal ECG is a good predictor of subsequent complications, stable patients with possible myocardial contusions but with a normal ECG tracing may be placed on telemetry for 24 h rather than monitored in an ICU.

159. The answer is d. (*Weissman, pp 308–327.*) Injury and sepsis result in accelerated protein breakdown with increased urinary nitrogen loss and increased peripheral release of amino acids. The negative nitrogen balance represents the net result of breakdown and synthesis (with breakdown increased and synthesis increased or diminished). Amino acids such as alanine are released by muscle and transported to the liver for incorporation into acute-phase proteins including fibrinogen, complement, haptoglobin, and ferritin. The amino acids also undergo gluconeogenesis to glucose, which is utilized primarily by the brain and other glycolytic tissues such as peripheral nerves, erythrocytes, and bone marrow. Other tissues receive energy from fat in the form of fatty acids or ketone bodies during starvation following major trauma; this helps to conserve body protein. Glutamine is the most abundant amino acid in the blood, and its levels in muscle and blood decrease following injury and sepsis, as it is consumed rapidly by replicating fibroblasts, lymphocytes, and intestinal endothelial cells. The use of glutamine may decrease protein catabolism in the intestine and may help prevent atrophy of the gastrointestinal tract in starved and parenterally nourished patients. Along with the counterregulatory hormones (glucagon, epinephrine, cortisol), interleukin 1 appears to mediate muscle breakdown. Recent studies have indicated that TNF (also called cachectin because of the role it plays in muscle wasting in septic or oncologic patients) also may be a principal catabolic cytokine in the traumatized patient. This protein is secreted by macrophages and further affects metabolism by inducing secretion of interleukin 1 and inhibiting synthesis and activity of lipogenic enzymes.

160. The answer is e. (*Moore, pp 745–750.*) Penetrating injury to the intraperitoneal or extraperitoneal rectum should be diagnosed by immediate sigmoidoscopy. Contrast studies of the rectum when sigmoidoscopy is inconclusive should use a water-soluble radiopaque medium such as Gastrografin. The use of barium is contraindicated because its spillage in the peritoneal cavity mixed with feces would increase the likelihood of subsequent intraabdominal abscesses. Instrumentation of the bullet track is also contraindicated because of the risk of injury to adjacent structures (e.g., bladder, ureters, iliac vessels). Angiography is not a sensitive method for demonstrating injury of the intestinal wall.

161. The answer is d. (*Moore, pp 637–653.*) A bile leak is a well-recognized complication after operative intervention for liver trauma, and a persistent bile leak should be treated with drainage and endoscopic retrograde cholangiopancreatography (ERCP) with sphincterotomy and/or stenting. Persistent bile leaks greater than 50 cc/d for over two weeks are considered biliary fistulas. Early biliary drainage greater than 300 cc/d warrants further evaluation to assess for injury to a main bile duct; major biliary injuries are treated with re-laparotomy and a hepatico-jejunostomy. Minor bile leaks can often be managed with drainage of the collection of bile, also known as a biloma, without further intervention. Bile leaks can also occur after nonoperative intervention for blunt liver trauma and should be suspected in a patient with nausea, vomiting, abdominal distention, and elevated liver function tests. Treatment consists of percutaneous drainage of the biloma, and ERCP if the bile leak persists.

162. The answer is a. (*Greenfield, pp 370–372.*) The presence of ischemic changes following vascular trauma is an indication for emergency exploration and repair. Nonsurgical management of arterial trauma when distal pulses are palpable may lead to delayed sequelae of embolization, occlusion, secondary hemorrhage, false aneurysm, and traumatic arteriovenous fistula. The presence of palpable pulses does not reliably exclude significant arterial injury. Injuries that may be missed if exploration is not performed include lacerations and partial transections containing hematomas, intramural or intraluminal thromboses, and intimal disruptions or tears. Injury to motor nerves would be apparent on neurologic examination. Injury to bone would be diagnosed by x-ray. Adjacent venous injury, in the absence of an expanding hematoma, would not by itself mandate exploration because there are numerous collateral venous channels in the extremities.

Prophylactic fasciotomy is not routinely performed for all arterial injuries but is indicated in the presence of an ischemic period exceeding 4 to 6 h, combined arterial and major venous injury, prolonged periods of hypotension, massive associated soft tissue trauma, and massive edema.

163. The answer is d. (*Greenfield, pp 202–203.*) The biochemical changes associated with shock result from tissue hypoperfusion, endocrine response to stress, and specific organ system failure. During shock, the sympathetic nervous system and adrenal medulla are stimulated to release catecholamines. Renin, angiotensin, antidiuretic hormone, adrenocorticotropin, and cortisol levels increase. Resultant changes include sodium and water retention and an increase in potassium excretion, protein catabolism, and gluconeogenesis. Potassium levels rise as a result of increased tissue release, anaerobic metabolism, and decreased renal perfusion. If renal function is maintained, potassium excretion is high and normal plasma potassium levels are restored.

164. The answer is d. (*Moore, pp 418, 434.*) Blowout orbital fractures require immediate operative intervention in the event of extraocular muscle entrapment. Inability to move the eye upward suggests entrapment of the inferior rectus muscle and mandates surgical release of the muscle. Patients with blowout fractures can have periorbital ecchymoses, pain, or diplopia. Surgery is indicated in patients with enophthalmos greater than 2 mm, diplopia on primary or inferior gaze, entrapment of extraocular muscles, or fracture greater than 50% of the orbital floor.

165. The answer is c. (*Greenfield, pp 252, 291.*) Infusion of lactated Ringer's solution is an effective immediate step, both clinically and experimentally, in managing hypovolemic shock. Use of this balanced salt solution helps correct the fluid deficit (in the extracellular, extravascular compartment) resulting from hypovolemic shock. This procedure may decrease requirements for whole blood in patients with hemorrhagic shock. If blood loss has been minimal and is controlled, whole blood transfusion may be avoided entirely. The theoretical objection to infusion of lactated Ringer's solution is that it will increase lactate levels and compound the problem of lactic acidosis. This has not been borne out in animal or clinical studies.

Along with the hemodynamic improvement that follows volume restitution, liver function improves, lactate metabolism is improved, excess lactate levels drop, and metabolic acidosis improves.

166. The answer is e. (*Cass, pp 213–220.*) In stable patients with suspected genitourinary tract injury, the first urologic study other than urinalysis should be the intravenous urogram. The technique of high-dose drip infusion is desirable because the high concentration of contrast achieved greatly facilitates interpretation in an unprepared patient. Intravenous pyelography should be performed before retrograde cystography to avoid obscuring visualization of the lower ureteral tract. The study also may preclude the need for retrograde urethrography in cases where, unlike the case presented, there is a suspicion of urethral injury. Renal arteriography is not indicated routinely but should be performed to rule out renal pedicle injury when no kidney function is demonstrated by drip infusion urography. Peritoneal lavage is not useful in the diagnosis of genitourinary injuries because the structures are retroperitoneal. Of patients with blunt renal trauma, 70 to 80% are successfully treated nonsurgically. Bed rest may reduce the likelihood of secondary hemorrhage; antibiotics may reduce the chance of an infection developing in a perirenal hematoma. Failure of conservative treatment is indicated by rising fever, increasing leukocytosis, evidence of secondary hemorrhage, and persistent or increasing pain and tenderness in the region of the kidney.

167. The answer is d. (*Moore, pp 820–821.*) If a urethral injury is suspected, a retrograde urethrogram should be performed before attempting to place a Foley catheter. If there is a urethral disruption, a suprapubic catheter should be placed. Urethral injuries can be associated with pelvic fractures, and suspicion of a urethral injury should be increased if any of the following signs are present: blood at the urethral meatus, a scrotal hematoma, or a free-floating prostate on rectal examination.

168. The answer is e. (*Moore, pp 724–728.*) Complications of pancreatic injury include fistula, pseudocyst, and abscess, but the cause of death in patients with pancreatic injury is most frequently exsanguination from associated injury to major vascular structures such as the splenic vessels, mesenteric vessels, aorta, or inferior vena cava. The majority of penetrating pancreatic injuries can be managed with simple drainage. Injury to the major pancreatic duct to the left of the mesenteric vessels is effectively treated with a distal pancreatectomy. The high morbidity and morality of pancreaticoduodenectomy for trauma limit its use to extensive blunt injuries to both pancreatic head and duodenum. For ductal injury in the region of the head of the pancreas (to the right of the mesenteric vessels), a Roux-en-Y limb of jejunum can be brought up and used to drain the transected duct. Finally, however small, all peripancreatic hematomas should be explored to search for pancreatic injury.

169. The answer is d. (*Dutky, pp 856–860.*) Rapid fluid administration is often the key to successful trauma resuscitation. Some of the important factors affecting the rate of fluid resuscitation include the diameter of the intravenous tubing, the size and length of the venous cannulas, the fluid viscosity, and the site of administration. According to Poiseuille's law, flow is proportional to the fourth power of the radius of a catheter and inversely proportional to its length. Therefore, the shorter a catheter and the larger its diameter, the faster a solution can be infused through it. Central venous placement alone does not ensure rapid flow. Importantly, the diameter of the intravenous tubing employed may be the rate-determining factor in fluid delivery: blood infusion tubing allows twice the flow of standard intravenous tubing and should be used when rapid fluid resuscitation is needed. Any patient suspected of having a major abdominal injury should immediately have at least two short, large-bore (16-gauge or larger) intravenous cannulas placed in peripheral veins. Longer, smaller catheters, such as standard 18-gauge central venous catheters, may take more time to place and will have lower flow rates. Once fluid resuscitation is under way, the physician may elect to place an 8 or 9 French pulmonary artery catheter-introducer via a central venous approach for further volume administration, as well as for measurement of central venous pressure or for Swan-Ganz catheter insertion. Lower-extremity venous cannulas, placed by saphenous vein cutdown or percutaneously into the femoral veins, are no longer advised as primary access for patients with abdominal trauma, since possible disruption of iliac veins or the inferior vena cava will render volume infusion ineffective. Studies have demonstrated that the flow rate of cold whole blood is roughly two-thirds that of whole blood at room temperature. Diluting and warming the blood by "piggybacking" it into infusion lines that are delivering crystalloid will decrease the blood's viscosity, enhance flow, and minimize hypothermia.

170. The answer is c. *(Flint, pp 703–707; Trunkey, pp 479–486.)* The pneumatic antishock garment (PASG) is composed of inflatable overalls with three compartments, two for the legs and one for the abdomen. It has now been convincingly demonstrated that the PASG elevates blood pressure by increasing peripheral vascular resistance rather than by an autotransfusion effect on venous return and increased cardiac output. The PASG is beneficial for controlling bleeding from pelvic fractures by reduction of pelvic volume and immobilization to restrict fracture movement. The suit pressure must be released very slowly because rapid deflation can lead to sudden, irreversible hypotension. This is probably due to a sudden decrease in peripheral vascular resistance and to the effects of vasodilation and washout of accumulated metabolites of capillary beds under the suit. On reperfusion of the lower body, a systemic metabolic acidemia with hyperkalemia may result and must be closely monitored. For these reasons, satisfactory intravenous volume must be attained prior to decompression of the PASG, a delay that may prevent adequate early evaluation of concealed injuries to the lower body.

171. The answer is c. *(Moore, pp 493–505.)* Although indications for thoracotomy in the emergency room are controversial, the procedure appears to be most beneficial when it is employed to (1) release cardiac tamponade in patients with penetrating thoracic trauma who are deteriorating too rapidly for a subxiphoid pericardial window to be created; (2) allow cross-clamping of the descending aorta in patients with intraabdominal bleeding for whom other measures are not effective in maintaining blood pressure; or (3) allow effective internal cardiac massage in patients who arrive in the emergency room with faint or absent pulses and distant heart sounds, and for whom other resuscitative efforts are unsuccessful. By contrast, existing evidence suggests that patients who are unsalvageable and do not benefit from emergency room thoracotomy include (1) those with no vital signs (pulse, pupillary reaction, spontaneous respiration) in the field and (2) those with blunt trauma to multiple organ systems and absent vital signs on arrival in the emergency room.

172. The answer is c. *(Way, p 189.)* In the absence of sepsis, patients with enterocutaneous fistulas should be treated initially nonoperatively with bowel rest, total parenteral nutrition (TPN), and correction of electrolyte abnormalities. Most enterocutaneous fistulas result from trauma sustained during surgical procedures. Irradiated, obstructed, and inflamed intestine is prone to fistulization. Complications of fistulas include fluid and electrolyte depletion, skin necrosis, and malnutrition. Fistulas are classified according to their location and the volume of output, because these factors influence prognosis and treatment. When the patient is stable, a small-bowel follow-through study can be obtained to determine (1) the location of the fistula, (2) the relation of the fistula to other hollow intraabdominal organs, and (3) whether there is distal obstruction. Proximal small-bowel fistulas (from the stomach to mid-ileum) tend to produce a high output of intestinal fluid and are less likely to close with conservative management than are distal, low-output fistulas (distal ileum or colon). Small-bowel fistulas that communicate with other organs (e.g., bladder) may need aggressive surgical repair because of the risk of associated infections. When these poor prognostic factors for stabilization and spontaneous closure are observed, early surgical intervention must be undertaken. The patient in the question, however, appears to have a low-output, distal enterocutaneous fistula. Antispasmodic drugs have not been proved effective; somatostatin has been used with mixed success in the setting of high-output fistulas. There is no indication for antibiotics in the absence of sepsis. Total parenteral nutrition (TPN) is given to maintain or restore the patient's nutritional balance while minimizing the quantity of dietary fluids and endogenous secretions in the gastrointestinal tract. Initial TPN therapy is warranted to allow for spontaneous closure of a low-output distal fistula, but often these patients can be subsequently placed on a low-residue diet. Should conservative management fail, surgical closure of the fistula is performed.

173. The answer is d. (*Greenfield, pp 365–366.*) Traumatic arterial injuries can be handled with several techniques. The basic principles of debridement of injured tissue and reestablishment of flow should be observed. Primary end-to-end anastomosis is preferable if this can be accomplished without tension. When 5 cm of artery has been destroyed, it is impossible to perform a tension-free primary anastomosis, and a reversed saphenous vein graft is the repair of choice. Ligation of the artery is to be avoided in order to prevent gangrene and limb loss. The use of prosthetic material (Gore-Tex) in a potentially infected field is also to be avoided, as infection at the suture line often leads to delayed hemorrhage. Harvesting an arterial graft of similar diameter from elsewhere in the body is hazardous and unnecessary when vein is available.

174. The answer is c. (*Moore, pp 622–626.*) Traumatic injuries to the diaphragm are associated with both blunt and penetrating trauma. The spleen, kidneys, intestines, and liver are the most frequently injured abdominal organs in blunt trauma; the diaphragm is the least. Missed injuries lead to problems with herniation and bowel strangulation with sufficient frequency that repair should not be delayed. All such injuries require repair once the diagnosis is made and the patient has been stabilized. Most acute defects in the diaphragm can be repaired via an abdominal approach, which allows exploration for coexisting injuries.

175. The answer is e. (*Moore, pp 671–673.*) Nonoperative management of a splenic injury is contraindicated if the physical examination is suggestive of an associated injury requiring operative intervention such as a blunt intestinal injury. The severity of the splenic injury can be graded based on the CT scan, but the grade of splenic injury does not always correlate to the need for operative intervention. Therefore, even the presence of a grade V injury (completely shattered spleen or hilar vascular injury) does not preclude a trial of nonoperative therapy. However, the opposite may also be true in that an apparently minor injury on CT scan may be much more significant on exploration. There may be a role for angiographic embolization of the splenic artery in the presence of a blush on CT scan, and there is evidence to suggest that the presence of a blush decreases the likelihood of success with nonoperative management. Patients who are hemodynamically unstable or who demonstrate clinical deterioration should undergo exploratory laparotomy. Although an RBC count greater than 100,000/μL constitutes a positive DPL in blunt abdominal trauma, a positive DPL in and of itself does not require exploratory laparotomy.

176. The answer is d. (*Moore, pp 575–580.*) There are multiple findings on chest x-ray that are suggestive of a thoracic aortic injury, such as widening of the mediastinum more than 8 cm, loss of the aortic knob, deviation of the nasogastric tube in the esophagus, depression of the left mainstem bronchus, an apical cap (apical pleural hematoma), sternal or scapular fracture, multiple left-sided rib fractures, and massive left hemothorax. However, a normal chest x-ray does not rule out a diagnosis of a thoracic great vessel injury. If clinical suspicion is high, then further diagnostic workup should be pursued. Aortography is the gold standard, but other imaging modalities such as transesophageal echocardiography or CT scan of the chest may be helpful in establishing the diagnosis as well.

177. The answer is c. (*Moore, pp 595–602.*) A positive DPL or a positive ultrasound exam in the hemodynamically unstable patient mandates exploratory laparotomy. A positive DPL for blunt abdominal trauma is characterized by aspiration of 10 cc of gross blood initially or more than 100,000/μL RBC, more than 500/μL WBC, or elevated amylase, bilirubin, or alkaline phosphatase.

178. The answer is b. (*Moore, pp 211–212.*) The patient is in neurogenic shock secondary to a spinal cord injury. In patients with cervical or thoracic injuries, loss of sympathetic regulation results in loss of vasomotor tone and hypotension. Patients with neurogenic shock are warm and pink, as opposed to patients who are hypovolemic, who are cold and clammy. Because of loss of the reflexive tachycardic response to hypotension, these patients are usually also bradycardic. Treatment is with fluid resuscitation initially and vasoconstrictors after the intravascular volume is restored. The patient in this scenario has a low central venous pressure suggesting intravascular volume depletion. Therefore, the patient requires further fluid resuscitation.

179. The answer is e. (*Moore, p 886.*) There are multiple sequelae of increased abdominal pressure or abdominal compartment syndrome. Because of decreased venous return, the intracranial pressure increases and cerebral perfusion pressure decreases. Compartment syndrome also results in increased peak airway pressures, decreased venous return and decreased cardiac output, increased systemic vascular resistance, decreased renal blood flow and glomerular filtration rate, and decreased portal venous flow with decreased liver function. Treatment requires decompressive laparotomy.

180. The answer is e. (*Moore, pp 1025–1026.*) Initial management should consist of isotonic crystalloid resuscitation with either normal saline or lactated Ringer's at a dose of 20 mL/kg body weight (800 mL). If the patient transiently responds, a second bolus should be administered. If the patient has a sustained response, fluids can be decreased to maintenance. If the patient does not respond, the bolus should be repeated and then blood transfusion initiated.

181–185. The answers are 181-b, 182-e, 183-a, 184-d, 185-c. (*Moore, pp 517–522, 526–530, 544–551, 556–562.*) Flail chest describes the paradoxical motion of the chest wall that occurs when consecutive ribs are broken in more than one place, usually following blunt trauma to the thorax. Respiratory distress may ensue when the noncompliant flail segment interferes with generation of adequate positive and negative intrathoracic pressure needed to move air through the trachea. In addition, a blow sufficiently violent to cause a flail chest may also contuse the underlying pulmonary parenchyma, which compounds the respiratory distress. Treatment consists of pain control and treatment of the underlying pulmonary contusion.

Airway obstruction denotes partial or complete occlusion of the tracheobronchial tree by foreign bodies, secretions, or crush injuries of the upper respiratory tract. Patients may present with symptoms ranging from cough and mild dyspnea to stridor and hypoxic cardiac arrest. An initial effort should be made to digitally clear the airway and to suction visible secretions; in selected stable patients, fiberoptic endoscopy may be employed to determine the cause of obstruction and to retrieve foreign objects. Unstable patients whose airways cannot be quickly reestablished by clearing the oropharynx must be intubated. An endotracheal intubation may be attempted, but cricothyroidotomy is indicated in the presence of proximal obstruction or severe maxillofacial trauma.

Blunt or penetrating trauma to the pericardium and heart will result in pericardial tamponade when fluid pressure in the pericardial space exceeds central venous pressure and thus prevents venous return to the heart. The result is shock, despite adequate volume and myocardial function. The treatment is pericardial decompression. A subxiphoid, supradiaphragmatic incision and creation of a pericardial window, ideally performed in the operating room, provides a rapid, safe means of confirming the diagnosis of tamponade and of relieving venous obstruction. If bleeding is encountered on opening the pericardial window, a sternotomy should be performed.

Tension pneumothorax occurs when a laceration of the visceral pulmonary pleura acts as a one-way valve that allows air to enter the pleural space from an underlying parenchymal injury but not to escape. Increasing intrapleural pressure causes collapse of the ipsilateral lung, compression of the contralateral lung due to mediastinal shift toward the opposite hemithorax, and diminished venous return. Treatment consists of relieving the pneumothorax. This is best accomplished via tube thoracostomy.

Open pneumothorax occurs when a traumatic defect in the chest wall permits free communication of the pleural space with atmospheric pressure. If the defect is larger than two-thirds of the tracheal diameter, respiratory efforts will move air in and out through the defect in the chest wall rather than through the trachea. The immediate treatment is placement of an occlusive dressing over the defect; subsequent interventions include placement of a thoracostomy tube (preferably through a separate incision), formal closure of the chest wall, and ventilatory assistance if needed.

Transplants, Immunology, and Oncology

Questions

DIRECTIONS: Each item below contains a question followed by suggested responses. Select the **one best** response to each question.

186. A 43-year-old man with a gangrenous gallbladder and gram-negative sepsis agrees to participate in a research study. An assay of tumor necrosis factor (TNF) is performed. Which of the following is the origin of this peptide?

a. Fibroblasts
b. Damaged vascular endothelial cells
c. Monocytes/macrophages
d. Activated T lymphocytes
e. Activated killer lymphocytes

187. A 49-year-old man who underwent liver transplantation five years ago for alcoholic cirrhosis presents with a gradually increasing bilirubin level. He undergoes a liver biopsy, which demonstrates a paucity of bile ducts. Which of the following is his best option for treatment?

a. Increase his immunosuppression
b. Administration of a monoclonal antibody against T-cells
c. Exploratory laparotomy with hepatic arterial reconstruction
d. Exploratory laparotomy with thrombectomy of the portal vein
e. Retransplantation

188. A 52-year-old woman in renal failure is listed as a transplant candidate. In order to assess the propriety of the transplant, which of the following combinations represents how a cross-match is performed?

a. Donor serum with recipient lymphocytes and complement
b. Donor lymphocytes with recipient serum and complement
c. Donor lymphocytes with recipient lymphocytes
d. Recipient serum with a known panel of multiple donor lymphocytes
e. Recipient serum with donor red blood cells and complement

189. A 39-year-old woman presents with generalized malaise and lymphadenopathy. Biopsy of a supraclavicular lymph node reveals non-Hodgkin's lymphoma. Forty-eight hours after initiation of chemotherapy, she develops a high-grade fever and her laboratory studies demonstrate hyperkalemia, hyperphosphatemia, and hypocalcemia. Which of the following cells mediates this syndrome?

a. Macrophages
b. Cytotoxic T lymphocytes
c. Natural killer cells
d. Polymorphonuclear leukocytes
e. Helper T lymphocytes

190. A 33-year-old diabetic man receives a renal allograft. The physicians choose cyclosporine as one of the antirejection medications. Which of the following functions does cyclosporine A primarily inhibit?

a. Macrophage function
b. Antibody production
c. Interleukin 1 production
d. Interleukin 2 production
e. Cytotoxic T cell effectiveness

191. A 24-year-old woman presents with lethargy, anorexia, tachypnea, and weakness. Laboratory studies reveal a BUN of 150 mg/dL, serum creatinine of 16 mg/dL, and potassium of 6.2 meq/L. Chest x-ray shows increased pulmonary vascularity and a dilated heart. Which of the following is the most appropriate management of this patient?

a. Emergency kidney transplantation
b. Creation and immediate use of a forearm arteriovenous fistula
c. Placement of a catheter in the internal jugular vein and initiation of hemodialysis
d. A 100-g protein diet
e. Renal biopsy

192. A 32-year-old woman with end-stage renal disease secondary to diabetic nephropathy is currently undergoing hemodialysis through a left arteriovenous fistula while awaiting a kidney transplant. Family immune profile studies reveal that both her mother and her father are haplotype identical with regard to HLA antigens and that her sister is a six-antigen match. Which of the following is the most appropriate next step in the patient's management?

a. Continue hemodialysis three times a week
b. Undergo cadaveric renal transplantation
c. Accept a kidney transplant from her sister
d. Accept a kidney transplant from her father
e. Accept a kidney transplant from her mother

193. A 56-year-old man has been given an orthotopic heart transplant because of severe cardiomyopathy. He has been doing well, but at the two-year mark, he begins to show signs of congestive heart failure. At this point, which of the following is the most common cause of death for patients such as this one?

a. Infection
b. Arrhythmia
c. Accelerated graft arteriosclerosis
d. Acute rejection episode
e. Cancer

194. A hypertensive 47-year-old man is proposed for kidney transplantation. He is anemic but is otherwise functional. Which of the following would preclude renal transplantation?

a. Positive cross-match
b. Donor blood type O
c. Two-antigen HLA match with donor
d. Blood pressure of 180/100 mmHg
e. Hemoglobin level of 8.2 g/dL

195. A 56-year-old woman undergoes a cadaveric renal transplant. After revascularization of the transplanted kidney, the parenchyma appears to become swollen and pale. The patient does not produce any urine postoperatively. Which of the following statements is true regarding the nonfunctioning of her kidney?

a. It is mediated by preformed donor antibodies against recipient HLA antigens
b. It can be prevented by performing lymphocytotoxicity cross-match testing
c. It is manifested grossly by a swollen, bluish kidney at the time of transplant surgery
d. This form of rejection is associated with disseminated intravascular coagulation (DIC)
e. The rejection process can be treated with a steroid bolus and OKT3

196. A 57-year-old man has end-stage heart failure due to atherosclerosis. He is first on the transplant list, and a donor becomes available. The harvest team is dispatched. Which of the following statements regarding heart transplantation is true?

a. Heart transplants are matched by size and ABO blood type rather than tissue typing
b. Cadaveric graft survival is significantly lower with heart transplants as compared with renal transplants
c. Cold ischemia time for donor hearts should not be more than 48 h
d. The upper age limit for heart transplant eligibility is 55 years
e. The leading cause of death after the first year of cardiac transplantation is chronic rejection

197. A 47-year-old man with hypertensive nephropathy develops fever, graft tenderness, and oliguria four weeks following cadaveric renal transplantation. Serum creatinine is 3.1 mg/dL. A renal ultrasound reveals mild edema of the renal papillae but normal flow in both the renal artery and the renal vein. Nuclear scan demonstrates sluggish uptake and excretion. Which of the following is the most appropriate next step?

a. Performing an angiogram
b. Decreasing steroid and cyclosporine dose
c. Beginning intravenous antibiotics
d. Performing renal biopsy, steroid boost, and immunoglobulin therapy
e. Beginning FK 506

198. Approximately six weeks following a heart transplant, a 59-year-old woman develops fever, malaise, and myalgias and is found to have a cytomegalovirus (CMV) infection. Which of the following is a potential sequela of CMV infection?

a. Pyelonephritis
b. GI ulceration and hemorrhage
c. Cholecystitis
d. Intraabdominal abscess
e. Parotitis

199. A 32-year-old man receives an orthotopic liver transplant. The center has an experienced liver transplant team that performs over 100 procedures per year. Which of the following indications for liver transplantation results in the best one-year survival rate?

a. Malignancy
b. Fulminant hepatic failure
c. Cholestatic liver disease
d. Biliary atresia
e. Alcoholic cirrhosis

200. A young woman who has received a transplant has posttransplant fever and malaise. Graft-versus-host disease is diagnosed. This has occurred most commonly with the transplantation of which of the following?

a. Kidney
b. Lung
c. Heart
d. Bone marrow
e. Pancreas

201. A brain-dead potential donor has become available. You must plan for the dispersal of the thoracic organs. Which of the following will necessitate a heart-lung transplant?

a. Primary pulmonary hypertension
b. Cystic fibrosis
c. End-stage emphysema
d. Idiopathic dilated cardiomyopathy with long-standing secondary pulmonary hypertension
e. End-stage pulmonary fibrosis secondary to sarcoidosis

202. A 19-year-old male who has had type I diabetes for many years has several stigmata, such as renal failure and retinopathy. Which of the following is true regarding successful whole-organ pancreas transplantation in type I diabetes?

a. It results in maintenance of normal serum glucose levels
b. Recurrence of diabetic nephropathy in simultaneously transplanted kidneys is not prevented
c. Oral glucose tolerance tests remain abnormal
d. The pathologic changes of diabetic retinopathy are reversed
e. The rate of diabetic ulcers and amputations in the lower extremities is reduced

203. A 55-year-old woman who has end-stage liver disease is referred to a hepatologist for evaluation. Which of the following would prevent her from being a transplantation candidate?

a. Use of alcohol three months ago
b. A diagnosis of Budd-Chiari syndrome
c. A 4-cm hepatocellular carcinoma in the right lobe of the liver
d. Development of hepatorenal syndrome requiring hemodialysis
e. History of breast cancer five years ago with no evidence of disease currently

204. A kidney transplant recipient presents with severe acute rejection that does not respond to steroid treatment. She is started on OKT3, which is a monoclonal antibody directed against the CD3 antigen complex on T cells. Which of the following statements is true regarding OKT3?

a. Binding of OKT3 to the CD3 antigen complex stimulates the T cells to proliferate
b. The most severe side effects of OKT3 are fever, chills, and headaches from cytokine release
c. OKT3 is an effective drug for acute rejection but cannot be used to prevent rejection
d. OKT3 should be used cautiously in patients with fluid overload because of the risk of pulmonary edema
e. OKT3 efficacy should be measured by checking drug levels in the blood

205. A 19-year-old college student presents with a testicular mass, and after treatment he returns for regular follow-up visits. Which of the following is the most useful serum marker for detecting recurrent disease after treatment of nonseminomatous testicular cancer?

a. Carcinoembryonic antigen (CEA)
b. Human chorionic gonadotropin (hCG)
c. Prostate-specific antigen (PSA)
d. CA125
e. p53 oncogene

206. An edentulous 72-year-old man with a 50-year history of cigarette smoking presents with a nontender, hard mass in the lateral neck. Which of the following is the best diagnostic test for establishing a diagnosis of malignancy?

a. Fine-needle aspiration cytology
b. Bone marrow biopsy
c. Nasopharyngoscopy
d. CT scan of the head and neck
e. Sinus x-ray

207. A 65-year-old man with a long-standing history of gastroesophageal reflux presents with symptoms of dysphagia. Upper endoscopy reveals a distal esophageal lesion which on biopsy is consistent with adenocarcinoma. Staging suggests that he has a $T_3N_0M_0$ lesion, and he is started on chemotherapy. Which of the following is true regarding intravenous administration of chemotherapy?

a. Subcutaneous extravasation of carmustine (BCNU) or 5-fluorouracil (5-FU) usually causes ulceration
b. Extravasation of doxorubicin rarely causes serious ulceration because the agent binds quickly to tissue nucleic acid
c. Serious and progressive ulceration can be expected following extravasation of vincristine or vinblastine
d. Problems of wound healing should be anticipated if systemic 5-FU therapy is begun less than two weeks postoperative
e. Administration of folinic acid prevents most of the toxicity of methotrexate, but does not help to normalize wound healing

208. A 49-year-old woman undergoes surgical resection of a malignancy. The family asks about the prognosis. The histopathology is available for review. For which of the following malignancies does histologic grade best correlate with prognosis?

a. Lung cancer
b. Melanoma
c. Colonic adenocarcinoma
d. Hepatocellular carcinoma
e. Soft tissue sarcoma

209. A mother notices an abdominal mass in her three-year-old son while giving him a bath. There is no history of any symptoms, but the boy's blood pressure is elevated at 105/85 mmHg. Metastatic workup is negative and the patient is explored. The mass shown here is found within the left kidney. Which of the following statements concerning this disease is correct?

a. This tumor is associated with aniridia, hemihypertrophy, and cryptorchidism
b. The majority of patients present with an asymptomatic abdominal mass and hematuria
c. Treatment with surgical excision, radiation, and chemotherapy results in survival of less than 60% even in histologically low-grade tumors
d. Surgical excision is curative and no further treatment is ordinarily advised
e. This tumor is the most common malignancy in childhood

210. An 11-year-old girl presents to your office because of a family history of medullary carcinoma of the thyroid. Physical examination is normal. Which of the following tests should you perform?

a. Urine vanillylmandelic acid (VMA) level
b. Serum insulin level
c. Serum gastrin level
d. Serum glucagon level
e. Serum somatostatin level

211. A 37-year-old woman has developed a 6-cm mass on her anterior thigh over the past 10 months. The mass appears to be fixed to the underlying muscle, but the overlying skin is movable. Which of the following is the most appropriate next step in her management?

a. Above-knee amputation
b. Excisional biopsy
c. Incisional biopsy
d. Bone scan
e. Abdominal CT scan

212. A 50-year-old man is incidentally discovered to have non-Hodgkin's lymphoma confined to the submucosa of the stomach during esophagogastroduodenoscopy for dyspepsia. Which of the following statements is true regarding his condition?

a. Surgery alone cannot be considered adequate treatment
b. Combined chemotherapy and radiation therapy, without prior resection, are not effective
c. Combined chemotherapy and radiation therapy, without prior resection, result in a high risk of severe hemorrhage and perforation
d. Outcome (freedom from progression and overall survival) is related to the histologic grade of the tumor
e. The stomach is the most common site for non-Hodgkin's lymphoma of the gastrointestinal tract

213. A patient with a hematologic malignancy seeks your advice. She has read on the commercial Internet that treatment with interferon might be helpful. Interferons are correctly characterized by which of the following statements?

a. They are a group of complex phospholipids
b. They are produced by virus-infected cells
c. They enhance viral replication
d. They cause Burkitt's lymphoma cell lines to divide
e. They have not been effective in the treatment of hairy cell leukemias

214. A 33-year-old woman seeks assistance because of a swelling of her right parotid gland. Biopsy is performed and reveals acinar carcinoma. In your discussion regarding surgery, which of the following statements regarding malignant parotid tumors is correct?

a. Acinar carcinoma is a highly aggressive malignant tumor of the parotid gland
b. Squamous carcinoma of the parotid gland exhibits only moderately malignant behavior
c. Regional node dissection for occult metastases is not indicated for malignant parotid tumors because of their low incidence and the morbidity of lymphadenectomy
d. Facial nerve preservation should be attempted when the surgical margins of resection are free of tumor
e. Total parotidectomy (superficial and deep portions of the gland) is indicated for malignant tumors

215. A 42-year-old man is undergoing chemotherapy after resection of a cecal adenocarcinoma with positive lymph nodes. You are asked to see him regarding a potential surgical complication. Which of the following potentially operable complications is a common occurrence among patients receiving systemic chemotherapy?

a. Acute cholecystitis
b. Perirectal abscess
c. Appendicitis
d. Incarcerated femoral hernia
e. Diverticulitis

216. A 28-year-old medical student seeks your attention because of a testicular mass. You recommend a biopsy. Subsequently, you must plan for optimal operative and perioperative therapy. Which of the following statements regarding testicular cancer is true?

a. Lymph node dissection after radical orchiectomy is useful for staging but does not increase survival
b. Seminomas and choriocarcinomas are best treated with orchiectomy and retroperitoneal lymph node dissection
c. Seminomas are extremely resistant to radiotherapy
d. Orchiectomy for a testicular mass is approached via the scrotum
e. Cryptorchidism is associated with an increased risk of testicular cancer

217. A young patient with type I diabetes and renal failure must decide between dialysis or possible transplantation. You must offer advice. Which of the following is an advantage of dialysis over renal transplantation?

a. Less expense if the treatment continues for less than two years
b. Increased number of pregnancies in female dialysis patients
c. Return of normal menses in female dialysis patients
d. Less anemia in dialysis patients
e. Increased one-year survival of dialysis patients

218. A 30-year-old previously healthy man presents with refractory hypertension on four medications. Urine analysis is positive for metanephrines. He was adopted as an infant and therefore does not know his family history. Which of the following inherited syndromes is not associated with this disease?

a. MEN IIA
b. MEN IIB
c. Von-Hippel Lindau disease
d. Neurofibromatosis I
e. Neurofibromatosis II

219. A 45-year-old man presents to his family physician to discuss screening colonoscopy. Which of the following is true about colorectal cancer screening?

a. In the absence of any family or personal history of colon cancer, he should begin screening at age 40
b. If a polyp is detected on screening colonoscopy, the patient should undergo repeat colonoscopy in one year
c. If no polyps are detected on screening colonoscopy, the patient should undergo repeat colonoscopy in three years
d. The sensitivity of air contrast barium enema for detecting polyps greater than 1 cm is only 70% and therefore should not be used in colorectal cancer screening
e. In patients with hereditary nonpolyposis colorectal cancer (HNPCC), screening colonoscopy should begin at either age 20 to 25 or 10 years younger than the youngest age at diagnosis in the family

220. A 53-year-old woman is submitted for breast lumpectomy and radiation therapy for breast cancer. You discuss this treatment with the radiation oncology attending in order to better understand the mechanism of action on your patient. Which of the following statements is true concerning radiation therapy?

a. Damage to DNA occurs primarily by the direct effect of ionizing radiation
b. Cellular hypoxia decreases sensitivity to radiation
c. Cells in the S phase of the cell cycle are most radiosensitive
d. Radiation therapy following lumpectomy of a breast cancer results in decreased survival when compared to modified radical mastectomy
e. Skin, gastrointestinal mucosa, and bone marrow are relatively insensitive to radiotherapy

221. You are responsible for recruiting patients into a new trial of interleukin 2 for cancer therapy. In choosing potential patients, which of the following statements regarding cancer therapy with interleukin 2 (IL-2) is true?

a. It is a B cell growth factor
b. It induces a major response in patients with metastatic breast cancer
c. It induces a major response in patients with metastatic colon cancer
d. It induces a major response in patients with metastatic melanoma
e. It induces a major response in patients with lymphoma

222. You are asked to provide a one-hour lecture to medical residents on the general topic of nutrition and cancer. You review a number of areas of interest. Which of the following statements concerning cancer and nutrition is correct?

a. Levels of nitrates in food and drinking water are positively correlated with the incidence of bladder cancer
b. Regular ingestion of vitamin D from childhood probably inhibits formation of carcinogens
c. Consumption of excessive amounts of animal dietary fats is associated with increased incidence of colon cancer
d. Nutritional support of cancer patients improves response of the tumor to chemotherapy
e. Alcohol ingestion is associated with pancreatic cancer

223. A patient requires both cardiac and renal transplantation. Preparation for the procedures is begun. How do cardiac allografts differ from renal allografts?

a. Cardiac allografts are matched by HLA tissue typing and renal allografts are not
b. Cardiac allografts can tolerate a longer period of cold ischemia than renal allografts
c. One-year graft survival for cardiac allografts is substantially lower than that for renal allografts
d. Cardiac allografts are matched only by size and ABO blood type
e. Cyclosporine is a critical component of the immunosuppressive regimen for cardiac allografts but not renal allografts

224. A patient with colon cancer has a mass in the upper lobe of his left lung 2.5 years following resection of his colon cancer and subsequent 12 months of chemotherapy. His carcinoembryonic antigen (CEA) level is rising. Which of the following predicts a five-year survival rate of greater than 20% following resection of pulmonary metastases?

a. Other organ metastases are present
b. Lung lesions are solitary
c. Local tumor recurrence is found
d. The tumor doubling time is less than 20 days
e. The patient has received prior chemotherapy

225. Preoperative preparations with your scrub team are under way prior to performing a thoracotomy for persistent pneumothorax on a patient who is known to have AIDS. Which of the following statements about transmission of HIV in the health care setting is true?

a. A freshly prepared solution of dilute chlorine bleach will not adequately decontaminate clothing
b. All needles should be capped immediately after use
c. Cuts and other open skin wounds are believed to act as portals of entry for HIV
d. Double gloving reduces the risk of intraoperative needle sticks
e. The risk of seroconversion following a needle stick with a contaminated needle is greater for HIV than for hepatitis B

226. A 57-year-old woman discovers a breast mass, which is biopsied and found to be carcinoma. After her treatment, she assembles her family and attempts to encourage them to obtain regular examinations and mammograms. Regarding the risk of breast cancer, which of the following statements is true?

a. Breast cancer occurs more commonly among women of the lower social classes
b. A history of breast cancer in a first-degree family relative is associated with a fourfold increase in risk
c. Women with a first birth after age 30 years have approximately twice the risk of those with a first birth before age 18
d. Cigarette smoking increases the risk of breast cancer
e. Hair dyes have been shown to increase the risk of breast cancer

227. A 42-year-old man is diagnosed with an osteosarcoma. His family history is significant for a 37-year-old sister with breast cancer and an uncle with adrenocortical carcinoma. His family physician suspects that he may have Li-Fraumeni syndrome and suggests genetic testing. Which of the following genes is most likely to be mutated if he has the syndrome?

a. APC gene
b. RET
c. p53
d. PTEN
e. p16

228. A patient with a solid malignancy is discussing chemotherapy with his oncologist. He is interested in the risks of the treatment. What is the primary toxicity of doxorubicin (Adriamycin)?

a. Cardiomyopathy
b. Pulmonary fibrosis
c. Peripheral neuropathy
d. Uric acid nephropathy
e. Hepatic dysfunction

229. A 25-year-old woman is diagnosed with bilateral breast cancer. She undergoes genetic testing to assess whether she has a mutation in either *BRCA1* or *BRCA2*. Which of the following statements is true regarding *BRCA* mutations?

a. Her risk, as a woman under the age of 40, for having a mutation in *BRCA1* or 2 is 40%
b. *BRCA1* tumors are more likely to be estrogen-receptor positive
c. A mutation in *BRCA2* is associated with an increased risk of colon cancer
d. A mutation in *BRCA1* is associated with an increased risk for pancreatic, bile duct, and gallbladder cancers
e. Both *BRCA1* and *BRCA2* are associated with an increased risk of ovarian cancer by age 70

230. A 56-year-old woman is undergoing chemotherapy. She presents today with complaints of burning on urination and bloody urine. Which of the following agents causes hemorrhagic cystitis?

a. Bleomycin
b. 5-fluorouracil
c. Cisplatin
d. Vincristine
e. Cyclophosphamide

231. A 38-year-old woman who underwent a cadaveric renal transplant eight years previously presents with fevers, fatigue, and weight loss. Evaluation included CT scans of the head, neck, chest, abdomen, and pelvis; she is noted to have diffuse lymphadenopathy and pulmonary nodules. A biopsy and histologic examination of a lymph node is performed. Which of the following viruses is most likely to be present in the lymph node?

a. Cytomegalovirus
b. Human papillomavirus
c. Human herpesvirus 8
d. Epstein-Barr virus
e. Coxsackie virus

232. A 41-year-old man underwent a successful living related kidney transplantation one year previously with good results. Preoperatively, he was noted to have an elevated calcium level; posttransplantation, he continues to have elevated calcium levels and associated symptoms. Which of the following is the most appropriate next step in management?

a. ^{99m}Tc-sestamibi scanning
b. Ultrasound of the neck
c. CT scan of the neck and mediastinum
d. Total parathyroidectomy with autotransplantation of a portion of a gland into the forearm
e. Measurement of urinary calcium levels

233. A 53-year-old man presents with constipation and a 20-lb weight loss over the course of six months. Colonoscopy reveals a fungating mass in the sigmoid colon; biopsy is consistent with adenocarcinoma. His metastatic workup is negative. A CEA level is obtained and is fourfold greater than normal. Which of the following is the appropriate use of this test?

a. As an indication for neoadjuvant chemotherapy
b. As an indication for postoperative radiation therapy
c. As an indication for preoperative PET scanning
d. As an indication for a more aggressive sigmoid resection
e. As a baseline measurement prior to monitoring postoperatively for recurrence

DIRECTIONS: Each group of questions below consists of lettered options followed by a set of numbered items. For each numbered item, select the **one** lettered option with which it is **most** closely associated. Each lettered option may be used once, more than once, or not at all.

Questions 234–236

For each stage in the patient's treatment, select the appropriate next step.

a. Left hemicolectomy
b. Right hemicolectomy
c. Subtotal colectomy
d. Total colectomy
e. Hepatic resection
f. External beam irradiation
g. 5-fluorouracil and leucovorin
h. External beam irradiation and chemotherapy
i. Abdominal MRI
j. No further treatment

234. A 65-year-old man is admitted to the hospital with complaints of inter-mittent constipation and microcytic anemia. Barium enema reveals a nonob-structing apple core lesion of the proximal sigmoid colon. Colonoscopy confirms the location of the mass and reveals no other synchronous lesions.

235. The patient undergoes surgery and recovers uneventfully. Pathology of the resected specimen is reported as Dukes C with negative surgical margins.

236. At six-month follow-up, an abdominal CT scan shows a 2-cm iso-lated lesion in the right lobe of the liver. Repeat colonoscopy shows no evi-dence of recurrent or metachronous lesions. Chest x-ray and bone scan are normal.

Questions 237–240

A 32-year-old man with diabetic nephropathy undergoes an uneventful renal transplant from his sister (two-haplotype match). His immunosuppressive regimen includes azathioprine, steroids, and cyclosporine. For each development in the postoperative period, select the most appropriate next step.

a. Begin gancyclovir
b. Administer steroid boost
c. Withhold steroids
d. Decrease cyclosporine
e. Increase cyclosporine
f. Decrease azathioprine
g. Obtain renal ultrasound
h. Begin broad-spectrum antibiotics
i. Administer filgrastim (Neupogen)
j. Administer FK50

237. On postoperative day 3 the patient is doing well, but you notice on his routine laboratory tests that his white blood cell count is 2.0.

238. The patient's WBC count gradually returns to normal, but on postoperative day 7 he develops a fever of 39.44°C (103°F) and a nonproductive cough. A chest x-ray reveals diffuse interstitial infiltrates, and a buffy coat is positive for viral inclusions.

239. The patient recovers from this illness and is discharged home on postoperative day 18. At three-month follow-up he is doing well, but you notice that his creatinine is 2.8 mg/dL. He has no fever, his graft is not tender, and his renal ultrasound is normal.

240. Six months following his transplant, the patient begins to develop fever, malaise, and pain of the right lower quadrant. On palpation, the graft is tender. Chest x-ray and urine and blood cultures are normal. Renal ultrasound shows an edematous graft.

Transplants, Immunology, and Oncology

Answers

186. The answer is c. (*Greenfield, pp 113–115.*) Tumor necrosis factor (TNF) is a peptide hormone produced by endotoxin-activated monocytes/macrophages and has been postulated to be the principal cytokine mediator in gram-negative shock and sepsis-related organ damage. Biologic actions of TNF include polymorphonuclear neutrophil (PMN) activation and degranulation; increased nonspecific host resistance; increased vascular permeability; lymphopenia; promotion of interleukins 1, 2, and 6; capillary leak syndrome; microvascular thrombosis; anorexia and cachexia; and numerous other protective and adverse effects in sepsis. Its role in sepsis provides a fertile field for research in critical care.

187. The answer is e. (*Brunicardi, pp 320–322.*) Chronic rejection is a late complication that manifests months to years after transplantation and is characterized by a paucity of bile ducts on biopsy—the "vanishing bile duct syndrome." Treatment options are limited, and the best option for treatment is retransplantation. Portal venous thrombosis that occurs early after transplantation should be treated with exploratory laparotomy and thrombectomy, but late portal venous thrombosis does not necessitate operative intervention due to the formation of collaterals. Hepatic arterial thrombosis, when detected early, should be treated with reexploration and thrombectomy with revision of the anastomosis. A late sequela of hepatic arterial thrombosis (HAT) is biliary strictures secondary to ischemia.

188. The answer is b. (*Greenfield, p 545.*) The purpose of a cross-match is to determine whether the recipient has circulating antibodies against donor HLA antigens. Such antibodies do not occur naturally, but rather are the result of prior sensitization during pregnancy, blood transfusions, or previous transplantation. A complement-dependent lymphocytotoxicity cross-match is performed by adding recipient serum and complement to donor cells (T cells, B cells, or monocytes). If specific antidonor antibodies are present, antibody binding results in complement fixation and cell lysis. This is detected by addition of a vital dye, which is taken up by the damaged cell membrane, resulting in a positive cross-match. If a positive cross-match is detected to donor T cells (HLA class I), transplantation will result in hyperacute rejection.

189. The answer is b. (*Greenfield, pp 539–543.*) The patient is manifesting symptoms of tumor lysis syndrome, which is mediated by cytotoxic T cells. Hyperkalemia and hyperphosphatemia are a result of tumor cell lysis, and hypocalcemia is a result of precipitation of phosphate and calcium. Unlike the granulocyte line, T lymphocytes express the T-cell receptor. This receptor imparts antigen specificity to T cells. The helper T cell, when stimulated by interleukin 1 and antigens, produces various lymphokines that ultimately produce effector cells. One of these effector cells is the cytotoxic T cell, which kills cells that express specific antigens, including viral, tumor, and nonbiologic antigens. Macrophages and natural killer cells have some tumoricidal activity; however, this is not specific for tumors.

190. The answer is d. (*Greenfield, pp 539–543.*) Cyclosporine is a highly effective immunosuppressive agent produced by fungi. It is more specific than the anti-inflammatory agents such as steroids or the antiproliferative agents such as azathioprine. The effectiveness of cyclosporine in preventing allograft rejection is related to its ability to inhibit interleukin 2 production. Without interleukin 2 from helper T cells, there is no clonal expansion of alloantigen-directed cytotoxic T cells and no stimulation of antibody production by B cells.

191. The answer is c. (*Townsend, pp 699–700.*) Hemodialysis, rather than management by dietary manipulation alone, should be instituted in patients with end-stage renal failure whose serum creatinine is over 15 mg/dL or whose creatinine clearance is less than 3 mL/min. It is important that hemodialysis be initiated prior to the onset of uremic complications. These complications include hyperkalemia, congestive heart failure, peripheral neuropathy, severe hypertension, pericarditis, bleeding, and severe anemia. The uremic hyperkalemic patient in congestive heart failure may require emergency dialysis in addition to the standard conservative measures, which include (1) limitation of protein intake to less than 60 g/d and restriction of fluid intake and (2) reduction of elevated serum potassium levels by insulin-glucose or sodium polystyrene sulfonate (Kayexalate) enema treatment. Arteriovenous fistulas require about two weeks to develop adequate size and flow. While awaiting maturation, temporary dialysis can be satisfactorily performed using a catheter placed in a central vein. Renal biopsy would be performed in an attempt to obtain a diagnosis of the underlying renal disease. Patients who are acceptable candidates for kidney transplantation usually should undergo this form of treatment, after they are stabilized, rather than chronic hemodialysis, the mortality for which is now higher than for transplantation. Despite adequate dialysis, problems of neuropathy, bone disease, anemia, and hypertension remain difficult to manage. Compared with chronic dialysis, transplantation restores more patients to happier and more productive lives.

192. The answer is c. (*Townsend, pp 702–703.*) The best graft survival rates for living related transplants are obtained when all six histocompatibility loci are identical. All family members of potential transplant recipients should be tissue typed and the donor should be selected on the basis of closest match, if psychological and medical evaluation makes this feasible. A patient receiving a living related renal transplant with no HLA matches still has a better outcome than a patient receiving a cadaveric transplant.

193. The answer is c. (*Greenfield, pp 597–607.*) Chronic graft rejection is manifested in cardiac allografts as chronic vascular rejection of main and intramuscular coronary arteries. Myointimal proliferation and medial scarring result in diffuse and eccentric arterial narrowing referred to as accelerated graft atherosclerosis. Infection remains the primary cause of death within the first year of cardiac transplant, but accelerated graft arteriosclerosis is the most common cause of mortality thereafter. Percutaneous transluminal coronary angioplasty, coronary artery bypass grafting, and retransplantation are the current options for combating this problem.

194. The answer is a. (*Greenfield, p 545.*) A positive cross-match means that the recipient has circulating antibodies that are cytotoxic to donor-strain lymphocytes. This incompatibility, which almost always leads to an acute humoral rejection of the graft, precludes transplantation. Blood type matching prior to organ allograft is similar to cross-matching prior to transfusion;

O is the universal donor and AB the universal recipient. Minor blood group factors do not appear to act as histocompatibility antigens. Matching of HLA antigens in cadaveric renal transplants may improve graft survival, but the impact is relatively minor. While attempts are made to pair recipient and donor by tissue typing, a two-antigen match is perfectly acceptable and even zero-antigen matches can be transplanted with good results. Neither hypertension nor anemia is a contraindication to transplantation; indeed, hypertension may be cured or ameliorated following successful transplantation. Patients with end-stage renal failure generally are anemic and can be transfused, if necessary, intraoperatively or postoperatively. Anemia generally also improves following transplantation because of increased erythropoietin production by the graft.

195. The answer is c. (*Townsend, p 713.*) Hyperacute rejection is mediated by cytotoxic antibodies with subsequent triggering of the complement, coagulation, and kinin systems. It can occur during surgery after the clamps are released from the vascular anastomosis and the recipient's antibodies are exposed to the donor's passenger lymphocytes and kidney tissue. Typically, the kidney will become swollen and bluish. Hyperacute rejection is the cause of immediate and early oliguria, and biopsies should be performed intraoperatively or early postoperatively. Hyperacute rejection is characterized pathologically by fibrin and platelet thrombosis and necrosis of the glomerular tufts, renal arterioles, and small arteries. Massive polymorphonuclear infiltrate with tubular necrosis occurs 24 to 36 h after transplantation. The intravascular coagulation rarely results in a systemic coagulopathy. Careful cross-matching can test for cytotoxic antibodies; in hyperacute rejection, preformed circulating antibodies are present against the donor antigens (not the recipient antigens). Although plasmapheresis and cyclophosphamide can transiently decrease the preformed antibody load, to date there exists no adequate prevention or treatment for hyperacute rejection.

196. The answer is a. (*Greenfield, pp 598–607.*) Cardiac transplantation is a treatment modality for selected patients with end-stage cardiac failure. Allograft survivals are approximately 80% at one year, while survival is about 96% at one year for renal cadaveric grafts. Although kidneys can be safely preserved by either hypothermic storage or hypothermic perfusion for periods up to 48 h, donor hearts protected by simple hypothermia should be transplanted within 4 h. For this reason the usual tissue-typing procedures used in kidney transplantation are impractical in cardiac transplantation, and indeed there is no correlation between match and outcome. In pairing donor and recipient for heart transplants, there must be at least ABO blood group compatibility. Cyclosporine has improved results in both cardiac and renal transplantation despite its major drawback of dose-related nephrotoxicity. Eligibility for cardiac transplantation has evolved from strict age criteria to more flexible guidelines based on a patient's likelihood of surviving and resuming a normally functional life after transplantation. Many centers, however, observe age 65 as the upper limit for transplantation. The leading causes of death in patients surviving more than one year after transplantation are infection and rejection.

197. The answer is d. (*Greenfield, p 575.*) The patient is experiencing an acute rejection episode. Acute rejection typically occurs between one week and three months posttransplantation and is characterized by an increasing creatinine, decreased urine output, and possible fevers or tenderness over the graft. Diagnosis is confirmed with a biopsy of the graft, and treatment includes high-dose steroids and an anti-T-cell antibody (e.g., OKT3, which is a murine monoclonal antibody to the human CD3 complex).

198. The answer is b. (*Greenfield, p 543.*) The most common posttransplantation viral infections are DNA viruses of the herpesvirus family and include cytomegalovirus (CMV), Epstein-Barr virus, herpes simplex virus, and varicella zoster virus. CMV infections may occur as either primary or reactive infections and have a peak incidence at about six weeks after transplant. The classic signs include fever, malaise, myalgia, arthralgia, and leukopenia. CMV infection can affect several organ systems and result in pneumonitis; ulceration and hemorrhage in the stomach, duodenum, or colon; hepatitis; esophagitis; retinitis; encephalitis; or pancreatitis. The risk of developing posttransplant CMV depends on donor-recipient serology, with the greatest risk in seronegative patients who receive organs from seropositive donors. Pyelonephritis, cholecystitis, intraabdominal abscesses, and parotitis are caused by bacterial infections or GI perforation and not primarily by CMV infection.

199. The answer is b. (*Greenfield, p 597.*) The prognosis after liver transplantation depends upon the etiology of the underlying liver disease.

Patients with cholestatic liver disease have the best survival rate (92%), while patients with fulminant hepatic failure have the worst (81%). Survival is also improved for patients who are not hospitalized just prior to transplantation.

200. The answer is d. (*Greenfield, p 544.*) Donor-type lymphoid cells transplanted within a graft may recognize the host's tissue as foreign and mount an immune response against the host. This response, termed graft-versus-host disease (GVHD), is common in bone marrow transplantation and is an important source of morbidity and mortality. Treatment requires more aggressive immunosuppression. Current clinical practice includes depletion of lymphocytes from the marrow graft in order to prevent the development of GVHD. GVHD has been documented following liver transplantation, presumably because of the large amount of lymphoid tissue in the donor liver. GVHD has not been described following heart, lung, pancreas, or kidney transplantation.

201. The answer is d. (*Greenfield, pp 608–616.*) Many causes of end-stage lung disease have been appropriately treated with lung transplantation. Whether one lung or both lungs are replaced at the time of transplantation depends on recipient factors. Patients with restrictive processes such as primary pulmonary fibrosis do well with a single lung transplant. For patients with primary pulmonary hypertension, unloading of the right ventricle with single lung transplantation has been adequate, and replacement of both lungs has not been necessary in most cases. Cystic fibrosis patients do well after lung transplantation, but double lung transplant is frequently necessary because of chronic infections. Secondary pulmonary hypertension is due to left ventricular failure with concomitant increases in pulmonary pressures secondary to increases in left ventricular end-diastolic pressures. Reactive secondary pulmonary hypertension is best treated with heart transplantation. Long-standing secondary pulmonary hypertension that is chiefly fixed is best treated with combined heart-lung transplantation.

202. The answer is a. (*Greenfield, pp 617–633.*) Whole-organ pancreas transplantation is the only therapy for type I insulin-dependent diabetes that maintains normal serum glucose levels and normal glucose tolerance tests. When the pancreas is transplanted along with a kidney, the tight glucose control generally prevents the recurrence of diabetic nephropathy. No series has shown the reversal of diabetic retinopathy or reduction in the rate of diabetic ulcers or of amputations, although some parameters of diabetic retinopathy may improve after pancreas transplantation.

203. The answer is a. (*Brunicardi, pp 316–318.*) The most common contraindication to liver transplantation is ongoing or recent substance abuse. Alcohol use within three months is a contraindication to liver transplantation. Patients with hepatocellular carcinoma (HCC) who would not tolerate resection because of portal hypertension and uncompensated liver disease can be treated with liver transplantation, which has the additional benefit of treating the underlying liver disease. Patients without vascular invasion or extrahepatic disease with a single lesion less than 5 cm in size or no more than three lesions, none of which are greater than 3 cm in size, are the best candidates. The presence of hepatorenal syndrome is an indication, not a contraindication, to liver transplantation. Presence of an extrahepatic malignancy should defer transplantation for two years after curative therapy for their malignancy.

204. The answer is d. (*Brunicardi, p 302.*) OKT3 is a monoclonal antibody against the CD3 antigen complex on mature T cells. In addition to minor side effects such as fevers and headaches that result from cytokine release after OKT3 administration, severe complications may occur such as noncardiogenic pulmonary edema, encephalopathy, aseptic meningitis, and nephrotoxicity. OKT3 administration results in clearance of T cells from the circulation, and thus drug efficacy can be measured by assessing the percentage of CD3 positive cells in the blood. OKT3 can be used as the primary treatment or second-line therapy for acute rejection, rejection prophylaxis, and induction therapy.

205. The answer is b. (*Brunicardi, p 1538.*) In following patients with non-seminomatous testicular tumors, elevated serum levels of the β subunit of human chorionic gonadotropin (hCG), alpha fetoprotein (AFP), and lactate dehydrogenase have been found to be useful indicators of tumor activity or recurrence. Prostate-specific antigen (PSA) has been utilized in screening for prostate cancer, although its role is controversial. CA125 has been used to follow ovarian cancers; it is fairly nonspecific but can alert the physician to the need for a more aggressive search for persistent disease when relative increases are noted in a patient after therapy. The p53 oncogenes have been found in soft tissue sarcomas, osteogenic sarcomas, and colon cancers; they have no role in the detection of recurrence.

206. The answer is a. *(Brunicardi, pp 530–531.)* Isolated enlarged cervical lymph nodes in the adult are malignant nearly 80% of the time (excluding benign tumors of the thyroid gland). They are usually metastatic squamous cell carcinomas arising from primary sources above the clavicles in the aerodigestive tract. Fine-needle aspiration cytology is commonly used to obtain histologic confirmation of suspected cancer. Aspiration cytology can usually diagnose carcinoma accurately, but lymphoma may be difficult to identify by this method, and open biopsy is often necessary. Bone marrow biopsy is not indicated prior to lymph node biopsy. It is done as part of the staging process after a diagnosis of lymphoma has been made. Endoscopy and scanning of the oropharynx and nasopharynx are part of the diagnostic workup of a suspected malignant cervical lymph node, but do not provide histologic proof of cancer.

207. The answer is d. *(Brunicardi, pp 276–281.)* Since chemotherapy is generally most effective in killing rapidly dividing cells, the rapidly dividing cells of a fresh surgical wound should be in jeopardy when chemotherapy is given in the early postoperative period. Each of the phases of normal wound healing is theoretically at risk from one or another class of chemotherapeutic agents. Immediately following wounding, inflammation and vascular permeability lead to fibrin deposition and polymorphonuclear neutrophil (PMN), monocyte, and platelet influx. Macrophages are attracted by the activated complement system. By the fourth day, the proliferative phase begins, and for the next 20 days fibroblasts produce mucopolysaccharides and collagen. Cross-linking of the collagen fibers then continues for several months in the maturation phase. It seems logical to delay antineoplastic agents for 10 to 14 days unless there are compelling clinical indications (e.g., superior vena cava syndrome) for more urgent treatment. Administration of folinic acid simultaneously with methotrexate normalizes wound healing. Extravasation of chemotherapeutic agents during intravenous administration may result in severe ulceration and sloughing. The nature of the injury is related largely to the nucleic acid–binding characteristics of the agent. Those agents that do not bind to tissue nucleic acid (vincristine, vinblastine, nitrogen mustard, BCNU, 5-FU) generally cause only local damage from the immediate injury. These substances are quickly metabolized or inactivated, and usual patterns of wound healing can be expected. On the other hand, agents that bind nucleic acid (doxorubicin, dactinomycin, mitomycin C, mithramycin, and daunorubicin) cause not only immediate toxic reaction in the tissues but, unless excised, continuing and progressive tissue damage. Though some authors have reported success with elevation and ice packs, most recommend surgical excision if there is severe pain, any sign of early necrosis, or significant blistering.

208. The answer is e. (*Brunicardi, pp 269–271.*) The management of malignant tumors may be guided by knowledge obtained by grading and staging the tumors. Histologic grading reflects the degree of anaplasia of tumor cells. Tumors in which histologic grading seems to have prognostic value include soft tissue sarcoma, transitional cell cancers of the bladder, astrocytoma, and chondrosarcoma. Grading has been of little predictive value in melanoma, hepatocellular carcinoma, or osteosarcoma. Staging is based on the extent of spread rather than histologic appearance and is more relevant in predicting the course of lung and colorectal cancers.

209. The answer is e. (*Brunicardi, pp 1508–1510.*) This is a nephroblastoma (Wilms tumor) adherent to the left kidney. These tumors are associated with aniridia (rarely) and with hemihypertrophy, cryptorchidism, or hypospadias in about 10% of cases. Most patients present with an asymptomatic mass found by a parent. Less than one-third of patients experience hematuria. As would be expected in over half such cases, this child is hypertensive, probably due to compression of the renal artery by the mass. Surgical treatment consists of resection of the kidney and ureter. Chemotherapy is indicated in patients with malignancy confined to one kidney, and chemoradiation is indicated after surgical excision for more advanced disease. Cure rates exceeding 80% are achieved in patients with hematogenous metastases. Computed tomography (CT) is used to assess the tumor characteristics and evaluate for metastases. Ultrasonography is utilized to assess for vascular invasion into the renal vein or vena cava. Wilms tumor is the most common abdominal malignancy of childhood, but represents only about 10% of childhood malignant tumors.

210. The answer is c. (*Greenfield, pp 1302–1305.*) Medullary carcinomas occur in families as part of syndromes called multiple endocrine neoplasia (MEN) type 2A and type 2B. MEN 2A consists of multicentric medullary thyroid cancer, pheochromocytomas or adrenal medullary hyperplasia, and hyperparathyroidism. MEN 2B consists of medullary cancer, pheochromocytoma and mucosal neuromas, gangliomas, and a Marfan-like habitus. These patients may develop medullary carcinoma at a very young age, and any patient with MEN 2B should be assumed to have medullary cancer until proved otherwise. Patients are followed carefully for pheochromocytoma with urine VMA, for hyperparathyroidism with serum calcium, and for medullary carcinoma with serum calcitonin. However, as some patients have a normal basal calcitonin, a pentagastrin or provocative calcium infusion test should be performed in these high-risk patients. Patients thought to have MEN 1 syndrome (pituitary, parathyroid, and pancreatic tumors) or Zollinger-Ellison syndrome should be assayed for serum gastrin, insulin, glucagon, and somatostatin. These assays may prove to be inappropriately high in MEN 1 syndrome due to pancreatic islet cell tumors.

211. The answer is c. (*Brunicardi, pp 1671–1673.*) Benign soft tissue tumors far outnumber their malignant counterparts. Because of this, prolonged delays are common before definitive treatment of soft tissue sarcomas is instituted. Risk for malignancy is increased for tumors greater than 5 cm in largest diameter, as well as for those lesions that are symptomatic or that have enlarged rapidly over a short period of time. Properly performed biopsy is critical in the initial treatment of any soft tissue mass. Improperly performed biopsies can complicate the care of the sarcoma patient and, in rare circumstances, even eliminate certain surgical options. Excisional biopsies should be reserved for small masses for which complete excision would not jeopardize subsequent treatment should a sarcoma be found. For all other masses, incisional biopsy should be performed. The incision should be placed directly over the mass and should be oriented along the long axis of the extremity.

212. The answer is e. (*Tondini, pp 831–837; Gobbi, pp 2528–2536.*) The stomach is the most common site in the gastrointestinal tract for non-Hodgkin's lymphoma, followed by the small intestine and the colon. Lymphomas constitute 3% of all malignant gastric tumors. Ninety percent of these lymphomas are of the non-Hodgkin's type. Surgery alone can be considered adequate treatment for patients with non-Hodgkin's lymphoma that does not infiltrate beyond the submucosa. However, gastric resection is not considered mandatory, and there are no substantial differences in response to therapy and survival when resection is compared with combined chemotherapy and radiation therapy, including in advanced cases. Moreover, chemotherapy and radiation therapy have been shown to be effective even in unresected bulky cases, and provide minimal risk of hemorrhage and perforation even in this setting.

213. The answer is b. (*Brunicardi, pp 281–284.*) The interferons are a group of glycoproteins first found as products of virus-infected cells that inhibited viral replication. Subsequently, they have been shown to have a variety of effects both on cells of the immune system and on malignant cells. Interferons cause Burkitt's lymphoma cell lines to differentiate and lose the capacity to divide. Hematologic malignancies are very responsive to interferons; up to 100% of hairy cell leukemias show some degree of remission. Interferon α has been used in the treatment of chronic active hepatitis B and C.

214. The answer is d. (*Greenfield, pp 650–652.*) Acinar, adenoid cystic, and low grades of mucoepidermoid carcinomas exhibit moderately malignant behavior. Undifferentiated, squamous, and high grades of mucoepidermoid carcinomas are considered highly malignant tumors. Regional node dissection is indicated for malignant tumors because of the high (up to 50%) incidence of occult regional metastases. Facial nerve preservation should be attempted when the margins are adequate and the tumor is well localized. The minimal appropriate procedure for parotid carcinoma is a superficial parotidectomy with nerve preservation. The nerve must be partially or totally sacrificed if the tumor directly involves the nerve trunk or its branches.

215. The answer is b. (*Brunicardi, pp 276–281.*) A surgeon is frequently asked to evaluate patients who are receiving systemic chemotherapy. Most complications of chemotherapy do not require surgical therapy. Perirectal abscesses are more common in these immunosuppressed patients. Gastrointestinal bleeding occurs secondary to mucosal irritation and thrombocytopenia. Pancreatitis is uncommon, but is associated with L-asparaginase use. Up to 20% of patients treated with floxuridine by continuous hepatic artery infusion develop some degree of inflammation and obstruction of the bile duct. Systemic chemotherapy does not increase the likelihood of acute cholecystitis, appendicitis, incarcerated femoral hernia, or diverticulitis.

216. The answer is e. *(Greenfield, pp 2194–2195.)* After radical orchiectomy, lymph node dissection is indicated in embryonal carcinoma, teratocarcinoma, and adult teratoma if there is no supradiaphragmatic spread. This dissection increases the five-year survival and helps in staging. Seminoma is extremely radiosensitive, and lymph node dissection is unnecessary. Choriocarcinoma are frequently associated with pulmonary metastases and are treated with chemotherapy. Orchiectomy for a testicular mass is approached via an inguinal incision in order to perform a high ligation of the cord and to eliminate spread of the tumor. Cryptorchidism (undescended testicle) is associated with decreased spermatogenesis and carries a lifelong risk of malignant degeneration even after being surgically corrected.

217. The answer is a. *(Greenfield, pp 575–576.)* Dialysis is less expensive than renal transplantation if the graft functions for less than two years. Recipients with functioning grafts are less anemic because of erythropoietin production by the graft. As more dialysis patients are treated with recombinant erythropoietin, this advantage may disappear. Transplanted females have more normal menses and an increased number of successful pregnancies. Patient survival in the two groups is comparable at one year.

218. The answer is e. *(Brunicardi, p 1460.)* Pheochromocytoma is associated with MEN IIA, MEN IIB, von Hippel-Lindau disease, and neurofibromatosis I. Hereditary pheochromocytomas are more likely to be multiple and bilateral.

219. The answer is e. *(Brunicardi, pp 1088–1090.)* In an average-risk patient, colorectal cancer screening should begin at age 50 and then an annual fecal occult blood test *or* flexible sigmoidoscopy every 5 years *or* annual fecal occult blood test and flexible sigmoidoscopy every 5 years *or* air contrast barium enema (which has a sensitivity of 90% for polyps greater than 1 cm in size) *or* colonoscopy every 10 years is recommended. If an adenomatous polyp is detected, then colonoscopy is recommended every three years. If no polyps are detected subsequently, colonoscopy can be performed every five years. If more than five polyps are detected, colonoscopy should occur annually. For patients with hereditary nonpolyposis colorectal cancer (HNPCC), screening should begin either between the ages of 20 and 25 or 10 years earlier than the youngest family member with colorectal cancer, whichever comes earlier.

220. The answer is b. *(Brunicardi, pp 285–286.)* Only about 30% of the biologic damage from x-rays is due to the direct effects on the target molecule. The remainder is due to an indirect action mediated by free radicals and can be modified by free radical scavengers such as sulfhydryl. The percentage of cells killed by a given dose of x-rays or gamma rays is greatly increased by molecular oxygen; cells deficient in oxygen are resistant to radiation. Among the basic principles of radiation biology is the observation that the sensitivity of mammalian cells to radiation varies with their position in the cell division cycle. M-phase (mitotic phase) cells are the most radiosensitive. Radiation is frequently employed for local control of disease. Overall and disease-free survival rates for breast lumpectomy and radiation are equivalent to those for mastectomy, in patients with Stage I and II breast cancers. Rapidly dividing cells of the gastrointestinal mucosa and bone marrow are particularly sensitive to the effects of radiation.

221. The answer is d. *(Greenfield, p 507.)* With the availability of recombinant interleukin 2, multiple trials of cancer therapy with this lymphokine have been undertaken. The most successful trials have documented complete or partial responses in patients with metastatic renal cell carcinoma and melanoma. However, IL-2 therapy has been ineffective in the treatment of breast cancer, colon cancer, and lymphoma. The therapy is not innocuous. All patients exhibit a marked lymphocytosis, eosinophilia, fluid retention, fever, and decrease in peripheral vascular resistance, effects similar to those of septic shock.

222. The answer is c. *(Heys, pp 614–623.)* Malignant tumors require energy substrates to grow and ordinarily claim these substrates from the host. In animal studies, withholding dietary proteins diminishes the rate of tumor growth. There is no evidence in the human to suggest acceleration of tumor growth when nutritional support is provided. There is also no evidence that nutritional therapy improves the response of the tumor to therapy. For nearly a century, the association of stomach cancer and diet has been recognized.

Among the wide variety of substances incriminated are nitrates and nitrosamides in food and drinking water. There is evidence that regular ingestion of vitamin C from childhood may reduce the formation of carcinogens, though reduction in the incidence of cancer has not been demonstrated. Excess amounts of dietary fat and deficiency of fiber have been clearly associated with colon cancer. Animal fats have also been associated with cancer of the exocrine pancreas, the prostate, and the endometrium. Alcohol consumption, especially when combined with cigarette smoking, increases the incidence of esophageal cancer. Consumption of alcohol also increases the incidence of pancreatitis, but not pancreatic cancer.

223. The answer is d. (*Greenfield, pp 575–576, 603–607.*) Cardiac allograft has become an accepted treatment for end-stage heart disease. One-year cardiac allograft survival exceeds 80%, which is comparable to renal allograft survival. Cardiac allografts have a cold ischemia preservation time of 4 to 5 h, and therefore tissue typing is not practical. Cardiac donors are matched to recipients only by size and ABO blood type. Tissue typing remains an important component of cadaveric kidney allograft matching. The mainstay of immunosuppression for both cardiac and renal allografts continues to include calcineurin inhibitors (FK506, cyclosporine), steroids, and antimitotic agents (azathioprine, mycophenylate mofetil).

224. The answer is b. (*Greenfield, pp 1128, 2155, 2279–2280.*) Resection of metastases of lung, liver, and brain can result in occasional five-year cures. In general, surgery should be undertaken only when the primary tumor is controlled, diffuse metastatic disease has been ruled out, and the affected patient's condition and the location of the metastasis permit safe resection. The best results have come from resection of pulmonary metastases, in which five-year survival rates exceed those for resection for primary bronchogenic carcinoma. For example, resection of pulmonary metastases in patients with osteogenic sarcoma can have survival rates up to 25 to 35%.

225. The answer is c. (*Rhame, pp 141–152; Wilson, pp 193–201.*) The risk of contracting HIV is much less than the risk of contracting hepatitis B from a patient. Although the risk of transmission of HIV in the health care setting is very low, there are reported cases of seroconversion after parenteral exposure. Particular precautions should be taken in operating on patients who are known to be seropositive for HIV or who have known risk factors. Recommendations include elimination of inexperienced personnel or personnel with open lesions on body surfaces from the operating room. Disposable gowns, drapes, masks, and eye shields should be used. Contaminated clothing should be soaked in a dilute solution (1:10) of chlorine bleach prior to washing. Double gloving does not reduce the major intraoperative risk of needle puncture, which is the primary source of risk to the operating team. Needles should never be capped; an uncapped needle is less dangerous than are the maneuvers to recap needles.

226. The answer is c. *(Brunicardi, pp 267–268.)* Risk factors for breast cancer include family history, nulliparity, previous breast cancer, early menarche, and late menopause. A late age at first birth (after age 30) increases the risk of breast cancer compared with early parity (age 18 or earlier). Having one first-degree relative (mother, sister, or daughter) with breast cancer also increases the risk. Women of the upper social classes, as measured by either education or income, have been found to have the highest incidence of breast cancer. Neither cigarette smoking nor the use of hair dye has been correlated with breast cancer.

227. The answer is c. *(Brunicardi, pp 260–267.)* Li-Fraumeni syndrome is associated most commonly with a mutation in the p53 tumor suppressor gene. Li-Fraumeni syndrome in an individual is based on (1) bone or soft tissue sarcoma in that person before the age of 45, (2) a first-degree relative with cancer before the age of 45, and (3) a first- or second-degree relative with sarcoma at any age or any cancer before the age of 45. The APC (adenomatous polyposis coli) gene is associated with familial adenomatous polyposis (FAP). The RET protooncogene is associated with multiple endocrine neoplasia (MEN) 2. The PTEN (phosphatase and tensin homologue) tumor suppressor gene is associated with Cowden disease, or multiple hamartoma syndrome. The p16 tumor suppressor gene is associated with hereditary malignant melanoma.

228. The answer is a. *(Brunicardi, pp 276–281.)* Doxorubicin, an antibiotic derived from *Streptomyces* species, has activity against sarcomas and carcinomas of the breast, liver, bladder, prostate, head and neck, esophagus, and lung. Its major side effect is production of a dilated cardiomyopathy. Patients receiving this agent should have echocardiography before and after treatment in order to monitor potential cardiac toxicity.

229. The answer is e. *(Brunicardi, pp 262–263.)* Both *BRCA1* and *BRCA2* are associated with an increased risk of ovarian cancer by age 70—44% and 27%, respectively. Approximately 10% of women under the age of 40 who develop breast cancer have a mutation in *BRCA1* or *2*. *BRCA1* is associated with an increased risk of colon cancer and prostate cancer in males. *BRCA2* is associated with an increased risk of gallbladder, bile duct, and pancreatic cancers as well as gastric cancer, malignant melanoma, and in men, prostate cancer. *BRCA1* breast cancers are more likely to be estrogen receptor–negative, and *BRCA2* breast cancers are more likely to be estrogen receptor–positive.

230. The answer is e. *(Brunicardi, pp 276–281.)* Cyclophosphamide is an alkylating agent used in the treatment of a variety of solid tumors. Its major side effect is hemorrhagic cystitis. Bleomycin can cause pulmonary fibrosis. Vincristine is an alkaloid that can cause peripheral and central neuropathies. Cisplatin is an alkylating agent that can lead to ototoxicity, neurotoxicity, and nephrotoxicity. 5-fluorouracil is an antimetabolite that can cause mucositis, dermatitis, and cerebellar dysfunction.

231. The answer is d. *(Townsend, pp 681–682.)* Posttransplant lymphoproliferative disorders (PTLD) are associated with the Epstein-Barr virus (EBV). PTLD has a range of clinical presentations, and treatment can include multiple modalities including withdrawal of immunosuppression, antiviral therapy with ganciclovir, chemotherapy, or immunotherapy with monoclonal antibodies. Other common posttransplantation malignancies include hepatocellular carcinomas, which are associated with hepatitis B and C; Kaposi's sarcoma, which is associated with human herpesvirus 8; and cervical cancers, which are associated with human papillomavirus. Although cytomegalovirus (CMV) infection can occur when CMV-seronegative recipients receive an organ from a CMV-seropositive donor, CMV does not predispose transplantation patients to malignancy.

232. The answer is d. *(Brunicardi, pp 1447–1448.)* The patient has tertiary hyperparathyroidism, which is manifested by persistent hypercalcemia secondary to autonomous parathyroid function after renal transplantation. Treatment is total parathyroidectomy with autotransplantation or subtotal parathyroidectomy. The imaging modalities described would be more appropriate in the workup of primary hyperparathyroidism—24-h urinary calcium levels are low in familial hypercalciuric hypercalcemia. Ultrasound, sestamibi scintigraphy, and CT scanning are all modalities that can be utilized to identify a parathyroid adenoma preoperatively.

233. The answer is e. *(Brunicardi, p 273.)* CEA is a glycoprotein that is present in early embryonic and fetal cells (an oncofetal antigen) and in colon cancer. It is not found in normal colon mucosa. It is not tumor-specific and may be elevated in a variety of benign and malignant conditions, including cirrhosis, ulcerative colitis, renal failure, pancreatitis, pancreatic cancer, stomach cancer, breast cancer, and lung cancer. However, the CEA assay is a sensitive serologic tool for identifying recurrent disease. In about two-thirds of patients with recurrent disease, an increased CEA level is the first indicator of tumor reappearance. A rising CEA following colon cancer surgery, in the absence of other conditions associated with an elevated CEA, predicts the appearance of liver metastases within one year with an accuracy approaching 70%. Although an elevated CEA level preoperatively predicts a higher risk of recurrence, the use of preoperative CEA levels as an indication for postoperative adjuvant chemotherapy is controversial and currently not supported by clinical practice guidelines.

234–236. The answers are 234-a, 235-g, 236-e. *(Greenfield, pp 1117–1129.)* The patient has a left colon cancer. In order to resect the tumor with an adequate margin (traditionally 5 cm) on its proximal and distal ends as well as to remove the draining lymph node basin, a left hemicolectomy should be performed. A Dukes C tumor is one that involves adjacent lymph nodes, regardless of extent of invasion into the wall of the colon. In patients with Stage III colon cancer (which corresponds to a Dukes C tumor), adjuvant chemotherapy is recommended. The liver is the most common site of bloodborne metastases from primary colorectal cancers. In a subgroup of patients, the liver may be the only site of disease. Overall, the pathologic stage is the most important determinant of prognosis.

237–240. The answers are 237-f, 238-a, 239-d, 240-b *(Greenfield, pp 571–576.)* Routine postoperative immunosuppression for a renal transplant recipient includes cyclosporine, azathioprine, and steroids. Cyclosporine is nephrotoxic and is frequently withheld in the postoperative period until the creatinine returns to normal following transplantation. Azathioprine has bone marrow toxicity as its major side effect, and both WBC and platelet counts need to be monitored in the immediate posttransplant period. The patient's decrease in WBCs is secondary to azathioprine toxicity, and the most appropriate step is to decrease the dose of azathioprine. Viral infections are a serious cause of morbidity following transplantation. A buffy coat is the supernatant of a centrifuged blood sample that contains the WBCs. Viral cultures from this supernatant as well as localization of inclusion bodies can identify transplant patients infected with cytomegalovirus (CMV). This patient has CMV pneumonitis and needs to be treated with high-dose gancyclovir.

An elevation in creatinine at three-month follow-up can be secondary to rejection, anastomotic problems, urologic complications, infection, or nephrotoxicity of various medications. With a normal ultrasound, no fever, and no graft tenderness, the most likely cause is cyclosporine-induced nephrotoxicity and the most appropriate step is a reduction in the cyclosporine dose. Finally, at six months with graft tenderness, fever, and an edematous kidney on ultrasound, rejection must be suspected. Negative cultures make infection unlikely, and a steroid boost is appropriate. Addition of monoclonal antibodies to CD3 (OKT3) or pooled antibodies against lymphocytes (ALG) is also appropriate in the treatment of a first rejection.

Endocrine Problems and the Breast

Questions

DIRECTIONS: Each item below contains a question followed by suggested responses. Select the **one best** response to each question.

241. A patient with mild skin pigmentation is admitted emergently to your service because of sudden abdominal pain, fever, and a rigid abdomen. Her blood work indicates a marked leukocytosis, a blood sugar of 55 mg/dL, a sodium value of 119 meq/dL, and a potassium value of 6.2 meq/dL. Her blood pressure is 88/58. She undergoes an exploratory laparotomy. Which of the following statements regarding her condition is true?

a. Treatment with exogenous steroids is usually ineffective
b. This condition is commonly seen as a consequence of metastasis of distant cancers, such as lung or breast, to the adrenal glands
c. Chronic adrenal insufficiency (Addison's disease) in the preoperative patient should be recognizable by a constellation of findings, including hyperglycemia, hypernatremia, and hypokalemia
d. Death from untreated chronic adrenal insufficiency may occur within hours of surgery
e. The most common underlying cause today is infection with resistant tuberculosis

242. A 45-year-old woman complains to her primary care physician of nervousness, sweating, tremulousness, and weight loss. The thyroid scan shown here exhibits a pattern that is most consistent with which of the following disorders?

a. Hypersecreting adenoma
b. Graves' disease
c. Lateral aberrant thyroid
d. Papillary carcinoma of thyroid
e. Medullary carcinoma of thyroid

243. A 35-year-old woman with a history of previous right thyroidectomy for a benign thyroid nodule now undergoes completion thyroidectomy for a suspicious thyroid mass. Several hours postoperatively, she develops progressive swelling under the incision, stridor, and difficulty breathing. Orotracheal intubation is successful. Which of the following is the most appropriate next step?

a. Fiberoptic laryngoscopy to rule out bilateral vocal cord paralysis
b. Administration of intravenous calcium
c. Administration of broad-spectrum antibiotics and debridement of the wound
d. Wound exploration
e. Administration of high-dose steroids and antihistamines

244. A 62-year-old woman presents with invasive ductal adenocarcinoma of the breast. Which of the following would not be an absolute contraindication to breast conservation therapy?

a. Diffuse suspicious microcalcifications throughout the breast
b. Multifocal disease in a single quadrant
c. Previous treatment of a breast cancer with lumpectomy and radiation
d. Two distinct tumors in two different quadrants of the breast
e. Persistently positive margins after multiple reexcisions of the breast cancer

245. A 29-year-old woman presents with a six-month history of right breast erythema and edema of the right breast with palpable axillary lymphadenopathy. A punch biopsy of the skin reveals neoplastic cells in the dermal lymphatics. Which of the following is the best next step in her management?

a. A course of nafcillin to treat the overlying cellulitis and then neoadjuvant chemotherapy for breast cancer
b. Modified radical mastectomy followed by adjuvant chemotherapy
c. Modified radical mastectomy followed by hormonal therapy
d. Combined modality chemotherapy and radiation therapy to the right breast with surgery reserved for residual disease
e. Combined modality therapy with chemotherapy, surgery, and radiation

246. A 15-year-old otherwise healthy female high school student begins to notice galactorrhea. A pregnancy test is negative. Which of the following is a frequently associated physical finding?

a. Gonadal atrophy
b. Bitemporal hemianopsia
c. Exophthalmos and lid lag
d. Episodic hypertension
e. Buffalo hump

247. A 52-year-old woman sees her physician with complaints of fatigue, headache, flank pain, hematuria, and abdominal pain. She undergoes a sestamibi scan that demonstrates persistent uptake in the right superior parathyroid gland at 2 h. Which of the following laboratory values is most suggestive of her diagnosis?

a. Serum acid phosphatase above 120 IU/L
b. Serum alkaline phosphatase above 120 IU/L
c. Serum calcium above 11 mg/dL
d. Urinary calcium below 100 mg/d
e. Parathyroid hormone levels below 5 pmol/L

248. A 53-year-old woman with MEN I syndrome presents with a dermatitic rash and is found to have an elevated fasting glucagon level. Which of the following statements is true regarding her need for further workup and treatment?

a. She should undergo visceral angiography as the initial test for localization of the lesion
b. Localization of the lesion is typically difficult because of its small size
c. Surgical treatment requires total pancreatectomy because there are usually multiple lesions
d. Metastatic disease is rare
e. Octreotide may be useful in the management of hyperglycemia in patients with unresectable disease

249. A 49-year-old man has become irritable, his facies have changed to a round configuration, he is impotent, he has developed purplish lines on his flanks, and he is hypertensive. His workup includes a CT scan that revealed a 3-cm right adrenal mass. Which of the following statements regarding his diagnosis and treatment is true?

a. Surgical intervention is indicated only for lesions greater than 6 cm in size
b. MRI and scintigraphic scans are not useful in distinguishing adenomas from carcinomas preoperatively
c. Operative exploration of both adrenal glands is indicated
d. Preoperative CT-guided biopsy of the adrenal lesion should be performed
e. Steroid replacement therapy may be required for up to 6 to 12 months postoperatively

250. A 40-year-old woman is found to have a 1- to 2-cm, slightly tender cystic mass in her breast; she has no perceptible axillary adenopathy. What of the following represents the best management option?

a. Reassurance and reexamination in the immediate postmenstrual period
b. Immediate excisional biopsy
c. Aspiration of the mass with cytologic analysis
d. Fluoroscopically guided needle localization biopsy
e. Mammography and reevaluation of options with new information

251. A 62-year-old Polynesian woman, who grew up in the South Pacific in the 1950s, has a lump in her neck. Which of the following statements concerning radiation-induced thyroid cancer is true?

a. It usually follows high-dose radiation to the head and neck
b. A patient with a history of radiation is safe if no cancer has been found 20 years after exposure
c. Approximately 25% of patients with a thyroid nodule and a history of head and neck irradiation develop thyroid cancer
d. Most radiation-induced thyroid cancers are follicular
e. The treatment of choice is a near-total (or total) thyroidectomy

252. A 55-year-old woman presents with a 6-cm right thyroid mass and palpable cervical lymphadenopathy. Fine-needle aspiration of one of the lymph nodes demonstrates the presence of calcified clumps of sloughed cells. Which of the following best describes the management of this thyroid disorder?

a. The patient should be screened for pancreatic endocrine neoplasms and hypercalcemia
b. The patient should undergo total thyroidectomy with modified radical neck dissection
c. The patient should undergo total thyroidectomy with frozen section intraoperatively, with modified radical neck dissection reserved for patients with extracapsular invasion
d. The patient should undergo right thyroid lobectomy followed by ^{131}I therapy
e. The patient should undergo right thyroid lobectomy

253. A 45-year-old woman is found to have lobular carcinoma in situ (LCIS) on a breast biopsy. Regarding counseling for her risk for invasive breast cancer, which of the following statements is true?

a. The most common type of invasive carcinoma after a diagnosis of LCIS is lobular carcinoma
b. Her risk of invasive carcinoma is greatest within 10 years after a diagnosis of LCIS, after which time the risk becomes minimal
c. Her risk of invasive carcinoma is equivalent in both breasts
d. Her risk of invasive carcinoma is significantly increased if a large focus of LCIS is present in the biopsy specimen
e. Early menarche and late menopause are associated with increased relative risks for breast cancer when compared to LCIS

254. A 14-year-old black girl has her right breast removed because of a large mass. The tumor weighs 1400 g and has a bulging, very firm, lobulated surface with a whorl-like pattern, as illustrated here. Which of the following is the most likely diagnosis?

a. Cystosarcoma phyllodes
b. Intraductal carcinoma
c. Malignant lymphoma
d. Fibroadenoma
e. Juvenile hypertrophy

255. As an incidental finding during an upper abdominal CT scan, a 3-cm mass in the adrenal gland is noted. Which of the following would not be an appropriate step in the patient's workup?

a. Laparoscopic adrenalectomy
b. Measurement of serum electrolytes
c. Measurement of plasma aldosterone and renin
d. Measurement of urine catecholamine excretion
e. Dexamethasone suppression test

256. A 53-year-old woman presents with complaints of weakness, anorexia, malaise, constipation, and back pain. While being evaluated, she becomes somewhat lethargic. Laboratory studies include a normal chest x-ray, serum albumin 3.2 mg/dL, serum calcium 14 mg/dL, serum phosphorus 2.6 mg/dL, serum chloride 108 mg/dL, BUN 32 mg/dL, and creatinine 2.0 mg/dL. Which of the following is the most appropriate initial management?

a. Intravenous normal saline infusion
b. Administration of thiazide diuretics
c. Administration of intravenous phosphorus
d. Use of mithramycin
e. Neck exploration and parathyroidectomy

257. Which of the following patients with primary hyperparathyroidism should undergo parathyroidectomy?

a. A 62-year-old asymptomatic woman
b. A 54-year-old woman with fatigue and depression
c. A 42-year-old woman with a history of kidney stones
d. A 59-year-old woman with mildly elevated 24-h urinary calcium excretion
e. A 60-year-old woman with mildly decreased bone mineral density measured at the hip of less than 2 standard deviations below peak bone density.

258. A woman sustains an injury to her chest after striking the steering wheel of her automobile during a collision. Which of the following statements concerning fat necrosis of the breast is true?

a. Most patients report a history of trauma
b. The lesion is usually nontender and diffuse
c. It predisposes patients to the development of breast cancer
d. It is difficult to distinguish from breast cancer
e. Excision exacerbates the process

259. Which of the following is the most likely diagnosis in a 45-year-old woman with hypertension, development of facial hair, and a 7-cm suprarenal mass?

a. Myelolipoma
b. Cushing's disease
c. Adrenocortical carcinoma
d. Pheochromocytoma
e. Carcinoid

260. A 36-year-old woman presents with palpitations, anxiety, and hypertension. Workup reveals a pheochromocytoma. Which of the following is the best approach to optimizing the patient preoperatively?

a. Fluid restriction 24 h preoperatively to prevent intraoperative congestive heart failure
b. Initiation of an alpha blocker 24 h prior to surgery
c. Initiation of an alpha blocker at one to three weeks prior to surgery
d. Initiation of a beta blocker one to three weeks prior to surgery
e. Escalating antihypertensive drug therapy with beta blockade followed by alpha blockade starting at least one week prior to surgery

261. A 31-year-old woman notices a breast lump during her second pregnancy. A biopsy confirms the presence of breast cancer. Which of the following statements is true?

a. Termination of a first-trimester pregnancy is mandatory
b. Radiation therapy is safe in the third trimester provided appropriate shielding is provided
c. Breast conservation is inappropriate for third-trimester pregnancies
d. Modified radical mastectomy should be delayed until after delivery
e. Administration of adjuvant chemotherapy is safe for the fetus during the second and third trimesters

262. A 40-year-old woman notices a skin rash around her areola. There is an erosive area about the nipple. There is tenderness, itching, and intermittent bleeding. Which of the following statements is true regarding this entity?

a. It usually precedes development of Paget's disease of bone
b. It presents with nipple-areolar eczematous changes
c. It does not involve axillary lymph nodes because it is a manifestation of intraductal carcinoma only
d. It accounts for 10 to 15% of all newly diagnosed breast cancers
e. It is adequately treated with wide excision when it presents as a mass

263. A 40-year-old man who has a long history of peptic ulcer disease that has not responded to medical therapy is admitted to the hospital. His serum gastrin levels are markedly elevated; at celiotomy, a small, firm mass is palpated in the tail of the pancreas. Correct statements concerning this patient's condition include which of the following?

a. Histamine or a protein meal will markedly increase basal acid secretion
b. Secretin administration will suppress acid secretion
c. The pancreatic mass will probably be benign
d. Distal pancreatectomy is the treatment of choice
e. H_2 receptor antagonists have not been beneficial in the treatment of this condition

264. A 29-year-old woman with a history of difficulty becoming pregnant presents to her primary care physician and is diagnosed with Graves' disease on iodine uptake scan; her TSH level is markedly suppressed and her free T4 level is elevated. She desires to conceive as soon as possible and elects to undergo thyroidectomy. After she is rendered euthyroid with medications preoperatively, which of the following management strategies should also be employed to reduce the risk of developing thyroid storm in the operating room?

a. Drops of Lugol's iodide solution daily beginning 10 days preoperatively
b. Preoperative treatment with phenoxybenzamine for three weeks
c. Preoperative treatment with propranolol for one week
d. Twenty-four hours of corticosteroids preoperatively
e. No other preoperative medication is required

265. This 30-year-old woman presented with weakness, bone pain, an elevated parathyroid hormone level, and a serum calcium level of 15.2 mg/dL. Skeletal survey films were taken, including the hand films and chest x-ray shown. Which of the following is the most likely cause of these findings?

a. Sarcoidosis
b. Vitamin D intoxication
c. Paget's disease
d. Metastatic carcinoma
e. Primary hyperparathyroidism

266. A 30-year-old woman presented with weakness, bone pain, an elevated parathyroid hormone level, and a serum calcium level of 15.2 mg/dL. Following correction of the patient's hypercalcemia with hydration and gentle diuresis with furosemide, which of the following is the best therapeutic approach?

a. Administration of maintenance doses of steroids
b. Radiation treatment for bony metastases
c. Neck exploration and resection of all four parathyroid glands
d. Neck exploration and resection of a parathyroid adenoma
e. Avoidance of sunlight, vitamin D, and calcium-containing dairy products

267. A 25-year-old woman is found to have an anterior neck mass. Her thyroid scan, shown here, exhibits findings that are consistent with which of the following disorders?

a. Carcinoma
b. Toxic adenoma
c. Toxic multinodular goiter
d. Graves' disease
e. de Quervain's (subacute) thyroiditis

268. Incisional biopsy of a breast mass in a 35-year-old woman demonstrates a cystosarcoma phyllodes at the time of frozen section. Which of the following is the most appropriate management strategy for this lesion?

a. Wide local excision with a rim of normal tissue
b. Lumpectomy and axillary lymphadenectomy
c. Modified radical mastectomy
d. Excision and postoperative radiotherapy
e. Excision, postoperative radiotherapy, and systemic chemotherapy

269. A 36-year-old woman, 20 weeks pregnant, presents with a 1.5-cm right thyroid mass. Fine-needle aspiration is consistent with a papillary neoplasm. The mass is cold on scan and solid on ultrasound. Which of the following methods of treatment is contraindicated?

a. Right thyroid lobectomy
b. Subtotal thyroidectomy
c. Total thyroidectomy
d. Total thyroidectomy with lymph node dissection
e. ^{131}I radioactive ablation of the thyroid gland

270. A 63-year-old woman notices lumps on both sides of her neck. A fine-needle aspirate is nondiagnostic, and she undergoes total thyroidectomy. On frozen section, pathology reveals Hürthle cell carcinoma. Correct statements concerning Hürthle cell carcinoma of the thyroid include which of the following?

a. It is a form of anaplastic thyroid cancer
b. It can be diagnosed by fine-needle aspiration
c. Treatment consists of a total thyroidectomy
d. Microscopically, it consists of clusters of cells separated by areas of collagen and amyloid
e. Once treated appropriately, it has a low rate of recurrence

271. A 51-year-old man presents with a 2-cm left thyroid nodule. Thyroid scan shows a cold lesion. Fine-needle aspiration cytology demonstrates follicular cells. Which of the following statements regarding this patient's condition is true?

a. Thyroid nodules in men are rarely malignant
b. Increased age is associated with improved prognosis in patients with follicular carcinomas
c. In the setting of abnormal cytology, an initial course of TSH suppression by thyroid hormone is recommended
d. In the setting of a possible follicular neoplasm, prophylactic neck dissection is indicated
e. Thyroid lobectomy is an acceptable treatment for this patient

272. A 41-year-old woman has noted bilateral thin serous discharge from her breasts. There seems to be no mass associated with it. Which of the following statements would be appropriate to tell the patient?

a. Intermittent thin or milky discharge can be physiologic
b. Expressible nipple discharge is an indication for open biopsy
c. Absence of a mass on mammogram rules out malignancy
d. Galactorrhea is indicative of an underlying malignancy
e. Pathologic discharge is usually bilateral

273. A 52-year-old woman is referred to you. She says that her doctor told her she had a condition called Cushing's. She has hypertension, obesity, and new skin striae. True statements regarding Cushing's disease and Cushing syndrome include which of the following?

a. Adrenocortical hyperplasia is the most common cause of Cushing's disease
b. Overproduction of ACTH is pathognomonic of Cushing syndrome
c. Clinical manifestations of Cushing's disease and Cushing's syndrome are identical
d. Cushing's syndrome is caused only by neoplasms of either the pituitary or adrenal glands
e. Cushing's disease is incurable

274. A 34-year-old woman has recurrent fainting spells induced by fasting. Her serum insulin levels during these episodes are markedly elevated. Correct statements regarding this patient's condition include which of the following?

a. The underlying lesion is more commonly located in the body or tail of the pancreas
b. The underlying lesion is usually multifocal
c. These lesions are usually malignant
d. Serum calcium levels may be elevated
e. She should be screened for a coexistent pheochromocytoma

275. A 36-year-old woman whose mother has just undergone treatment for breast cancer is asking about how this affects her and what can be done to lessen her chances of having the disease. Which of the following is not a significant risk factor for breast cancer?

a. Dietary fat intake
b. Paternal relative with *BRCA1* mutation
c. Excessive estrogen exposure—early menarche, late menopause, nulliparity
d. Previous biopsy with atypical hyperplasia
e. Exposure to ionizing radiation

DIRECTIONS: Each group of questions below consists of lettered options followed by a set of numbered items. For each numbered item, select the **one** lettered option with which it is **most** closely associated. Each lettered option may be used once, more than once, or not at all.

Questions 276–280

For each clinical description, select the appropriate stage of breast cancer.

a. Stage I
b. Stage II
c. Stage III
d. Stage IV
e. Inflammatory carcinoma

276. Tumor not palpable, clinically positive lymph nodes fixed to one another, no evidence of metastases

277. Tumor 5.0 cm; clinically positive, movable ipsilateral lymph nodes; no evidence of metastases

278. Tumor 2.1 cm, clinically negative lymph nodes, no evidence of metastases

279. Tumor not palpable, but breast diffusely enlarged and erythematous, clinically positive supraclavicular nodes, and evidence of metastases

280. Tumor 0.5 cm, clinically negative lymph nodes, pathological rib fracture

Questions 281–285

A 43-year-old man presents with signs and symptoms of peritonitis in the right lower quadrant. The clinical impression and supportive data suggest acute appendicitis. At exploration, however, a tumor is found; frozen section suggests carcinoid features. For each tumor described, choose the most appropriate surgical procedure.

a. Appendectomy
b. Segmental ileal resection
c. Cecectomy
d. Right hemicolectomy
e. Hepatic wedge resection and appropriate bowel resection

281. A 2.5-cm tumor at the base of the appendix

282. A 1.0-cm tumor at the tip of the appendix

283. A 0.5-cm tumor with serosal umbilication in the ileum

284. A 1.0-cm tumor of the midappendix; a 1-cm firm, pale lesion at the periphery of the right lobe of the liver

285. A 3.5-cm tumor encroaching onto the cecum and extensive liver metastases

Questions 286–290

For each clinical problem outlined, select acceptable treatment options.

a. No further surgical intervention
b. Wide local excision
c. Wide local excision with adjuvant radiation therapy
d. Wide local excision with axillary lymph node dissection and radiation therapy
e. Simple mastectomy (without axillary lymph node dissection)
f. Modified radical mastectomy (simple mastectomy with in-continuity axillary lymph node dissection)
g. Radical mastectomy
h. Bilateral prophylactic simple mastectomies

286. A 49-year-old woman undergoes biopsy of a 5.0-cm left breast mass; she has no palpable axillary lymph nodes. Biopsy of the mass shows cystosarcoma phyllodes

287. A 42-year-old woman has a mammogram that demonstrates diffuse suspicious mammographic calcifications suggestive of multicentric disease. Biopsy of one of the lesions reveals ductal carcinoma in situ.

288. A 51-year-old (premenopausal) woman undergoes needle localization biopsy for microcalcifications. Pathology reveals sclerosing adenosis.

289. A 49-year-old woman has a 6-cm palpable mass that is biopsy-proven ductal adenocarcinoma. She undergoes neoadjuvant chemotherapy which reduces the tumor to 3 cm in size. However, she has palpable axillary lymph nodes; fine-needle aspirate demonstrates adenocarcinoma. She desires breast conservation therapy if possible.

290. A neglected 82-year-old woman presents with a locally advanced breast cancer that is invading the pectoralis major muscle over a broad base. She is otherwise in good health.

Endocrine Problems and the Breast

Answers

241. The answer is d. *(Townsend, pp 1050–1051.)* Failure to recognize adrenal cortical insufficiency, particularly in the postoperative patient, may be a fatal error that is especially regrettable because therapy (exogenous steroids) is effective and easy to administer. Adrenal insufficiency may occur in a host of settings including infections (e.g., tuberculosis—formerly the most common cause, HIV-associated infections), autoimmune states, adrenal hemorrhage (classically, during meningococcal septicemia), pituitary insufficiency, after burns, in the setting of coagulopathy, and—most commonly today—after interruption of chronically administered exogenous steroids. Although the adrenal gland is an occasional site for distant metastases, such as from lung or breast, it is rare to have enough destruction of the glands to produce clinical adrenal insufficiency. Chronic adrenal insufficiency (classic Addison's disease) should be recognizable preoperatively by the constellation of skin pigmentation, weakness, weight loss, hypotension, nausea, vomiting, abdominal pain, hypoglycemia, hyponatremia, and hyperkalemia. Death may occur within hours of surgery if a patient with Addison's disease is operated on without cognizance of adrenal insufficiency and pretreatment with exogenous steroids. Patients who have adrenal insufficiency as a result of interruption of chronically administered exogenous steroids may not develop the classic electrolyte abnormalities until the preterminal period. Adrenal insufficiency may also develop insidiously in the postoperative period, progressing over a course of several days. This insidious course is seen when adrenal injury occurs in the perioperative period, as would be the case with adrenal damage from hemorrhage into the gland in a patient receiving postoperative anticoagulant therapy. The adrenocorticotropic hormone (ACTH) stimulation test is the best test for establishing the diagnosis of adrenal insufficiency.

242. The answer is a. *(Brunicardi, pp 1405–1410.)* The thyroid scan shows a single focus of increased isotope uptake, often referred to as a hot nodule; the remainder of the thyroid gland has not taken up radioactive iodine.

Hyperfunctioning adenomas become independent of thyroid stimulating hormone (TSH) control and secrete thyroid hormone autonomously, which results in clinical hyperthyroidism. The elevated thyroid hormone levels ultimately diminish TSH levels severely and thus depress function of the remaining normal thyroid gland. An isolated focus of increased uptake on a thyroid scan is virtually diagnostic of a hyperfunctioning adenoma. Carcinomas usually display diminished uptake and are called cold nodules. Graves' disease would probably manifest as a diffusely hyperactive gland without nodularity. Multinodular goiter would display many nodules with varying activity.

243. The answer is d. (*Brunicardi, p 1429.*) The clinical presentation is consistent with a wound hematoma and necessitates exploration of the wound, drainage of the hematoma, and identification and control of any bleeding vessels. If airway control is unable to be obtained prior to the operating room, the wound should be opened at the bedside. Bilateral vocal cord dysfunction can be a cause of postoperative stridor and difficulty breathing, particularly after reoperative surgery; however, bilateral vocal cord dysfunction should manifest immediately after extubation. Hypocalcemia can occur postthyroidectomy due to ischemia or accidental removal of parathyroid tissue but is typically transient. Symptoms of hypocalcemia are usually neuromuscular and cardiac in nature.

244. The answer is b. (*Greenfield, pp 1358–1360.*) There is strong evidence from multiple randomized trials that there is no difference in survival in patients receiving modified radical mastectomy versus lumpectomy and axillary node dissection followed by radiation (breast conservation therapy) for Stages I and II breast cancer. Absolute contraindications to breast conservation therapy include diffuse microcalcifications suspicious for malignancy, persistently positive margins in the face of multiple reexcisions, pregnancy (except in the third trimester with radiation therapy deferred until after delivery), multiple tumors in separate quadrants, and a previous history of therapeutic radiation to the breast. Relative contraindications include multifocal disease within a single quadrant and expected poor cosmetic results (e.g., large tumor, small breast).

245. The answer is e. (*Townsend, p 912.*) Currently, treatment of inflammatory breast cancer consists of multimodality therapy with chemotherapy, surgery, and radiation, which results in a 50% five-year survival rate.

The clinical description of peau d'orange results from neoplastic invasion of dermal lymphatics with resultant edema of the breast; this clinical presentation and the skin biopsy findings are diagnostic for inflammatory breast cancer. Although the clinical picture may resemble that of a bacterial infection of the breast (mastitis), care must be taken to differentiate between the two pathologies.

246. The answer is b. (*Townsend, pp 1031–1032.*) Increased prolactin levels may be due to a variety of etiologies including but not limited to medications, pregnancy, cirrhosis, or tumors. Prolactin-secreting tumors in the pituitary gland may cause bitemporal hemianopsia due to compression of the optic chiasm. They are typically associated with amenorrhea and galactorrhea in women. In both sexes, lack of libido and impotence or infertility may be noted. Sexual vigor is usually restored after removal of the adenomas. Observation alone is recommended for asymptomatic patients. Symptomatic relief can be afforded by dopaminergic agonists (e.g., bromocriptine), which usually cause tumor shrinkage. Surgery is reserved for those individuals with persistent symptoms despite adequate therapy or who do not desire long-term medical therapy.

247. The answer is c. (*Greenfield, pp 1293–1298.*) Primary hyperparathyroidism is a common disease, with approximately 50,000 new cases diagnosed each year in the United States. Essential to the diagnosis of hyperparathyroidism is the finding of hypercalcemia. Though there are many causes of hypercalcemia, hyperparathyroidism is by far the most prevalent. The majority of patients with primary hyperparathyroidism have a single parathyroid adenoma, which can be localized in 75 to 80% of patients with sestamibi scanning. Elevated parathyroid hormone (PTH) levels in conjunction with elevated calcium levels is diagnostic for hyperparathyroidism. Patients with primary hyperparathyroidism have either normal or elevated urinary calcium. As the name suggests, patients with familial hypocalciuric hypercalcemia (FHH) have hypercalcemia. They also usually have elevated PTH, but urine calcium excretion is low (as opposed to normal to high as with a parathyroid adenoma). Surgery is not indicated in this relatively rare setting of hypercalcemia.

248. The answer is e. (*Greenfield, p 909.*) Glucagonomas are usually solitary and large, and as such are easily identifiable on CT scanning of the abdomen. Usually located in the body or tail of the pancreas, resection requires distal pancreatectomy. Metastases are common and should be resected whenever feasible. Octreotide may be useful in the treatment of hyperglycemia in patients with unresectable disease.

249. The answer is e. *(Greenfield, pp 1320–1321.)* After adrenalectomy for a functioning adenoma, steroid replacement therapy may be required for up to 6 to 12 months postoperatively, even with a normally functioning contralateral adrenal gland. Primary adrenal pathology causes 10 to 20% of all cases of Cushing's syndrome. In 10 to 15% of cases, adenomas are bilateral. All functioning adenomas should be resected, while nonfunctioning adenomas should be resected if the lesion is greater than 6 cm in size or carcinoma is suspected. A hyperfunctioning adrenal adenoma can usually be lateralized by preoperative radiologic studies, eliminating the need to explore both adrenal glands—CT scanning is a sensitive, but not specific, initial study. MRI or scintigraphic studies (using radiolabeled norcholesterol, NP-59) are more specific and can be utilized to aid in distinguishing adrenal adenomas from carcinomas. Surgical approaches include transabdominal laparoscopy or a posterior unilateral flank route. The anterior transperitoneal approach is usually reserved for complicated cases such as large or obviously malignant lesions.

250. The answer is c. *(Brunicardi, pp 465–466, 476.)* Most clinicians would recommend aspiration and cytologic examination of the cyst fluid in this situation. Cysts are common lesions in the breasts of women in their thirties and forties; malignancies are relatively rare. All such lesions justify attention, however, and physicians must not underestimate the fear associated with the discovery of a mass in the breast, even in low-risk situations. If the lesion does not completely disappear after aspiration, excision is advised. In young women, the breast parenchyma is dense, which limits the diagnostic value of mammography. The National Cancer Center Network recommends a breast exam every three years for women 20 years of age and older and a yearly mammogram and breast exam for women over the age of 40.

251. The answer is e. *(Brunicardi, pp 1413–1420.)* Treatment of radiation-induced thyroid cancer, which is usually of the papillary type, consists of a near-total (or total) thyroidectomy for multiple reasons: (1) a high incidence of bilaterality, (2) a greater incidence of complications if a second operation is necessary, (3) better detection of recurrent or persistent disease (using thyroglobulin levels), and (4) more effective use of radioactive iodine therapy postoperatively. The latent period for these tumors is 20 to 30 years or longer. Approximately 40% of patients with a history of radiation and a thyroid nodule are found to have thyroid cancer.

252. The answer is b. *(Brunicardi, pp 1417–1420.)* Papillary carcinoma of the thyroid frequently metastasizes to cervical lymph nodes, but distant metastasis is uncommon. Overall, survival at 10 years is greater than 95%. Several scoring systems for determining prognosis have been developed; one of the more common systems takes into account age, grade, extrathyroidal invasion and metastases, and size (AGES). Treatment of high-risk papillary carcinomas consists of near-total (or total) thyroidectomy. If patients have lymph node metastases in the lateral neck, concomitant modified radical neck dissection should be performed with total thyroidectomy. The surgical management of low-risk papillary thyroid cancers is controversial (lobectomy versus total thyroidectomy). Medullary, but not papillary, thyroid carcinoma is associated with multiple endocrine neoplasia syndrome.

253. The answer is c. *(Greenfield, pp 1352–1353.)* Lobular carcinoma in situ (LCIS) is considered to be a risk factor for invasive breast carcinoma, most commonly ductal carcinoma. The risk for breast cancer is equivalent in both breasts, lasts indefinitely, and is not correlated to the amount of LCIS in the biopsy specimen. The relative risk for invasive breast cancer is less than 2 for early menarche and late menopause, while the relative risk is greater than 5 for patients with a diagnosis of LCIS.

254. The answer is d. *(Brunicardi, p 466.)* Fibroadenomas occur infrequently before puberty but are the most common breast tumors between puberty and the early thirties. They usually are well demarcated and firm. Although most fibroadenomas are no larger than 3 cm in diameter, giant or juvenile fibroadenomas frequently are very large. The bigger fibroadenomas (greater than 5 cm) occur predominantly in adolescent black girls. The average age at onset of juvenile mammary hypertrophy is 16 years. This disorder involves a diffuse change in the entire breast and does not usually manifest clinically as a discrete mass; it may be unilateral or bilateral and can cause an enormous and incapacitating increase in breast size. Regression may be spontaneous and sometimes coincides with puberty or pregnancy. Cystosarcoma phyllodes may also cause a large lesion. Together with intraductal carcinoma, it characteristically occurs in older women. Lymphomas are less firm than fibroadenomas and do not have a whorl-like pattern. They display a characteristic fish flesh texture.

255. The answer is a. *(Brunicardi, pp 1462–1463.)* Adrenal "incidentalomas" are an uncommon finding on CT scans (<5%). Nonfunctional adrenal lesions greater than 6 cm in size, functional adrenal lesions, or lesions suspicious for malignancy should be excised. Appropriate workup may include a dexamethasone suppression test to rule out Cushing's syndrome, 24-h urine collection to rule out pheochromocytoma, and measurement of serum electrolytes and plasma rennin and aldosterone to rule out an aldosteronoma in hypertensive patients. MRI or scinitigraphic studies (norcholesterol—NP 59) may be useful in predicting malignancy.

256. The answer is a. *(Brunicardi, pp 1434–1440.)* Acute management of the hypercalcemic state includes vigorous hydration to restore intravascular volume, which is invariably diminished. This will establish renal perfusion and thus promote urinary calcium excretion. The patient described is exhibiting classic signs and symptoms of hyperparathyroidism. In addition, if a history is obtainable, frequently the patient will relate a history of renal calculi and bone pain—the syndrome characterized as "groans, stones, and bones." Thiazide diuretics are contraindicated because they frequently cause patients to become hypercalcemic. Instead, diuresis should be promoted with the use of loop diuretics such as furosemide (Lasix). The use of intravenous phosphorus infusion is no longer recommended because precipitation in the lungs, heart, or kidney can lead to serious morbidity. Mithramycin is an antineoplastic agent that in low doses inhibits bone resorption and thus diminishes serum calcium levels; it is used only when other maneuvers fail to decrease the calcium level. Calcitonin is useful at times. Bisphosphonates are used for lowering calcium levels in resistant cases, such as those associated with humoral malignancy. Emergency neck exploration is seldom warranted. In unprepared patients, the morbidity is unacceptably high.

257. The answer is c. *(Brunicardi, pp 1438–1439.)* Patients with symptomatic primary hyperparathyroidism as manifested by kidney stones, renal dysfunction, or osteoporosis should undergo parathyroidectomy. However, management of "asymptomatic" patients is controversial. Indications for surgical intervention for asymptomatic primary hyperparathyroidism include age less than 50 years, markedly elevated urine calcium excretion, kidney stones on radiography, decreased creatinine clearance, markedly elevated calcium or one episode of life-threatening hypercalcemia, and substantially decreased bone mass.

258. The answer is d. *(Townsend, p 889.)* Injury to breast tissue may cause necrosis of mammary adipose tissue and lead to the formation of a tender, localized, firm mass. A history of trauma is often elicited from affected patients, but less apparent factors, such as prolonged pressure, may also produce fat necrosis. Half the patients in whom the diagnosis is made do not recall a history of trauma. The pathophysiology of this lesion seems to involve early development of liquefaction of mammary fat with the formation of a cystic mass. Through a process of fibrosis, this lesion evolves into a firm, sometimes calcified lump that may be difficult to distinguish from carcinoma. There is, however, no relation between fat necrosis and the subsequent development of breast cancer. Excisional biopsy is usually required for definitive diagnosis; if the diagnosis of fat necrosis is confirmed, simple excision removes and terminates the process.

259. The answer is c. *(Brunicardi, pp 1458–1460.)* The constellation of symptoms in this patient is typical of a functional adrenocortical tumor (androgens). Approximately 50% of adrenocortical tumors are functional and can secrete cortisol, androgens, estrogens, aldosterone, or multiple hormones. The single most important determinant of malignancy is the size of the tumor. Treatment consists of en bloc resection of the tumor and involved adjacent organs, such as the kidney or the tail of the pancreas. Symptoms related to hormone production can be minimized by complete resection despite the inability to cure advanced disease. Mitotane has been utilized as adjuvant therapy for unresectable or metastatic disease, but has not been proven to decrease mortality. Cushing's disease refers to hypercortisolism due to a pituitary tumor and subsequent bilateral adrenal hyperplasia. Pheochromocytomas are characterized by hypertension and symptoms of excessive catecholamine production. Myelipomas are benign adrenal lesions.

260. The answer is c. *(Brunicardi, pp 1461–1462.)* Patients with pheochromocytomas should be treated preoperatively with alpha-blockade using phenoxybenzamine one to three weeks before surgery. Beta blockade may be necessary in addition to alpha blockade for optimal blood pressure control, but should not be started in the absence of alpha blockade because of the risk of cardiovascular collapse. With alpha blockade, patients also require volume expansion.

261. The answer is e. *(Greenfield, p 1365.)* Chemotherapy can be administered to a pregnant patient but should be delayed until after the first trimester due to the increased risk of fetal abnormalities. Elective termination of pregnancy has not been demonstrated to improve survival. Since radiation exposure endangers the fetus and there is no evidence that general anesthesia and nonabdominal surgery increase premature labor, modified radical mastectomy is recommended for stage I or II carcinoma (tumor less than 4 cm in diameter). Patients in later stages of pregnancy, however, can start radiation therapy shortly after delivery, and some may be candidates for breast-conserving surgery and adjuvant radiotherapy. Radiation therapy is contraindicated in all trimesters of pregnancy. Chemotherapy does not appear to increase the risk of congenital malformation when given in the second or third trimester of pregnancy. Patients who require adjuvant chemotherapy during the first trimester may opt for a therapeutic abortion, however, since there is a slightly increased risk of fetal malformation in that circumstance.

262. The answer is b. *(Townsend, p 912.)* Paget's disease of the breast is unrelated to Paget's disease of bone. It represents a small percentage (1 to 3%) of all breast cancers and is thought to originate in the retroareolar lactiferous ducts. It progresses toward the nipple-areola complex in most patients, where it causes the typical clinical finding of nipple eczema and erosion. Up to 20% of patients with Paget's disease have an associated breast mass, and these patients are more likely to have involvement of axillary nodes. Nipple-areolar disease alone usually represents in situ cancer; these patients have a 10-year survival rate of over 80%. In contrast, if Paget's disease presents with a mass, the mass is likely to be an infiltrating ductal carcinoma. The generally recommended surgical procedure for Paget's disease is currently a modified radical mastectomy. The validity of breast-saving surgery and adjuvant radiation therapy for patients without an associated mass is under investigation.

263. The answer is d. *(Brunicardi, pp 969–971.)* Zollinger-Ellison syndrome refers to hyergastrinemia resulting from an endocrine tumor of the pancreas. Over 50% of the tumors are malignant, and 40% have metastases at the time of surgery. Until recently, total gastrectomy was the primary operation for this tumor; however, it is now believed that operative exploration of the patient with resection of the tumor should be done if possible. H_2 receptor antagonists have also proved very promising in the management of these patients. Patients with Zollinger-Ellison tumors have very high basal levels of gastric acid (greater than 35 meq/h) and serum gastrin (usually greater than 200 pg/mL). A protein meal or histamine usually does not increase acid and gastrin levels as it would in conventional duodenal ulcer patients. A paradoxical rise in serum gastrin after intravenous secretin is diagnostic of Zollinger-Ellison syndrome.

264. The answer is a. *(Brunicardi, p 1410.)* Drops of Lugol's iodide solution daily beginning 10 days preoperatively should be prescribed to decrease the likelihood of postoperative thyroid storm, a manifestation of severe thyrotoxicosis. Propylthiouracil or methimazole can also be used preoperatively but are contraindicated in pregnant women. If thyroid storm occurs, treatment is beta blockade, for example, propranolol.

265. The answer is e. *(Brunicardi, pp 1436–1437.)* This patient's presentation and films are consistent with primary hyperparathyroidism. The elevated parathyroid hormone level (PTH) confirms the diagnosis. Her chest film demonstrates marked osteopenia, and the hand films are classic for this disease, with severe demineralization and periosteal bone resorption most prominent in the middle phalanges (osteitis fibrosa cystica). The films show no evidence of malignant lesions or mediastinal adenopathy consistent with sarcoidosis, and an elevated PTH level is not found in Paget's disease or vitamin D intoxication.

266. The answer is d. *(Brunicardi, pp 1440–1444.)* Treatment for primary hyperparathyroidism in this setting is resection of the diseased parathyroid glands after initial correction of the severe hypercalcemia. Neck exploration will yield a single parathyroid adenoma in about 85% of cases. Two adenomas are found less often (approximately 5% of cases) and hyperplasia of all four glands occurs in about 10 to 15% of patients. If hyperplasia is found, treatment includes resection of 3½ glands. The remnant of the fourth gland can be identified with a metal clip in case reexploration becomes necessary. Alternatively, all four glands can be removed with autotransplantation of a small piece of parathyroid tissue into the forearm or sternocleidomastoid muscle. Subsequent hyperfunction, should it develop, can then be treated by removal of this tissue. Patients often need calcium supplementation postoperatively. Vitamin D supplementation may also be necessary if hypocalcemia develops and persists despite treatment with oral calcium.

267. The answer is a. *(Brunicardi, pp 1405–1416.)* This patient's thyroid scan shows a discrete area of decreased radioactive iodine uptake with the remainder of the gland accepting iodine normally. This means the tissue that composes the nodule is not endocrinologically active for thyroid hormone. The two major mass lesions of the thyroid that can produce this pattern are a nonfunctioning follicular adenoma and a carcinoma. Carcinomas seldom produce thyroid hormone. Adenomas may be very active (toxic) and suppress the remaining gland. Most thyroid adenomas, however, are not hormone-producing and appear as cold nodules on thyroid scan. Graves' disease produces a diffusely hyperactive gland without nodularity. De Quervain's thyroiditis presents as a painful, swollen thyroid gland rather than as a discrete nodule. A large parathyroid adenoma could conceivably displace the thyroid gland and produce a pattern similar to the one shown, but it would be unusual. A localized infectious process also could produce such a pattern. The essential point is that a cold thyroid nodule may represent a carcinoma, and needle biopsy or surgical excision is indicated to rule out this possibility.

268. The answer is a. *(Greenfield, p 1368.)* Cystosarcoma phyllodes is a tumor most often seen in younger women. It can grow to enormous size and at times ulcerate through the skin. Still, it is a lesion with low propensity toward metastasis. Local recurrence is common, especially if the initial resection was inadequate. Simple reexcision with adequate margins is curative. Very large lesions may necessitate simple mastectomy to achieve clear margins. Axillary lymphadenectomy, however, is seldom indicated without biopsy-positive demonstration of tumor in the nodes. The low incidence of metastatic disease suggests that adjunctive therapy is indicated only for known metastatic disease, even when the tumors are quite large and ulcerated.

269. The answer is e. *(Brunicardi, pp 1417–1423.)* This patient has cytologic evidence of a papillary lesion, possibly papillary carcinoma. Papillary carcinoma is a relatively nonaggressive lesion with 10-year survival of 95%. The lesion is frequently multicentric, which argues for more complete resection. Metastases, when they occur, are usually responsive to surgical resection or radioablation therapy. Removal of the involved lobe, and possibly the entire thyroid gland, is appropriate. Central and lateral lymph node dissection is performed for clinically suspect lymph nodes. Papillary carcinoma is frequently multifocal. Bilateral disease mandates total thyroidectomy. However, radioactive ^{131}I is contraindicated in pregnancy and should be used with caution in women of childbearing age.

270. The answer is c. *(Brunicardi, p 1421.)* Hürthle cell cancer is a type of follicular cancer, but differs from follicular neoplasms in that it is more often multifocal and bilateral, is more likely to spread to local nodes and distant sites, and has a higher mortality rate. Lobectomy can be performed for unilateral adenomas, but carcinomas (as evidenced by extracapsular or vascular invasion) should be treated with total thyroidectomy and central lymph node dissection. Because invasion cannot be determined by fine-needle aspiration, Hürthle cell cancer cannot be diagnosed on FNA. Amyloid deposits in the stroma of a thyroid tumor are diagnostic of medullary carcinoma.

271. The answer is e. *(Brunicardi, pp 1420–1421.)* Thyroid nodules are somewhat less common in men and should always suggest malignancy. Follicular carcinomas cannot be diagnosed by FNA; capsular or vascular invasion on histology confirms a diagnosis of malignancy. For lesions less than 4 cm in size, thyroid lobectomy is adequate because at least 80% of follicular lesions are adenomas. For confirmed carcinomas or lesions greater than 4 cm in size, total thyroidectomy should be performed. There is no role for prophylactic neck dissection for follicular carcinomas. Age, tumor size, and tumor grade are all associated with increased mortality. Suppression with thyroid hormone (Synthroid) in the setting of abnormal cytology is not recommended.

272. The answer is a. *(Greenfield, pp 1343–1344.)* Nipple discharge from the breast may be classified as pathologic, physiologic, or galactorrhea. Galactorrhea may be due to hormonal imbalance (hyperprolactinemia, hypothyroidism), drugs (oral contraceptives, phenothiazines, antihypertensives, tranquilizers), or trauma to the chest. Physiologic nipple discharge is intermittent, nonlactational (usually serous), and due to stimulation of the nipple or to drugs (estrogens, tranquilizers). Both galactorrhea and physiologic discharge are frequently bilateral and arise from multiple ducts. Pathologic nipple discharge may be caused by benign lesions of the breast (duct ectasia, papilloma, fibrocystic disease) or by cancer. It may be bloody, serous, or gray-green. It is spontaneous and unilateral and can often be localized to a single nipple duct. When pathologic discharge is diagnosed, an effort should be made to identify the source. If an associated mass is present, it should be biopsied. If no mass is found, a terminal duct excision of the involved duct(s) should be performed.

273. The answer is c. *(Brunicardi, pp 1455–1456.)* Cushing's disease is caused by hypersecretion of ACTH by the pituitary gland. This hypersecretion, in turn, is caused by either a pituitary adenoma (90% of cases) or diffuse pituitary corticotrope hyperplasia (10% of cases) due to hypersecretion of CRH (corticotropin-releasing hormone) by the hypothalamus. A high cure rate is achieved with surgery, occasionally followed by adjuvant radiotherapy for large pituitary adenomas. Cushing's syndrome refers to the clinical manifestations of glucocorticoid excess due to any cause (Cushing's disease, administration of exogenous glucocorticoids, adrenocortical hyperplasia, adrenal adenoma, adrenal carcinoma, ectopic ACTH-secreting tumors) and includes truncal obesity, hypertension, hirsutism, moon facies, proximal muscle wasting, ecchymoses, skin striae, osteoporosis, diabetes mellitus, amenorrhea, growth retardation, and immunosuppression. The most common cause of Cushing's syndrome is iatrogenic, via administration of synthetic corticosteroids.

274. The answer is d. *(Greenfield, pp 903–905.)* Insulin-secreting endocrine tumors of the pancreas produce paroxysmal nervous system manifestations that may be a consequence of hypoglycemia, although the blood glucose level may bear little relation to the severity of the symptoms, even in the same patient from episode to episode. Most insulinomas are single discrete tumors (90%). They are evenly distributed between the head, body, and tail of the pancreas. Patients with insulinoma in the setting of the MEN 1 syndrome (synchronous islet cell tumors of the pancreas, pituitary hyperplasia or adenomas, and parathyroid chief cell hyperplasia) are more likely to have multiple tumors throughout the pancreas. If a careful examination of the pancreas reveals one or more specific adenomas, these can be enucleated. The finding of an elevated serum calcium level would raise the suspicion of MEN 1 and parathyroid hyperplasia. Insulinomas are not associated with MEN 2, which consists of coexistent medullary thyroid cancer, parathyroid hyperplasia, and pheochromocytoma. Approximately 10% of insulinomas are malignant. Streptozotocin, a potent antibiotic that selectively destroys islet cells, can be useful in controlling symptoms from unresectable malignant tumors of the islet cells but probably has little to offer in the definitive management of the typical benign islet cell insulinoma.

275. The answer is a. (*Greenfield, pp 1349–1353.*) Studies have failed to demonstrate a correlation between diet and breast cancer risk. Age is the most common risk factor. Another important risk factor is family history in a first-degree relative or presence of a genetic mutation such as *BRCA 1* or *2*, which can be inherited through either the maternal or the paternal side of the family. Other risk factors include excessive estrogen exposure, obesity, alcohol use, hormone replacement, ionizing radiation, and a history of a prior breast cancer or abnormal breast biopsy (LCIS or atypical hyperplasia).

276–280. The answers are 276-c, 277-b, 278-b, 279-e, 280-d. (*Greenfield, p 1358.*) The American Joint Committee on Cancer has defined a four-tiered staging system for breast cancer based on the clinical criteria of tumor size, involvement of lymph nodes, and metastatic disease. In one version of this system, a separate category is reserved for inflammatory breast cancer. While the grouping of breast cancers into stages provides a useful shorthand for expressing a patient's survival probability, it is noteworthy that considerable heterogeneity exists with respect to tumor size and nodal characteristics among tumors that are classified within a given stage. The TNM stage of breast cancer is assigned by measuring the greatest diameter of the tumor (T), assessing the axillary and clavicular lymph nodes for enlargement and fixation (N), and judging whether metastatic disease is present (M). In general, the worst of the three TNM parameters will determine the stage assignment. Tumors that are not palpable are classified as T_0; tumors 2 cm or less as T_1; tumors greater than 2 but not more than 5 cm as T_2; tumors greater than 5 cm as T_3; and tumors with extension into the chest wall or skin as T_4. Clinically negative lymph nodes are classified as N_0; positive, movable ipsilateral axillary nodes as N_1; fixed ipsilateral axillary nodes as N_2; and ipsilateral internal mammary nodes as N_3. Absence of evidence of metastatic disease is classified as M_0 and distant metastatic disease as M_1. The patient in question 276 has a $T_0N_2M_0$ lesion. This is stage III (fixed or matted nodes are a poor prognostic sign). The patient in question 277 has a $T_2N_1M_0$ lesion. This is stage II. The patient in question 278 has a $T_2N_0M_0$ lesion. Though smaller than the tumor in question 277 and without clinically involved nodes, this tumor is also stage II. The patient in question 279 has findings compatible with inflammatory breast cancer. A biopsy of the involved skin and a mammogram would confirm the diagnosis. The patient in question 280 has a $T_1N_0M_1$ lesion. This is stage IV (stage IV is any T, any N, M_1).

281–285. The answers are 281-d, 282-a, 283-b, 284-e, 285-c. (*Greenfield, pp 839–841.*) Carcinoid tumors are most commonly found in the appendix and small bowel, where they may be multiple. They have a tendency to metastasize, which varies with the size of the tumor. Tumors less than 1 cm uncommonly metastasize. Tumors greater than 2.0 cm are more often found to be metastatic. Metastasis to the liver and beyond may give rise to the carcinoid syndrome. The tumors cause an intense desmoplastic reaction. Spread into the serosal lymphatics does not imply metastatic disease; local resection is potentially curative. When metastatic lesions are found in the liver, they should be resected when technically feasible to limit the symptoms of the carcinoid syndrome. When extensive hepatic metastases are found, the disease is not curable. Resection of the appendix and cecum may be performed to prevent an early intestinal obstruction by locally encroaching tumor.

286–290. The answers are 286-b, 287-e, 288-a, 289-d, 290-g. (*Townsend, pp 896–924.*) Generally accepted treatment for stage I breast cancer in premenopausal women includes lumpectomy (wide excision, partial mastectomy, quadrantectomy), combined with axillary lymph node dissection (or sentinel lymph node biopsy) and adjuvant radiation therapy, or modified radical mastectomy. Both approaches offer equivalent chances of cure; there is a higher incidence of local recurrence with lumpectomy, axillary dissection, and radiation, but this observation has not been found to affect the overall cure rate in comparison with mastectomy. Patients with familial breast cancer (multiple first-degree relatives and penetrance of breast cancer through several familial generations) have extremely high risks of developing breast cancer in the course of their lifetimes. A subset of patients with familial breast cancer has been identified by a specific gene mutation (BRCA1); however, the genetic basis of most cases of familial breast cancer has yet to be elucidated. A patient with a history of familial breast cancer and multiple biopsies showing atypia may reasonably request bilateral prophylactic simple mastectomies. Alternatively, she may continue with routine surveillance. Lobular carcinoma in situ is a histologic marker that identifies patients at increased risk for the development of breast cancer. It is not a precancerous lesion in itself, and there is no benefit to widely excising it because the risk of subsequent cancer is equal for both breasts. As the risk for the future development of breast cancer is now estimated to be approximately 1% per year, prophylactic mastectomy is no longer recommended. Proper management consists of close surveillance for cancer by twice-yearly examinations and yearly mammography. Sclerosing adenosis is a benign lesion. Ductal carcinoma in situ is the precursor of invasive ductal carcinoma. It is described in four histologic variants (papillary, cribriform, solid, and comedo), of which the comedo subtype shows the greatest tendency to recur after wide excision alone. Ductal carcinoma in situ is treated with wide excision alone (for small noncomedo lesions) or wide excision plus radiation therapy. For multicentric DCIS, simple mastectomy is recommended. Cystosarcoma phyllodes is treated with wide local excision with at least 1-cm margins; axillary lymphadenectomy is not routinely recommended in the absence of clinically suspicious nodes. There are few indications for radical mastectomy, as it is both more traumatic and more disfiguring than any other method of local control of breast cancer and offers no greater survival benefit. However, one indication for radical mastectomy is locally advanced breast cancer with wide invasion of the pectoralis major in a patient who is physiologically able to tolerate general anesthesia.

Gastrointestinal Tract, Liver, and Pancreas

Questions

DIRECTIONS: Each item below contains a question followed by suggested responses. Select the **one best** response to each question.

291. A 74-year-old woman is admitted with upper GI bleeding. She is started on H$_2$ blockers, but experiences another bleeding episode. Endoscopy documents diffuse gastric ulcerations. Omeprazole is added to the H$_2$ antagonists as a therapeutic approach to the management of acute gastric and duodenal ulcers. Which of the following is the mechanism of action of omeprazole?

a. Blockage of the breakdown of mucosa-damaging metabolites of NSAIDs
b. Provision of a direct cytoprotective effect
c. Buffering of gastric acids
d. Inhibition of parietal cell hydrogen-potassium ATPase
e. Inhibition of gastrin release and parietal cell acid production

292. A 35-year-old woman presents with frequent and multiple areas of cutaneous ecchymosis. Workup demonstrates a platelet count of 15,000/µL, evaluation of the bone marrow reveals a normal number of megakaryocytes, and ultrasound examination demonstrates a normal-sized spleen. Based on the exclusion of other causes of thrombocytopenia, she is given a diagnosis of immune (idiopathic) thrombocytopenic purpura (ITP). Which of the following is the most appropriate treatment on diagnosis?

a. Expectant management with close follow-up of platelet counts
b. Immediate platelet transfusion to increase platelet counts to greater than 50,000/µL
c. Glucocorticoid therapy
d. Intravenous immunoglobulin therapy
e. Referral to surgery for laparoscopic splenectomy

293. A 59-year-old woman presents with right lower quadrant pain, nausea, and vomiting. She undergoes an uncomplicated laparoscopic appendectomy. Postoperatively, the pathology reveals a 2.5-cm mucinous adenocarcinoma with lymphatic invasion. Staging workup, including colonoscopy, chest x-ray, and CT scan of the abdomen and pelvis, is negative. Which of the following is the best next step in her management?

a. No further intervention at this time; follow-up every six months for two years.
b. Chemotherapy alone
c. Neoadjuvant chemotherapy followed by right hemicolectomy
d. Ileocecectomy
e. Right hemicolectomy

294. A 41-year-old man complains of regurgitation of saliva and of ingested but undigested food. An esophagram reveals a bird's-beak deformity. Which of the following statements is true about this condition?

a. Chest pain is common in the advanced stages of this disease
b. More patients are improved by forceful dilatation than by surgical intervention
c. Manometry can be expected to show high resting pressures of the lower esophageal sphincter
d. Surgical treatment consists primarily of resection of the distal esophagus with reanastomosis to the stomach above the diaphragm
e. Patients with this disease are at no increased risk for the development of carcinoma

295. A 32-year-old man with a three-year history of ulcerative colitis (UC) presents for discussion for surgical intervention. Which of the following is true regarding total proctocolectomy for ulcerative colitis?

a. Patients with UC should consider surgery after five years because the risk of carcinoma increases to greater than 50%
b. Symptoms relating to peripheral arthritis or ankylosing spondylitis will improve or resolve after proctocolectomy
c. Early proctocolectomy can prevent the development of primary sclerosing cholangitis in UC patients
d. Proctocolectomy is not advised in younger patients because of the need for a permanent ileostomy
e. Preservation of the rectum is a surgical option in the definitive management of UC

296. A 39-year-old previously healthy male is hospitalized for two weeks with epigastric pain radiating to his back, nausea, and vomiting. Initial laboratory values initially revealed an elevated amylase level consistent with acute pancreatitis. Five weeks following discharge, he complains of early satiety, epigastric pain, and fevers. On presentation, his temperature is 38.9°C (102°F) and his heart rate is 120 beats per minute; his white blood cell count is 24,000/mm³, and his amylase level is normal. He undergoes a CT scan demonstrating a 6-cm by 6-cm rim-enhancing fluid collection in the body of the pancreas. Which of the following would be the most definitive management of the fluid collection?

a. Antibiotic therapy alone
b. CT-guided aspiration with repeat imaging in two to three days
c. Antibiotics and CT-guided aspiration with repeat imaging in two to three days
d. Antibiotics and percutaneous catheter drainage
e. Surgical internal drainage of the fluid collection with a cyst-gastrostomy or Roux-en-Y cyst-jejunostomy

297. A previously healthy 79-year-old woman presents with early satiety and abdominal fullness. CT scan of the abdomen, pictured here, reveals a cystic lesion in the body and tail of the pancreas. CT-guided aspiration demonstrates an elevated carcinoembryonic antigen level. Which of the following is the best treatment option for this patient?

a. Distal pancreatectomy
b. Serial CT scans with resection if the lesion increases significantly in size
c. Internal drainage with Roux-en-Y cyst-jejunostomy
d. Percutaneous drainage of the fluid-filled lesion
e. Endoscopic retrograde pancreaticocholangiography (ERCP) with pancreatic stent placement

298. A 29-year-old male is diagnosed with familial adenomatous polyposis (FAP) and undergoes a total proctocolectomy with ileoanal j-pouch reconstruction. Regarding his future prognosis, which of the following is he least at risk for?

a. Cholangiocarcinomas
b. Gastric polyps
c. Periampullary malignancies
d. Abdominal desmoid tumors
e. Benign osteomas

299. A 56-year-old woman is referred to you about three months after a colostomy subsequent to a sigmoid resection for cancer. She complains that her stoma is not functioning properly. Which of the following is the most common serious complication of an end colostomy?

a. Bleeding
b. Skin breakdown
c. Parastomal hernia
d. Colonic perforation during irrigation
e. Stomal prolapse

300. A 56-year-old previously healthy physician notices that his eyes are yellow and he has pain in the right upper quadrant. Ultrasound and CT scan demonstrate a mass in the head of the pancreas. Endoscopic ultrasound suggests involvement of the superior mesenteric vein. Which of the following statements regarding his treatment and prognosis is true?

a. Total pancreatectomy is associated with improved survival
b. Involvement of the superior mesenteric vein is a contraindication to pancreaticoduodenectomy
c. Involvement of the superior mesenteric artery is a contraindication to pancreaticoduodenectomy
d. Pylorus preservation is never indicated at the time of pancreaticoduodenectomy
e. Preoperative biliary stenting is associated with improved survival after pancreaticoduodenectomy.

301. A 45-year-old woman is explored for a perforated duodenal ulcer 6 h after onset of symptoms. She has a history of chronic peptic ulcer disease treated medically with minimal symptoms. Which of the following is the procedure of choice to treat her perforation?

a. Simple closure with omental patch
b. Truncal vagotomy and pyloroplasty
c. Antrectomy and truncal vagotomy
d. Highly selective vagotomy
e. Hemigastrectomy

302. A 45-year-old man with a history of chronic peptic ulcer disease undergoes a truncal vagotomy and antrectomy with a Billroth II reconstruction for gastric outlet obstruction. Six weeks after surgery, he returns, complaining of postprandial weakness, sweating, lightheadedness, crampy abdominal pain, and diarrhea. Which of the following would be the best initial management strategy?

a. Treatment with a long-acting somatostatin analogue
b. Dietary advice and counseling that symptoms will probably abate within three months of surgery
c. Dietary advice and counseling that symptoms will probably not abate but are not dangerous
d. Workup for neuroendocrine tumor (e.g., carcinoid)
e. Preparation for revision to Roux-en-Y gastrojejunostomy

303. A 60-year-old male patient with hepatitis C with a previous history of variceal bleeding is admitted to the hospital with hematemesis. His blood pressure is 80/60 mmHg, physical examination reveals splenomegaly and ascites, and initial hematocrit is 25%. Prior to endoscopy, which of the following is the best initial management of the patient?

a. Administration of intravenous octreotide
b. Administration of a beta blocker (e.g., propranolol)
c. Measurement of prothrombin time and transfusion with cryoglobulin if elevated
d. Empiric transfusion of platelets given splenomegaly
e. Gastric and esophageal balloon tamponade (Sengstaken-Blakemore tube)

304. A 32-year-old alcoholic with end-stage liver disease has been admitted to the hospital three times for bleeding esophageal varices. He has undergone banding and sclerotherapy previously. He admits to currently drinking a six-pack of beer per day. On his abdominal examination, he has a fluid wave. Which of the following is the best option for long-term management of this patient's esophageal varices?

a. Orthotopic liver transplantation
b. Transection and reanastomosis of the distal esophagus
c. Distal splenorenal shunt
d. End-to-side portocaval shunt
e. Transjugular intrahepatic portosystemic shunt (TIPS)

305. A 55-year-old man complains of chronic intermittent epigastric pain, and gastroscopy demonstrates a 2-cm prepyloric ulcer. Endoscopic biopsy yields no malignant tissue. After a six-week trial of medical therapy, the ulcer is unchanged. Which of the following is the best next step in his management?

a. Repeat trial of medical therapy
b. Local excision of the ulcer
c. Highly selective vagotomy
d. Partial gastrectomy with vagotomy and Billroth I reconstruction
e. Vagotomy and pyloroplasty

306. During an operation for carcinoma of the hepatic flexure of the colon, an unexpected discontinuous 3-cm metastasis is discovered in the edge of the right lobe of the liver. Which of the following is the most appropriate next step for the surgeon?

a. Terminate the operation, screen the patient for evidence of other metastases, and plan further therapy after the reevaluation
b. Perform a right hemicolectomy and a right hepatic lobectomy
c. Perform a right hemicolectomy and a wedge resection of the metastasis
d. Perform a cecostomy and schedule reoperation after a course of systemic chemotherapy
e. Perform local resection of the primary colon cancer and plan radiation therapy for the lesion on the liver

307. A 42-year-old man with no history of use of nonsteroidal antiinflammatory drugs (NSAIDs) presents with recurrent gastritis. Infection with *Helicobacter pylori* is suspected. Which of the following statements is true?

a. Morphologically, the bacteria is a gram-positive, tennis-racket-shaped organism
b. Diagnosis can be made by serologic testing or urea breath tests
c. Diagnosis is most routinely achieved via culturing endoscopic scrapings
d. The most effective way to treat and prevent recurrence of this patient's gastritis is through the use of single-drug therapy aimed at eradicating *H. pylori*
e. The organism is easily eradicated

308. A 22-year-old college student notices a bulge in his right groin. It is accentuated with coughing, but is easily reducible. Which of the following hernias follows the path of the spermatic cord within the cremaster muscle?

a. Femoral
b. Direct inguinal
c. Indirect inguinal
d. Spigelian
e. Interparietal

309. A spry octogenarian who has never before been hospitalized is admitted with signs and symptoms typical of a small-bowel obstruction. Which of the following clinical findings would provide the most help in ascertaining the diagnosis?

a. Coffee-grounds aspirate from the stomach
b. Aerobilia
c. A leukocyte count of 40,000/μL
d. A pH of 7.5, P_{CO_2} of 50 kPa, and paradoxically acid urine
e. A palpable mass in the pelvis

310. A 42-year-old man has had bouts of intermittent crampy abdominal pain and diarrhea. Colonoscopy is performed. You must discuss the problem with the patient. Which of the following colonic pathologies is thought to have no malignant potential?

a. Ulcerative colitis
b. Villous adenomas
c. Familial polyposis
d. Peutz-Jeghers syndrome
e. Crohn's colitis

311. A 70-year-old woman has nausea, vomiting, abdominal distention, and episodic crampy midabdominal pain. She has no history of previous surgery but has a long history of cholelithiasis for which she has refused surgery. Her abdominal radiograph reveals a spherical density in the right lower quadrant. Which of the following is the definitive treatment for this patient's bowel obstruction?

a. Ileocolectomy
b. Cholecystectomy
c. Ileotomy and extraction
d. Nasogastric tube decompression
e. Intravenous antibiotics

312. A 53-year-old man presents to the emergency room with left lower quadrant pain, fever, and vomiting. CT scan of the abdomen and pelvis reveals a thickened sigmoid colon with inflamed diverticula and a 7-cm by 8-cm rim-enhancing fluid collection in the pelvis. After percutaneous drainage and treatment with antibiotics, the pain and fluid collection resolve. He returns as an outpatient to clinic one month later. He undergoes a colonoscopy, which demonstrates only diverticula in the sigmoid colon. Which of the following is the most appropriate next step in this patient's management?

a. Expectant management with sigmoid resection if symptoms recur
b. Cystoscopy to evaluate for a fistula
c. Sigmoid resection with end colostomy and rectal pouch (Hartmann's procedure)
d. Sigmoid resection with primary anastomosis
e. Long-term suppressive antibiotic therapy

313. A 29-year-old woman complains of postprandial right upper quadrant pain and fatty food intolerance. Ultrasound examination reveals no evidence of gallstones or sludge. Upper endoscopy is normal, and all of her liver function tests are within normal limits. She then undergoes a CCK-HIDA scan, which reveals that her gallbladder ejection fraction is 15% at 20 min. Which of the following is true regarding her treatment options?

a. Avoidance of fatty foods is the only therapeutic option
b. Ultrasound examination should be repeated immediately, since the false negative rate for ultrasound in detecting gallstones is 10 to 15%
c. Treatment with ursodeoxycholic acid results in improvement in symptoms in 35% of patients
d. Laparoscopic cholecystectomy results in improvement in symptoms in 85% of patients
e. Surgical intervention should be reserved for patients whose symptoms do not resolve with conservative treatment

314. A 47-year-old asymptomatic woman is incidentally found to have a 5-mm polyp and no stones in her gallbladder on ultrasound examination. Which of the following is the best management option?

a. Aspiration of the gallbladder with cytologic examination of the bile
b. Observation with repeat ultrasound examinations to evaluate for increase in polyp size
c. Laparoscopic cholecystectomy
d. Open cholecystectomy with frozen section
e. En bloc resection of the gallbladder, wedge resection of the liver, and portal lymphadenectomy

315. A 59-year-old man undergoes orthotopic heart transplantation for ischemic cardiomyopathy and has a prolonged postoperative course with multiple organ failure. Two weeks postoperatively, while still requiring inotropes and mechanical ventilation, he develops fevers and right upper quadrant pain. Ultrasound examination demonstrates a thickened gallbladder wall but no stones. A HIDA scan demonstrates nonfilling of the gallbladder. Which of the following is the best initial treatment?

a. Antibiotics alone
b. Emergent laparoscopic cholecystectomy
c. Antibiotics for 7 to 10 days followed by delayed laparoscopic cholecystectomy after the patient has recovered
d. Antibiotics and percutaneous cholecystostomy tube
e. CT-guided aspiration of the gallbladder

316. A 48-year-old woman develops pain in the right lower quadrant while playing tennis. The pain progresses and the patient presents to the emergency room later that day with a low-grade fever, a white blood count of 13,000, and complaints of anorexia and nausea as well as persistent, sharp pain of the right lower quadrant. On examination, she is tender in the right lower quadrant with muscular spasm, and there is a suggestion of a mass effect. An ultrasound is ordered and shows an apparent mass in the abdominal wall. Which of the following is the most likely diagnosis?

a. Acute appendicitis
b. Cecal carcinoma
c. Hematoma of the rectus sheath
d. Torsion of an ovarian cyst
e. Cholecystitis

317. A 32-year-old alcoholic man, recently immigrated from Mexico, presents with right upper quadrant pain and fevers for two weeks. CT scan of the abdomen demonstrates a non-rim-enhancing fluid collection in the periphery of the right lobe of the liver. The patient's serology is positive for antibodies to *Entamoeba histolytica*. Which of the following is the best initial management option for this patient?

a. Treatment with antiamebic drugs
b. Percutaneous drainage of the fluid collection
c. Marsupialization of the fluid collection
d. Surgical drainage of the fluid collection
e. Liver resection

318. A 45-year-old executive experiences increasingly painful retrosternal heartburn, especially at night. He has been chewing antacid tablets. An esophagogram shows a hiatal hernia. In determining the proper treatment for a sliding hiatal hernia, which of the following is the most useful modality?

a. Barium swallow with cinefluoroscopy during Valsalva maneuver
b. Flexible endoscopy
c. 24-h monitoring of esophageal pH
d. Measurement of the size of the hernia on upper GI
e. Assessment of the patient's smoking and drinking history

319. A 56-year-old man presents with acholic stools, dark urine, and scleral icterus. His laboratory values reveal an elevated conjugated bilirubin level. Which of the following statements regarding the etiology of obstructive jaundice is true?

a. A markedly elevated SGOT and SGPT are usually associated with obstructive jaundice
b. When extrahepatic biliary obstruction is suspected, the first test should be endoscopic ultrasonography (EUS)
c. A Klatskin tumor will result in extrahepatic ductal dilation only
d. A liver-spleen scan will add significantly to the diagnostic workup for obstructive jaundice
e. Carcinoma of the head of the pancreas can cause deep epigastric or back pain in as many as 80% of patients

320. A 22-year-old truck driver presents with a painful fluctuant mass between his gluteal folds, which has been present for two days. Which of the following is the most likely diagnosis?

a. Pilonidal cyst
b. Perianal hidradenitis suppurativa
c. Crohn's disease of the anus
d. Fistula in ano
e. Ischiorectal abscess

321. A 72-year-old man status post CABG five years ago presents with hematochezia, abdominal pain, and fevers. Colonoscopy reveals patches of dusky-appearing mucosa at the splenic flexure without active bleeding. Which of the following is the most appropriate management of this patient?

a. Angiography with administration of intraarterial papaverine
b. Emergent laparotomy with left hemicolectomy and transverse colostomy
c. Aortomesenteric bypass
d. Exploratory laparotomy with thrombectomy of the inferior mesenteric artery
e. Expectant management

322. A 62-year-old man has been diagnosed by endoscopic biopsy as having a sigmoid colon cancer. He is otherwise healthy and presents to your office for preoperative consultation. He asks a number of questions regarding removal of a portion of his colon. Which of the following statements is true regarding the effects of colon resection?

a. Net absorption of water by the rectum has been demonstrated in humans
b. Patients who undergo major colon resections suffer little change in their bowel habits following operation
c. The left colon is better adapted for water absorption than the right colon
d. The right colon is better adapted for electrolyte absorption than the left colon
e. The role of the ileocecal valve in normal fluid homeostasis is well established

323. A 64-year-old woman has been experiencing pain with each bowel movement and is found to have a large, fixed rectal mass. Biopsy confirms rectal adenocarcinoma. Chest x-ray is normal. Which of the following tests would be least helpful in the operative planning and preoperative counseling for this patient?

a. Rigid proctoscopy
b. Barium enema
c. MRI of the pelvis
d. CT scan of the chest
e. Rectal endosonography

324. A 45-year-old man is involved in a motor vehicle accident and requires laparotomy. At surgery, the mesentery is torn and the distal small bowel is devitalized. Extensive resection is performed. Postoperative nutritional status is an issue. Which of the following statements regarding absorption by the small intestine is true?

a. All but the fat in milk is digested and absorbed in humans by the end of the duodenum
b. Complete absorption of carbohydrates in a normal meal occurs in the ileum
c. In short gut syndrome, much of the dietary carbohydrate appears in the stool
d. Aldosterone markedly decreases sodium transport across the gut mucosa
e. Enzymes of the brush border of the small intestine can digest and absorb less than 5% of an average protein meal in the absence of the pancreas

325. A 39-year-old woman with no significant past medical history and whose only medication is oral contraceptive pills presents to the emergency room with right upper quadrant pain. CT scan demonstrates a 6-cm hepatic adenoma in the right lobe of the liver. Which of the following describes the definitive treatment of this lesion?

a. Cessation of oral contraceptives and serial CT scans
b. Intraarterial embolization of the hepatic adenoma
c. Embolization of the right portal vein
d. Resection of the hepatic adenoma
e. Systemic chemotherapy

326. A 43-year-old man without symptoms is incidentally noted on CT scan to have a 4-cm lesion in the periphery of the left lobe of the liver. The lesion enhances on the arterial phase of the CT scan and has a central scar suggestive of focal nodular hyperplasia (FNH). Which of the following is the recommended treatment of this lesion?

a. No further treatment is necessary
b. Wedge resection of the lesion
c. Formal left hepatectomy
d. Intraarterial embolization of the lesion
e. Radiofrequency ablation of the liver lesion

327. A 57-year-old previously alcoholic man with a history of chronic pancreatitis presents with hematemesis. Endoscopy reveals isolated gastric varices in the absence of esophageal varices. His liver function tests are normal and he has no stigmata of end-stage liver disease. Ultrasound examination demonstrates normal portal flow but a thrombosed splenic vein. He undergoes banding, which is initially successful, but he subsequently rebleeds during the same hospitalization. Attempts to control the bleeding endoscopically are unsuccessful. Which of the following is the most appropriate next step in management?

a. Transjugular intrahepatic portosystemic shunt (TIPS)
b. Surgical portocaval shunt
c. Surgical mesocaval shunt
d. Splenectomy
e. Placement of a Sengstaken-Blakemore tube

328. A previously healthy 15-year-old boy is brought to the emergency room with complaints of about 12 h of progressive anorexia, nausea, and pain of the right lower quadrant. On physical examination, he is found to have a rectal temperature of 38.18°C (100.58°F) and direct and rebound abdominal tenderness localizing to McBurney's point as well as involuntary guarding in the right lower quadrant. At operation through a McBurney-type incision, the appendix and cecum are found to be normal, but the surgeon is impressed by the marked edema of the terminal ileum, which also has an overlying fibrinopurulent exudate. Which of the following is the most appropriate next step?

a. Close the abdomen after culturing the exudate
b. Perform a standard appendectomy
c. Resect the involved terminal ileum
d. Perform an ileocolic resection
e. Perform an ileocolostomy to bypass the involved terminal ileum

329. A 32-year-old woman undergoes a cholecystectomy for acute chole-cystitis and is discharged home on the sixth postoperative day. She returns to the clinic eight months after the operation for a routine visit and is noted by the surgeon to be jaundiced. Laboratory values on readmission show total bilirubin 5.6 mg/dL, direct bilirubin 4.8 mg/dL, alkaline phos-phatase 250 IU (normal 21 to 91 IU), SGOT 52 kU (normal 10 to 40 kU), and SGPT 51 kU (normal 10 to 40 kU). An ultrasonogram shows dilated intrahepatic ducts. The patient undergoes the transhepatic cholangiogram seen here. Which of the following is the most appropriate next manage-ment step?

a. Choledochoplasty with insertion of a T tube
b. End-to-end choledochocholedochal anastomosis
c. Roux-en-Y hepaticojejunostomy
d. Percutaneous transhepatic dilatation
e. Choledochoduodenostomy

330. After complete removal of a sessile polyp of 2.0-cm by 1.5-cm found one fingerlength above the anal mucocutaneous margin, the pathologist reports it to have been a villous adenoma that contained carcinoma in situ. Which of the following is the most appropriate next step in management?

a. Reexcision of the biopsy site with wider margins
b. Abdominoperineal rectosigmoid resection
c. Anterior resection of the rectum
d. External radiation therapy to the rectum
e. No further therapy

331. A 55-year-old woman with cancer of the cervix undergoes hysterectomy and is found to have pelvic lymph nodes involved with cancer. She receives a course of external beam radiation (4500 rads). When the physician counsels her prior to her radiation treatment, she should be told of all the possible complications of radiation enteritis. Which of the following is generally not associated with radiation injury?

a. Malabsorption
b. Intussusception
c. Ulceration
d. Fistulization
e. Perforation

332. Prolonged ileus is noted in a postoperative patient subsequent to a small-bowel lysis of adhesions. Which of the following would be expected to stimulate intestinal motility?

a. Fear
b. Gastrin
c. Secretin
d. Acetylcholine
e. Cholecystokinin

333. A 62-year-old man has been noticing progressive difficulty swallowing first solid food and now liquids as well. A barium study shows a ragged narrowing just below the carinal level. Endoscopic biopsy confirms squamous cell carcinoma. Which of the following statements concerning carcinoma of the esophagus is true?

a. Alcohol has not been implicated as a precipitating factor
b. Squamous carcinoma is the most common type at the cardioesophageal junction
c. It has a higher incidence in males
d. It occurs more commonly in patients with corrosive esophagitis
e. Surgical excision is the only effective treatment

334. A 53-year-old woman with a history of a vagotomy and antrectomy with Billroth II reconstruction for peptic ulcer disease presents with recurrent pain. She undergoes an EGD, which demonstrates an ulcer. Serum gastrin levels are measured and found to be over 1000 pg/mL (normal is 40 to 150) on three separate determinations. Which of the following is the best test for confirming a diagnosis of gastrinoma?

a. An arteriogram
b. A secretin stimulation test
c. A total gastrectomy
d. A subtotal gastrectomy
e. A highly selective vagotomy

335. A 52-year-old man with a family history of MEN I has an elevated gastrin level and is suspected to have a gastrinoma. Which of the following is the most likely location for his tumor?

a. Fundus of the stomach
b. Antrum of the stomach
c. Within the triangle formed by the junction of the second and third portions of the duodenum, the junction of the neck and body of the pancreas, and the junction of the cystic and common bile duct
d. The tail of the pancreas
e. Within the triangle formed by the inferior edge of the liver, the cystic duct, and the common hepatic duct

336. A 73-year-old woman presents to the emergency room complaining of severe epigastric pain radiating to her back, nausea, and vomiting. CT scan of the abdomen demonstrates inflammation and edema of the pancreas. A right upper quadrant ultrasound demonstrates the presence of stones in the gallbladder and a dilated common bile duct; her liver function tests are elevated. Which of the following is true regarding her prognosis?

a. An amylase level greater than 1000 mg/dL correlates with an increased risk for complications
b. Her age is a negative prognostic factor
c. A total bilirubin greater than 3.0 mg/dL is the most important predictor of outcome
d. Use of the first 5 of Ranson's criteria only is as good a predictor of outcome as all 11
e. A base deficit of more than 5meq/L at admission is a negative prognostic factor

337. A 55-year-old man who is extremely obese reports weakness, sweating, tachycardia, confusion, and headache whenever he fasts for more than a few hours. He has prompt relief of symptoms when he eats. These symptoms are most suggestive of which of the following disorders?

a. Diabetes mellitus
b. Insulinoma
c. Zollinger-Ellison syndrome
d. Carcinoid syndrome
e. Multiple endocrine neoplasia, type II

338. A 57-year-old woman sees blood on the toilet paper. Her doctor notes the presence of an excoriated bleeding 2.8-cm mass at the anus. Biopsy confirms the clinical suspicion of anal cancer. In planning the management of a 2.8-cm epidermoid carcinoma of the anus, which of the following is the best initial management strategy?

a. Abdominoperineal resection
b. Wide local resection with bilateral inguinal node dissection
c. Local radiation therapy
d. Systemic chemotherapy
e. Combined radiation therapy and chemotherapy

339. An 80-year-old man is admitted to the hospital complaining of nausea, abdominal pain, distention, and diarrhea. A cautiously performed transanal contrast study reveals an apple core configuration in the rectosigmoid area. Which of the following is the most appropriate next step in his management?

a. Colonoscopic decompression and rectal tube placement
b. Saline enemas and digital disimpaction of fecal matter from the rectum
c. Colon resection and proximal colostomy
d. Oral administration of metronidazole and checking a *Clostridium difficile* titer
e. Evaluation of an electrocardiogram and obtaining an angiogram to evaluate for colonic mesenteric ischemia

340. Patients with Crohn's disease are frequently seen in your office. A 46-year-old woman asks about the need for surgery, since she was recently diagnosed with the disease. Indications for operation in Crohn's disease include all but which of the following?

a. Intestinal obstruction
b. Enterovesical fistula
c. Ileum–ascending colon fistula
d. Enterovaginal fistula
e. Free perforation

341. A 50-year-old man presents to the emergency room with a 6-h history of excruciating abdominal pain and distention. The abdominal film shown here is obtained. Which of the following is the most appropriate next diagnostic maneuver?

a. Emergency celiotomy
b. Upper gastrointestinal series with small-bowel follow-through
c. CT scan of the abdomen
d. Barium enema
e. Sigmoidoscopy

342. A 37-year-old stockbroker consults you because of increasing epigastric pain. You perform upper endoscopy and confirm a duodenal ulcer as the cause of his symptoms. Biopsy is performed and is benign. In addition to antisecretory therapy, antibiotics should be started. Which of the following organisms is most closely associated with gastric and duodenal ulcer disease?

a. *Campylobacter*
b. Cytomegalovirus
c. *Helicobacter*
d. *Mycobacterium avium-intracellulare*
e. *Yersinia enterocolitica*

343. On Monday morning, a septuagenarian man has a moderate-sized abdominal aneurysm resected. On Friday, he is noted to be markedly distended, with an abdominal radiograph demonstrating an air-filled, kidney-bean-shaped structure in the left upper quadrant. Which of the following is the most appropriate management at this time?

a. Decompression of the large bowel via colonoscopy
b. Replacement of the nasogastric tube and administration of low-dose cholinergic drugs
c. Continued nothing-by-mouth orders, administration of a gentle saline enema, and encouragement of ambulation
d. Immediate return to the operating room for operative decompression by transverse colostomy
e. Right hemicolectomy

344. A visitor from abroad presents with abdominal pain and fever. CT scan shows a large, calcified cystic mass in the right lobe of the liver. Echinococcus is suggested by the CT findings. Which of the following is the most appropriate management of echinococcal liver cysts?

a. A large cyst should be treated by percutaneous aspiration of its contents
b. Medical treatment with albendazole usually preempts the need for surgical drainage
c. Negative serologic tests suggest that the cyst is chronic and inactive and that no treatment is indicated
d. Leakage of cyst fluid puts the patient at risk for anaphylactic reaction
e. Coexistent extrahepatic cysts are uncommon

345. A 28-year-old woman who is 15 weeks pregnant has new onset of nausea, vomiting, and right-sided abdominal pain. She has been free of nausea since early in her first trimester. The pain has become worse over the past 6 h. Which of the following statements regarding appendicitis during pregnancy is correct?

a. Appendicitis is the most prevalent extrauterine indication for celiotomy during pregnancy
b. Appendicitis occurs more commonly in pregnant women than in nonpregnant women of comparable age
c. Suspected appendicitis in a pregnant woman should be managed with a period of observation due to the risks of laparotomy to the fetus
d. Noncomplicated appendicitis results in a 20% fetal mortality and premature labor rate
e. The severity of appendicitis correlates with increased gestational age of the fetus

346. A 56-year-old woman has nonspecific complaints that include an abnormal sensation when swallowing. An esophagram is obtained. Which of the following is most likely to require surgical correction?

a. Large sliding esophageal hiatal hernia
b. Paraesophageal hiatal hernia
c. Traction diverticulum of esophagus
d. Schatzki's ring of distal esophagus
e. Esophageal web

347. A 65-year-old man who is hospitalized with pancreatic carcinoma develops abdominal distention and obstipation. The following abdominal radiograph is obtained. Which of the following is the most appropriate management of this patient?

a. Urgent colostomy or cecostomy
b. Discontinuation of anticholinergic medications and narcotics and correction of metabolic disorders
c. Digital disimpaction of fecal mass in the rectum
d. Diagnostic and therapeutic colonoscopy
e. Detorsion of volvulus and colopexy or resection

348. An elderly nursing home patient complains of swallowing difficulty and choking on food. The physician on call orders a barium swallow, and an outpouching in the right neck is observed. Which of the following is true regarding this abnormality?

a. Aspiration pneumonitis is unlikely
b. It is a congenital abnormality
c. The most common symptom is a sensation of high obstruction on swallowing
d. It is a traction-type diverticulum
e. Treatment is restriction of certain foods

349. A 48-year-old man presents with jaundice and right upper quadrant pain. Endoscopy shows blood coming from the ampulla of Vater. True statements regarding hemobilia include which of the following?

a. The classic presentation includes biliary colic, jaundice, and gastrointestinal bleeding
b. Spontaneous bleeding secondary to hematologic disorders is the major cause of this disorder
c. Percutaneous transhepatic catheter placement of an absorbable gelatin sponge (Gelfoam) is the preferred treatment in cases of significant intrahepatic bleeding
d. Angiography and endoscopy have no role in the treatment of intrahepatic bleeding
e. Arterial embolization is advocated for hemobilia from the extrahepatic bile ducts

350. A 30-year-old female patient who presents with bleeding per rectum is found at colonoscopy to have colitis confined to the transverse and descending colon. A biopsy is performed. Which of the following statements is true about this patient?

a. The inflammatory process is likely to be confined to the mucosa and submucosa
b. The inflammatory reaction is likely to be continuous
c. Superficial as opposed to linear ulcerations can be expected
d. Noncaseating granulomas can be expected in up to 50% of patients with similar disease
e. Microabcesses within crypts are common

351. A 24-year-old man presents to the emergency room with abdominal pain and fevers. CT scan of the abdomen reveals inflammation of the terminal ileum. He is referred to a gastroenterologist, where he is given the new diagnosis of Crohn's disease. Regarding the risk of complications from this disease, which of the following statements is true?

a. The occurrence of toxic megacolon is common
b. Perforation occurs in about 25% of patients with similar disease
c. Fistulas between the colon and segments of intestine, bladder, vagina, urethra, and skin may develop
d. Extraintestinal manifestations including uveitis and erythema nodosum would be exceedingly rare in this patient
e. This patient would be at no increased risk for the development of cancer of the colon as compared with an age-matched population

352. An upper GI series is performed on a 71-year-old woman who presented with several months of chest pain that occurs when she is eating. The film shown here is obtained. Investigation reveals a microcytic anemia and erosive gastritis on upper endoscopy. Which of the following statements about the patient's condition is true?

a. It is congenital
b. The gastroesophageal junction is above the diaphragm
c. Ulceration, gastritis, and anemia are common
d. It usually is controlled by medical therapy
e. Surgical treatment, if indicated, should be delayed up to three months to allow inflammation around the gastroesophageal junction to subside

353. A 54-year-old man complains that his eyes are yellow. His bilirubin is elevated. His physical exam is unremarkable. A CT of the abdomen shows a mass in the head of the pancreas. Cytology from the ERCP is positive for cancer. Which of the following statements regarding adenocarcinoma of the pancreas is true?

a. It occurs most frequently in the body of the gland
b. It carries a 1 to 2% five-year survival rate
c. It is nonresectable if it presents as painless jaundice
d. It can usually be resected if it presents in the body or tail of the pancreas and does not involve the common bile duct
e. It is associated with diabetes insipidus

354. A 28-year-old woman presents with hematochezia. She is admitted to the hospital and undergoes upper endoscopy that is negative for any lesions. Colonoscopy is performed and no bleeding sources are identified, although the gastroenterologist notes blood in the right colon and old blood coming from above the ileocecal valve. Which of the following is the test of choice in this patient?

a. Angiography
b. Small-bowel enteroclysis
c. CT scan of the abdomen
d. ^{99m}Tc pertechnate scan
e. Small-bowel endoscopy

355. A 32-year-old woman presents to the hospital with a 24-h history of abdominal pain of the right lower quadrant. She undergoes an uncomplicated appendectomy for acute appendicitis and is discharged home on the fourth postoperative day. The pathologist notes the presence of a carcinoid tumor (1.2 cm) in the tip of the appendix. Which of the following statements is true?

a. The patient should be advised to undergo ileocolectomy
b. The most common location of carcinoids is in the appendix
c. The carcinoid syndrome occurs in more than half of patients with carcinoid tumors
d. The tumor is an apudoma
e. Carcinoid syndrome is seen only when the tumor is drained by the portal venous system

356. A 58-year-old man notices a bulge in his groin, associated with mild discomfort. It is easily reducible when he is examined in your office. It does not descend into the scrotum. Which of the following statements regarding direct inguinal hernias is true?

a. They are the most common inguinal hernias in women
b. They protrude medially to the inferior epigastric vessels
c. They should be opened and ligated at the internal ring
d. They commonly protrude into the scrotal sac in men
e. They incarcerate more commonly than indirect hernias

357. A 35-year-old woman presents with pancreatitis. Subsequent endoscopic retrograde cholangiopancreatography (ERCP) reveals the congenital cystic anomaly of her biliary system illustrated in the film shown here. Which of the following statements regarding this problem is true?

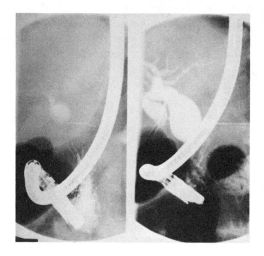

a. Treatment consists of internal drainage via choledochoduodenostomy
b. Malignant changes may occur within this structure
c. Most patients present with the classic triad of epigastric pain, an abdominal mass, and jaundice
d. Cystic dilation of the intrahepatic biliary tree may coexist and is managed in a similar fashion
e. Surgery should be reserved for symptomatic patients

358. A 36-year-old man is in your intensive care unit following thoracotomy for a 24-hour-old esophageal perforation. His WBC is markedly elevated, and he is febrile and hypotensive. His NG tube fills with blood and continues to bleed. Emergency upper endoscopy documents diffuse gastric erosions. Which of the following statements regarding stress ulceration is true?

a. It is true ulceration, extending into and through the muscularis mucosa
b. It classically involves the antrum
c. Increased secretion of gastric acid has been shown to play a causative role
d. It frequently involves multiple sites
e. It is seen following shock or sepsis, but for some unknown reason does not occur following major surgery, trauma, or burns

359. A patient with known gallstones presents with right upper quadrant pain, fever, jaundice, and shaking chills. He is febrile. Cholangitis is suspected. Which of the following statements concerning cholangitis is correct?

a. The most common infecting organism is *Staphylococcus aureus*
b. The diagnosis is suggested by the Charcot triad
c. The disease occurs primarily in young, immunocompromised patients
d. Cholecystostomy is the procedure of choice in affected patients
e. Surgery is indicated once the diagnosis of cholangitis is made

360. An 88-year-old man with a history of end-stage renal failure, severe coronary artery disease, and brain metastases from lung cancer presents with acute cholecystitis. His family wants "everything done." Which of the following is the best management option in this patient?

a. Tube cholecystostomy
b. Open cholecystectomy
c. Laparoscopic cholecystectomy
d. Intravenous antibiotics followed by elective cholecystectomy
e. Lithotripsy followed by long-term bile acid therapy

361. After a weekend drinking binge, a 45-year-old alcoholic man presents to the hospital with abdominal pain, nausea, and vomiting. On physical examination, the patient is afebrile and is noted to have a palpable tender mass in the epigastrium. Laboratory tests reveal an amylase of 250 U/dL (normal < 180). A CT scan done on the second hospital day is pictured here. Which of the following statements concerning this patient's condition is true?

a. The mass may cause gastric outlet or extrahepatic biliary obstruction
b. Spontaneous resolution almost never occurs
c. The mass is seen only with acute pancreatitis
d. The mass has an epithelial lining
e. Malignant degeneration occurs in about 25% of cases if left untreated

362. Upper endoscopy is performed on a patient with recurrent small upper GI bleeding episodes. A lesion is seen in the proximal stomach that is characterized as a bleeding vessel. Dieulafoy's lesion of the stomach is suspected. Which of the following best characterizes this lesion?

a. A large mucosal defect with underlying friable vascular plexus
b. Frequent rebleeding after endoscopic treatment
c. Massive bleeding that requires subtotal gastrectomy
d. Location in the proximal stomach
e. Acid-peptic changes of the gastric mucosa

363. During an appendectomy for acute appendicitis, a 4-cm mass is found in the midportion of the appendix. Frozen section reveals this lesion to be a carcinoid tumor. Which of the following statements is true?

a. No further surgery is indicated
b. A right hemicolectomy should be performed
c. There is about a 50% chance that this patient will develop the carcinoid syndrome
d. Carcinoid tumors arise from islet cells
e. Carcinoid syndrome can occur only in the presence of liver metastases

364. A 45-year-old man is examined for a yearly executive physical. A small mass is palpated in the rectum, and sigmoidoscopy demonstrates it to be a 2-cm mass covered by normal rectal mucosa. Biopsy suggests carcinoid. Which of the following is true regarding rectal carcinoid tumors?

a. Endoscopic resection is sufficient for tumors smaller than 2 cm
b. Patients frequently present with the carcinoid syndrome
c. They are rapidly growing tumors
d. Local recurrence is rare with complete resection of the primary lesion
e. Patients can develop the carcinoid syndrome even in the absence of liver metastases

365. An ultrasound is performed on a patient with right upper quadrant pain. It demonstrates a large gallstone in the cystic duct but also a polypoid mass in the fundus. Which of the following is an indication for cholecystectomy for a polypoid gallbladder lesion?

a. Size greater than 0.5 cm
b. Presence of clinical symptoms
c. Patient age of over 25 years
d. Presence of multiple small lesions
e. Absence of shadowing on ultrasound

366. An alcoholic man has been suffering excruciating pain recalcitrant to analgesics and splanchnic block. A surgeon recommends total pancreatectomy. A patient who has a total pancreatectomy might be expected to develop which of the following complications?

a. Diabetes mellitus
b. Hypercalcemia
c. Hyperphosphatemia
d. Constipation
e. Weight gain

367. A 28-year-old previously healthy woman arrives in the emergency room complaining of 24 h of anorexia, nausea, and lower abdominal pain that is more intense in the right lower quadrant than elsewhere. On examination, she has peritoneal signs of the right lower quadrant and a rectal temperature of 38.8°C (101.8°F). At exploration through incision of the right lower quadrant, she is found to have a small, contained perforation of a cecal diverticulum. Which of the following statements regarding this situation is true?

a. Cecal diverticula are acquired disorders
b. Cecal diverticula are usually multiple
c. Cecal diverticula are mucosal herniations through the muscularis propria
d. Diverticulectomy, closure of the cecal defect, and appendectomy may be indicated
e. An ileocolectomy is indicated even with well-localized inflammation

368. Incidental finding of a liver mass that enhances with intravenous contrast prompts a surgical consultation. MRI is suggestive of a hemangioma. The patient's platelet count is 75,000. Which of the following is true regarding cavernous hemangiomas of the liver in adults?

a. The majority become symptomatic
b. They may undergo malignant transformation
c. They enlarge under hormonal stimulation
d. They should be resected to avoid spontaneous rupture and life-threatening hemorrhage
e. A liver-spleen radionucleotide scan is the most sensitive and specific way to make the diagnosis

369. A right hemicolectomy is performed on a 57-year-old woman with adenocarcinoma who had a preoperative elevation of carcinoembryonic antigen (CEA) to 123. After falling to normal levels postoperatively, her most recent (24-month) follow-up level was 85. Correct statements regarding CEA and colorectal tumors include which of the following?

a. Elevated CEA is indicative of a tumor of gastrointestinal origin
b. A low CEA level after resection of a colon tumor is a poor marker of disease control
c. Ninety percent of colorectal tumors produce CEA
d. There is a high likelihood of liver involvement if the CEA level is high (greater than 100 ng/mL)
e. CEA levels are unusually low in cigarette smokers

370. A 61-year-old woman with a history of unstable angina complains of hematemesis after retching and vomiting following a night of binge drinking. Endoscopy reveals a longitudinal mucosal tear at the gastroesophageal junction, which is not actively bleeding. Which of the following is the next recommended step in the management of this patient?

a. Angiography with embolization
b. Balloon tamponade
c. Exploratory laparotomy, gastrotomy, and oversewing of the tear
d. Systemic vasopressin infusion
e. Expectant management

DIRECTIONS: Each group of questions below consists of lettered options followed by a set of numbered items. For each numbered item, select the **one** lettered option with which it is **most** closely associated. Each lettered option may be used once, more than once, or not at all.

Questions 371–374

Select the appropriate surgical procedure for each patient.

a. Vagotomy and antrectomy
b. Antrectomy alone
c. Vagotomy and pyloroplasty
d. Vagotomy and gastrojejunostomy
e. Proximal gastric vagotomy

371. A 72-year-old patient with an intractable type I ulcer along the incisura with a significant amount of scarring along the entire length of the lesser curvature

372. A 46-year-old patient with gastric outlet obstruction secondary to ulcer disease and severe inflammation around the pylorus and first and second portions of the duodenum

373. A 90-year-old patient with a bleeding duodenal ulcer

374. A 36-year-old patient with a type III (pyloric) ulcer that is refractory to medical treatment

Questions 375–378

Select the appropriate surgical procedure for each patient.

a. Low anterior resection
b. Abdominoperineal resection
c. Subtotal colectomy with end ileostomy
d. Total proctocolectomy with ileoanal j-pouch
e. Sigmoid resection with end colostomy (Hartmann's procedure)
f. Transanal excision
g. Diverting colostomy

375. A 37-year-old man with a 10-year history of ulcerative colitis who has a sessile polyp 10 cm from the anal verge with high-grade dysplasia

376. A 60-year-old woman with recurrent squamous cell carcinoma of the anus after chemoradiation

377. A 68-year-old woman with fecal incontinence who presents with a large fixed adenocarcinoma 3 cm from the anal verge

378. A 33-year-old man with a history of Crohn's disease presents with severe abdominal pain and fever. On examination, his heart rate is 130 beats per minute, blood pressure 105/62, and temperature 38.9°C (102°F). Workup reveals a leukocytosis of 32,000/mm³. Plain films reveal a markedly dilated large colon.

Questions 379–380

For each patient, select the likely diagnosis.

a. Spontaneous bacterial peritonitis
b. Perforated hollow viscus
c. Ruptured spleen
d. Ruptured echinococcal liver cyst
e. Gallstone ileus
f. Emphysematous cholecystitis
g. Sigmoid volvulus
h. Cecal volvulus

379. A 65-year-old previously healthy man presents with severe abdominal pain that came on suddenly. He has abdominal tenderness and guarding in all four quadrants on physical examination. A radiograph is obtained and demonstrates a radiolucency under the right hemidiaphragm.

380. An 82-year-old nursing home patient presents to the emergency room with vomiting, abdominal pain, and distention. A radiograph is obtained and demonstrates a grossly dilated loop of intestine overlying the sacrum in the shape of an upside-down U.

Gastrointestinal Tract, Liver, and Pancreas

Answers

291. The answer is d. (*McQuaid, pp 285–316.*) Omeprazole (Prilosec) irreversibly inhibits the hydrogen-potassium-ATPase (proton pump) in the secretory canaliculus of the gastric parietal cell. This blocks the last step in the acid-secretory process. Omeprazole's duration of action exceeds 24 h, and doses of 20 to 30 mg/d inhibit more than 90% of 24-h acid secretion. Omeprazole provides excellent suppression of meal-stimulated and nocturnal acid secretion and seems very safe for short-term therapy. Prolonged administration in laboratory animals has been associated with significant hypergastrinemia, hyperplasia of enterochromaffin-like cells, and carcinoid tumors.

292. The answer is c. (*Townsend, pp 1682–1685.*) Patients with ITP who are asymptomatic and have a platelet count greater than 30,000/μL can be treated expectantly with follow-up. Of these patients, those with a platelet count between 30,000 and 50,000/μL have an increased risk for more severe thrombocytopenia. Patients with a platelet count lower than 30,000/μL or less than 50,000/μL with significant bleeding or risk factors for bleeding should be treated. Initial medical treatment is with prednisone (1 mg/kg), and intravenous immunoglobulin (IVIG) is used in patients with severe bleeding or preoperatively prior to splenectomy. Platelet transfusions are reserved for patients with acute bleeding. Splenectomy is indicated in patients who have severe symptomatic thrombocytopenia, patients in whom remission is achieved only with toxic doses of steroids, patients with a relapse after initial steroid therapy, patients with persistent thrombocytopenia for more than three months and a platelet count less than 30,000/μL, and possibly in patients with a persistent platelet count of less than 10,000/μL after six weeks of therapy. The platelet count can be expected to rise shortly after splenectomy, and prolonged remissions are expected in approximately two-thirds of cases.

293. The answer is e. (*Townsend, pp 1395–1396; Brunicardi, p 1134.*) Patients with appendiceal adenocarcinoma, a rare neoplasm accounting for less than 0.5% of gastrointestinal tumors, should undergo formal right hemicolectomy. Often affecting older patients, they may present with symptoms mimicking those of acute appendicitis. A thorough initial workup and follow-up are necessary because of the high rate of synchronous and metachronous tumors. Five-year survival is 55% but depends on the tumor stage.

294. The answer is c. *(Townsend, pp 1099–1102.)* Patients with achalasia, which is a functional disorder caused by failure of relaxation of the lower esophageal sphincter (LES), typically present with dysphagia, chest pain, and regurgitation of saliva and undigested food. The characteristic appearance of the esophagram is the tapered bird's-beak deformity at the level of the esophagogastric junction; the esophagus is often dilated and may contain an air-fluid level. Manometry yields high resting pressures of the LES, which fails to relax or only partially relaxes. The absence of peristaltic deglutitory contractions in the body of the esophagus is also noted during manometry. Initial management of achalasia includes medications (calcium channel blockers or long-acting nitrates), and other management options include endoscopic dilation or injection of botulinum toxin (Botox) into the LES. Surgery results in improvement in over 90% of patients, compared with only 70% of patients treated by forceful dilatation. Surgical treatment is an esophagomyotomy. Patients with achalasia have seven times the risk of developing squamous cell carcinoma as the general population. This dreaded complication can occur even after successful treatment for the disease.

295. The answer is b. *(Townsend, pp 1425–1435.)* Although total proctocolectomy may relieve or resolve extraintestinal manifestations of UC such as peripheral arthritis or ankylosing spondylitis, surgery is not preventative or curative for primary sclerosing cholangitis (PSC). The risk of colon cancer in pancolitis is 0 to 3% at 5 and 10 years and increases to 50% after 30 years with the disease. In patients with both PSC and UC, the risk of cancer is increased fivefold from that for patients with UC alone. Indications for operative intervention in UC include acute management of toxic megacolon or fulminant colitis and definitive management for intractable disease or presence of high-grade dysplasia or carcinoma. Definitive surgical management options for UC include total proctocolectomy with end ileostomy (typically reserved for older or incontinent patients) and total proctocolectomy with ileoanal pouch anastomosis. In patients undergoing emergent colectomy for toxic megacolon, total abdominal colectomy without resection of the rectum can be performed initially. However, given that UC always involves the rectum, definitive management of UC requires resection of most of the rectal mucosa, although controversy exists regarding retention of the very distal rectal mucosa such as with a stapled ileoanal anastomosis.

296. The answer is d. (*Townsend, pp 1658–1660.*) The patient most likely has an infected pancreatic pseudocyst. Pseudocysts are nonepithelialized fluid collections that can present at earliest four to six weeks after an episode of acute pancreatitis. The treatment for infected pancreatic pseudocysts is similar to that for pancreatic abscesses—percutaneous catheter drainage with antibiotics. Aspiration of the fluid can be diagnostic but is not a definitive treatment, even with the addition of antibiotics. Internal drainage of pancreatic pseudocysts is contraindicated in the presence of infection.

297. The answer is a. (*Brunicardi, pp 1289–1290.*) This woman has a cystadenocarcinoma arising from the pancreatic body and tail; the treatment is surgical resection. About 90% of primary malignant neoplasms of the exocrine pancreas are adenocarcinomas of duct cell origin. The remaining neoplasms include serous and mucinous cystadenomas/cystadenocarcinomas, solid pseudopapillary tumors, and intraductal mucinous papillary adenomas/tumors. Cystadenocarcinomas may be several times the size of typical ductal cancers and often arise in the body or tail of the pancreas. They may become very large without invading adjacent viscera and do not generally cause significant pain or weight loss. The clinical presentation is usually quite subtle, with symptoms related primarily to the enlarging mass. There are no diagnostic laboratory findings, and definitive preoperative diagnosis is rare. An elderly patient with no history of pancreatitis is unlikely to have a pseudocyst, and a benign neoplasm is also less likely in this age group. Endoscopic ultrasound and aspiration of the cyst fluid can assist with the diagnosis; a high CEA level and low amylase level in the cyst fluid can be suggestive of malignancy. Aggressive surgical resection is indicated for cystic neoplasms of the pancreas. Internal drainage is the treatment of choice for noninfected pancreatic pseudocysts but is contraindicated if malignancy is suspected. ERCP with stent placement may be indicated in patients with pancreatic pseudocyst with fistula and proximal ductal stricture, but it has no role in the treatment of pancreatic malignancies. Percutaneous drainage is contraindicated in malignancies as well.

298. The answer is a. *(Townsend, pp 1451–1455.)* Familial adenomatous polyposis (FAP) is an autosomal dominant disorder that results in a nearly 100% risk of colorectal cancer, and therefore definitive surgical therapy consists of removal of all affected colonic and rectal mucosa. Associated lesions include fundic gland hyperplasia in the stomach with limited malignant potential, adenomatous polyps in the duodenum and periampullary region which are premalignant, extraintestinal malignancies, retroperitoneal and abdominal wall desmoid tumors, and benign osteomas.

299. The answer is c. *(Townsend, pp 321–322.)* According to the United Ostomy Association Data Registry, the most frequent serious complication of end colostomies is parastomal herniation, which commonly occurs when the stoma is placed lateral to, rather than through, the rectus muscle. Symptomatic herniation requires operative relocation of the stoma or mesh herniorrhaphy. Minor problems are frequently encountered with colostomies. They include irregularity of function, irritation of the skin due to leakage of enteric contents, or bleeding from the exposed mucosa following trauma. Prolapse occurs most frequently with transverse loop colostomies and is likely due to the use of the transverse loop to decompress distal colon obstructions. As the intestine decompresses, it retracts from the edge of the surrounding fascia, which allows prolapse or herniation of the mobile transverse colon. Optimal treatment of stomal prolapse is restoration of intestinal continuity or conversion to an end colostomy. Perforation of a stoma is usually due to careless instrumentation with an irrigation catheter.

300. The answer is c. *(Blumgart, pp 1074, 1084.)* Involvement of the superior mesenteric artery by a pancreatic tumor precludes resection for cure and therefore is a contraindication to proceeding with a Whipple procedure of pancreaticoduodenectomy. Involvement of the superior mesenteric vein does not necessarily preclude resection for cure, as 2 to 3 cm of the portal vein/superior mesenteric vein can be resected and an end-to-end anastomosis or venous bypass can be performed. Pyloric preservation is a well-accepted modification of the Whipple procedure. Total pancreatectomy is reserved for patients with extensive low-grade or extensive intraductal papillary lesions involving most of the pancreas. Preoperative biliary stenting is controversial with regard to the risk of increased infectious complications postoperatively; preoperative stenting does not improve survival.

301. The answer is c. (*Greenfield, pp 750–766.*) Perforation of a duodenal ulcer is an indication for emergency celiotomy and closure of the perforation. In patients with no prior history of peptic ulcer disease, simple closure with an omental patch is recommended. Patients with long-standing ulcer disease require a definitive acid-reducing procedure, except in high-risk situations. The choice of procedure is made by weighing the risk of recurrence against the incidence of undesirable side effects of the procedure, and considerable controversy persists about this issue. Antrectomy and truncal vagotomy offers a recurrence rate of 1%, but carries a 15 to 25% incidence of sequelae such as diarrhea, dumping syndrome, bloating, and gastric stasis. Highly selective vagotomy, if technically feasible, offers a 1 to 5% incidence of side effects but carries a recurrence rate of 10 to 13% in some series, although results are better when gastric and prepyloric ulcers are excluded. In general, definitive acid-reducing procedures should be postponed if the perforation is more than 12 h old or if there is extensive peritoneal soilage. Pyloroplasty and truncal vagotomy carries intermediate rates of recurrence and side effects, but has the advantage of speed in the setting of very ill patients with acute perforation.

302. The answer is b. (*Townsend, pp 1295–1297.*) Though reminiscent of the carcinoid syndrome, this patient's complaints in the context of recent gastric surgery are highly suggestive of the dumping syndrome, which is characterized by intestinal symptoms (bloating, cramping, diarrhea) and vasomotor symptoms (weakness, flushing, palpitations, diaphoresis, and dizziness) after ingestion of a meal following surgical removal of part of the stomach or alteration of the pyloric sphincter. Early dumping occurs within 20 to 30 min of eating and is attributed to the rapid influx of fluid with a high osmotic gradient into the small intestine from the gastric remnant. Late dumping syndrome occurs 2 to 3 h after a meal; symptoms resemble those of hypoglycemic shock. Medical management consists of reassurance and dietary measures (avoidance of large amounts of sugars, frequent small meals, and separation of fluids and solids). The majority of cases will resolve within three months of operation on this regimen.

Octreotide, a long-acting somatostatin analogue, can be used as well, but cost is a limiting factor. Surgery for intractable dumping consists of creation of an antiperistaltic limb of jejunum distal to the gastrojejunostomy.

303. The answer is a. (*Townsend, pp 1580–1593.*) Restoration of circulating blood volume is the first priority in patients with an acute variceal bleed. Initial resuscitation should be with isotonic crystalloids followed by transfusion of blood. Elevated prothrombin times should be corrected with fresh-frozen plasma, and although mild hypersplenism and thrombocytopenia are associated with portal hypertension, platelet transfusion is indicated only for platelet counts less than 50,000/μL. Medical therapy consists of either octreotide or vasopressin to decrease splanchnic blood flow. Because of coronary vasoconstrictive effects, nitroglycerin is usually administered concomitantly with vasopressin. Beta blockade (e.g., propranolol), with or without a long-acting nitrate, has been used to prevent recurrent variceal bleeding, but is not indicated in the acutely bleeding patients who are hemodynamically unstable. Balloon tamponade controls variceal hemorrhage immediately in more than 85% of patients. However, although balloon tamponade (Sengstaken-Blakemore tube) has reduced the mortality and morbidity from variceal hemorrhage in good-risk patients, an increased awareness of the associated complications (aspiration, asphyxiation, and ulceration at the tamponade site), as well as a rebleeding rate of 40%, have reduced its use. Balloon tamponade is indicated as a temporary measure when vasopressin or octreotide and sclerotherapy fail.

304. The answer is e. (*Townsend, pp 1584–1591.*) Patients with poorly compensated liver disease who develop recurrent variceal bleeds should undergo transjugular intrahepatic portosystemic shunting (TIPS). Beta blockade and endoscopic therapy are typically used as initial therapeutic options for patients with variceal bleeds. In patients with well-compensated liver disease, portosystemic shunts can be used to prevent recurrent variceal bleeds. Portocaval, mesocaval, and splenorenal shunts are considered nonselective shunts and are associated with the development or worsening of encephalopathy postoperatively. The distal splenorenal shunt is a selective shunt procedure and is associated with a lower rate of encephalopathy. However, in patients with Child's C cirrhosis (poorly compensated liver disease), surgical shunting should be avoided because of increased operative mortality. Hepatic transplantation is contraindicated in a patient who is actively drinking. Esophageal transection and reanastomosis, or the Suguira procedure, are typically reserved for patients with splanchnic venous thrombosis who are not shunt candidates.

305. The answer is c. (*Greenfield, pp 762–766.*) Benign gastric ulcers have a peak incidence in the fifth decade, with male predominance. About 95% of gastric ulcers are located near the lesser curvature. The initial management of a gastric ulcer consists of antimicrobial therapy directed against *Helicobacter pylori*. Indications for surgical intervention are hemorrhage, perforation, disease refractory to medical therapy, and inability to rule out a malignancy. Therefore, this patient with a persistent gastric ulcer should undergo surgical resection via either a distal gastrectomy with gastroduodenostomy (Billroth I reconstruction) or with gastrojejunostomy (Billroth II reconstruction). Only ulcers associated with acid hypersecretion require a vagotomy as well (type II—body of stomach, with concomitant duodenal ulcer, or type III—prepyloric). Type I (in the body and along the lesser curvature) and type IV (near the gastroesophageal junction) ulcers do not require vagotomy.

306. The answer is c. (*Greenfield, p 1128.*) Because approximately 5% of colorectal cancers are associated with resectable hepatic metastases, appropriate preoperative discussion should include obtaining permission for removal of synchronous peripheral hepatic lesions if they are found. If gross tumor is removed, a 25% cure rate can be anticipated. Adequate local resection, either by wedge or by limited partial hepatectomy, may be carried out whenever no extrahepatic disease is found and the hepatic lesion is technically removable. Any option that leaves the potentially obstructing primary cancer unremoved would be unacceptable. Radiation therapy has little to offer in colon cancer or its hepatic metastases. Because hepatic metastases receive most of their perfusion from the hepatic artery, local infusion of floxuridine (FUDR) via an implantable hepatic artery pump has been reported to provide palliation in selected patients with unresectable hepatic lesions.

307. The answer is b. (*Schwesinger, pp 411–416.*) *Helicobacter pylori* infections have become extremely common: nearly one-third of all American adults are now infected. Morphologically, the organism is a gram-negative, corkscrew-shaped, motile bacillus with three to seven flagella. Noninvasive approaches with simple, relatively inexpensive serologic and urea breath tests can establish the diagnosis of *H. pylori* infection. Culturing endoscopic scrapings or biopsy specimens has proved to be impractical because of the need for special media and elaborate growth conditions. A rapid urease test is used when endoscopy provides a specimen for analysis. Therapy is problematic because the organism is not easily eradicated. Monotherapy is largely ineffective. However, dual- and triple-drug therapy can achieve eradication in 80 to 90% of patients. Unfortunately, compliance rates with multidrug therapy are low.

308. The answer is c. (*Greenfield, pp 1200–1203.*) An indirect inguinal hernia leaves the abdominal cavity by entering the dilated internal inguinal ring and passing along the anteromedial aspect of the spermatic cord. The internal inguinal ring is an opening in the transversalis fascia for the passage of the spermatic cord; an indirect inguinal hernia, therefore, lies within the fibers of the cremaster muscle. A femoral hernia passes directly beneath the inguinal ligament at a point medial to the femoral vessels, and a direct inguinal hernia passes through a weakness in the floor of the inguinal canal medial to the inferior epigastric artery. Each is dependent on defects in Hesselbach's triangle of transversalis fascia and neither lies within the cremaster muscle fibers. Spigelian hernias, which are rare, protrude through an anatomic defect that can occur along the lateral border of the rectus muscle at its junction with the linea semilunaris. An interparietal hernia is one in which the hernia sac, instead of protruding in the usual fashion, makes its way between the fascial layers of the abdominal wall. These unusual hernias may be preperitoneal (between the peritoneum and transversalis fascia), interstitial (between muscle layers), or superficial (between the external oblique aponeurosis and the skin).

309. The answer is b. (*Greenfield, pp 806–807.*) The finding of air in the biliary tract of a nonseptic patient is diagnostic of a biliary enteric fistula. When the clinical findings also include small-bowel obstruction in an elderly patient without a history of prior abdominal surgery (a virgin abdomen), the diagnosis of gallstone ileus can be made with a high degree of certainty. In this condition, a large chronic gallstone mechanically erodes through the wall of the gallbladder into adjacent stomach or duodenum. As the stone moves down the small intestine, mild cramping symptoms are common. When the gallstone arrives in the distal ileum, the caliber of the bowel no longer allows passage, and obstruction develops. Surgical removal of the gallstone is necessary. The diseases suggested by the other response items (bleeding ulcer, peritoneal infection, pyloric outlet obstruction, pelvic neoplasm) are common in elderly patients, but each would probably present with symptoms other than those of small-bowel obstruction.

310. The answer is d. (*Brunicardi, pp 1078–1080, 1084–1088.*) Cancer of the colon in patients with chronic ulcerative colitis is 10 times more frequent than in the general population. Duration of disease is very important; the risk of developing cancer is low in the first 10 years but thereafter rises about 4% per year. The average age of cancer development in patients with chronic ulcerative colitis is 37 years; idiopathic carcinoma of the colon, however, develops at an average age of 65 years. Crohn's colitis is currently felt to be a precancerous condition as well. The chance of development of carcinoma of the colon in patients with familial polyposis is essentially 100%. Treatment of the patient with familial polyposis generally consists of total proctocolectomy with ileoanal j-pouch. Villous adenomas have been demonstrated to contain malignant portions in about one-third of affected persons and invasive malignancy in another one-third of removed specimens. Anterior resection is performed for large lesions or those containing invasive carcinomas when the lesion is above the peritoneal reflection. Abdominal-perineal resection is indicated for low-lying rectal villous adenomas when they have demonstrated invasive carcinomas. Transrectal excision with regular follow-up examinations is sufficient for lesions without invasive carcinomas. Peutz-Jeghers syndrome is characterized by intestinal polyposis and melanin spots of the oral mucosa. Unlike the adenomatous polyps seen in familial polyposis, the lesions in this condition are hamártomas, which have no malignant potential.

311. The answer is c. (*Greenfield, pp 806–807.*) Gallstone ileus is due to erosion of a stone from the gallbladder into the gastrointestinal tract (most commonly the duodenum). The stone becomes lodged in the small bowel (usually in the terminal ileum) and causes small-bowel obstruction. Plain films of the abdomen that demonstrate small-bowel obstruction and air in the biliary tract are diagnostic of the condition. Treatment consists of ileotomy, removal of the stone, and cholecystectomy if it is technically safe. If there is significant inflammation of the right upper quadrant, ileotomy for stone extraction followed by an interval cholecystectomy is often a safer alternative. Operating on the biliary fistula doubles the mortality rate compared with simple removal of the gallstone from the intestine.

312. The answer is d. *(Brunicardi, pp 1081–1084.)* The indications for surgical intervention for diverticular disease include hemorrhage secondary to diverticulosis, recurrent episodes of diverticulitis, intractability to medical therapy, and complicated diverticulitis. The latter includes perforated diverticulitis with or without abscess and fistulous disease. Diverticular abscesses are treated with percutaneous drainage initially followed by definitive resectional therapy. Initial percutaneous drainage allows for a one-stage procedure that consists of resection of the affected colon with primary anastomosis. Perforated diverticulitis is typically treated with either the Hartmann's procedure (sigmoid resection with end colostomy and rectal stump) or sigmoid resection, anastomosis, and diverting loop ileostomy.

313. The answer is d. *(Townsend, p 1612.)* Cholecystectomy results in improvement in symptoms in 85 to 94% of patients with biliary dyskinesia. The diagnosis is confirmed by CCK-HIDA scan. Technetium labeled hydroxyiminodiacetic acid (HIDA) is injected intravenously, which is subsequently excreted into the biliary tract. After filling of the gallbladder, cholecystokinin (CCK), a hormone that is normally released by the duodenum after ingestion of a meal, is infused intravenously to stimulate gallbladder contraction. A gallbladder ejection fraction of less than 35% at 20 min is diagnostic of biliary dyskinesia. There is no role for oral dissolutional therapy with ursodeoxycholic acid in the treatment of biliary colic, since no gallstones are present.

314. The answer is b. *(Brunicardi, p 1044.)* Gallbladder polyps can be observed with serial ultrasounds if they are less than 1 cm in size. Patients with suspected gallbladder carcinoma should undergo cholecystectomy with intraoperative frozen section, and if there is invasion of the serosa and no evidence of metastatic or extensive local disease, they should undergo a radical cholecystectomy (portal lymphadenectomy and either wedge or formal resection of the liver surrounding the gallbladder fossa in addition to the cholecystectomy). Bile aspiration does not have a role in the workup of gallbladder polyps or gallbladder carcinoma.

315. The answer is d. (*Brunicardi, p 1208.*) The initial treatment of choice in patients with acute acalculous cholecystitis who are not good candidates for surgical intervention is antibiotic therapy and placement of a percutaneous cholecystostomy tube. Risk factors for acute acalculous cholecystitis include trauma, major operations, and prolonged illness with multiple organ failure. Ultrasonography may demonstrate a thickened gallbladder wall or pericholecystic fluid. However, the diagnostic test of choice is a HIDA scan; nonvisualization of the gallbladder is diagnostic for acute cholecystitis, calculous or acalculous. Because patients who develop acalculous cholecystitis are typically not good surgical candidates, laparoscopic cholecystectomy is deferred in those patients until after resolution of the underlying problem(s). If the patient fails to improve with these measures, then cholecystectomy may be necessary. Antibiotics alone or aspiration alone are not adequate treatment options for acute acalculous cholecystitis.

316. The answer is c. (*Brunicardi, p 1320.*) Hematomas of the rectus sheath are more common in the elderly, and a history of trauma, sudden muscular exertion, or anticoagulation can usually be elicited. The pain is of sudden onset and is sharp in nature. The hematoma typically presents as an abdominal mass that does not change with contraction of the rectus muscles. The diagnosis can be established preoperatively with an ultrasound or CT scan showing a mass within the rectus sheath. Management is conservative unless symptoms are severe and bleeding persists, in which case surgical evacuation of the hematoma and ligation of bleeding vessels may be required.

317. The answer is a. (*Blumgart, pp 1147–1157.*) Amebic liver abscesses should be treated initially with metronidazole monotherapy, as opposed to pyogenic liver abscesses, which are treated initially with percutaneous catheter drainage and antibiotics against gram-negative and anaerobic organisms (e.g., *Esherischia coli, Klebisella pneumoniae,* bacteroides, enterococcus, and anaerobic streptococci). If improvement fails to occur, then other antimicrobial agents can be added. Abscesses that are refractory to medical therapy may require laparotomy.

318. The answer is b. *(Brunicardi, pp 911–918.)* Surgical treatment for sliding esophageal hernias (Type I paraesophageal hernias) should be considered only in symptomatic patients with objectively documented esophagitis or stenosis. The overwhelming majority of sliding hiatal hernias are totally asymptomatic, even many of those with demonstrable reflux. Even in the presence of reflux, esophageal inflammation rarely develops because the esophagus is so efficient at clearing the refluxed acid. Symptomatic hernias should be treated vigorously by the variety of medical measures that have been found helpful. Patients who do have symptoms of episodic reflux and who remain untreated can expect their disease to progress to intolerable esophagitis or fibrosis and stenosis. Neither the presence of the hernia nor its size is important in deciding on surgical therapy. Once esophagitis has been documented to persist under adequate medical therapy, manometric or pH studies may help determine the optimum surgical treatment.

319. The answer is b. *(Greenfield, pp 897–898, 1027–1029.)* While elevation of SGOT and SGPT is indicative of hepatocellular disease, elevated alkaline phosphatase is indicative of biliary obstruction. Based on safety and cost, ultrasonography is the initial diagnostic procedure. Once ductal dilation is identified, a percutaneous transhepatic cholangiogram or ERCP may be performed to localize and characterize the obstruction. If a distal common bile duct obstruction is noted, a CT scan is recommended to image the head of the pancreas. In most instances, a liver-spleen scan adds little to the diagnostic workup. This also applies to the upper gastrointestinal series. Cancer of the head of the pancreas is associated with painless jaundice.

320. The answer is a. *(Townsend, pp 1496–1506.)* The patient has an infected pilonidal cyst, which typically presents as a painful fluctuant mass between the gluteal clefts and is usually a disease of young obese and/or hirsute men. Perianal hidradenitis suppurativa is a disease of the apocrine glands that results in chronic inflammation and multiple sinuses and abscesses in the perianal region. Crohn's disease of the anus can present as multiple fissures, fistulas, and abscesses and may or may not be associated with inflammation of the rectum. A fistula-in-ano can present as a perianal abscess or a chronically draining track in the perianal region. An ischiorectal abscess often presents with pain and fever before manifestation of a palpable fluctuant mass on rectal examination.

321. The answer is e. (*Townsend, pp 1441–1443.*) Ischemic colitis presents as hematochezia, fever, and abdominal pain. Unlike acute mesenteric ischemia, which affects the small intestine and requires emergent intervention, ischemic colitis rarely requires surgical intervention unless full-thickness necrosis, perforation, or refractory bleeding are present. Expectant management with intravenous fluids, bowel rest, and supportive care is the treatment of choice.

322. The answer is b. (*Greenfield, pp 1063–1069.*) Because the reserve capacity of the colon for water absorption greatly exceeds the normal requirements for maintaining stable bowel function, patients may undergo resection of a large fraction of the colon and suffer little change in bowel habits. Neither the right nor the left colon appears to be a site of preferential water and electrolyte absorption, nor does the ileocecal valve play a noticeable role in fluid homeostasis. However, in diseases characterized by increased fluid secretion of the small bowel, the colon is more likely to be overwhelmed by the absorptive demand following partial colectomy than in the intact state. The rectum does not appear to play a role in fluid absorption.

323. The answer is d. (*Brunicardi, pp 1091–1094.*) Workup of a patient with a diagnosed rectal cancer can include rigid proctoscopy to assess the distance of the lesion from the anal verge, barium enema or colonoscopy to rule out synchronous colon lesions, CT abdomen/pelvis to rule out liver metastases and evaluate pelvic lymphadenopathy, MRI to evaluate the extent of local invasion for large rectal tumors, and endorectal ultrasonography to assess depth of invasion through the rectal wall and perirectal lymphadenopathy. Neoadjuvant chemoradiation is administered in patients with T_{3-4} and/or nodal disease and in appropriate candidates for potential sphincter preservation. Chest CT is indicated if the preoperative chest x-ray is abnormal.

324. The answer is a. (*Greenfield, pp 792–795.*) Digestion and absorption of dietary carbohydrate by the duodenum and small intestine are so avid that complete absorption has already occurred by the time ingested food has traversed 200 cm of jejunum. Most fat absorption occurs in the duodenum and proximal jejunum. Simple fluids that require minimal digestion, such as milk, are entirely absorbed, save for their fat content, within the duodenum. Even in the short gut syndrome, virtually all dietary carbohydrate is absorbed within the residual jejunum. While pancreatic peptidases are important to protein digestion, redundant digestive enzymes are so widely distributed within the duodenal and jejunal brush border that 95% of a protein meal can be absorbed in the absence of the pancreas. Salt and water flux in the small intestine is influenced by a variety of hormones; aldosterone markedly increases sodium uptake, while prostaglandins stimulate fluid and electrolyte secretion.

325. The answer is d. *(Brunicardi, pp 1160–1161.)* Hepatic adenomas are associated with oral contraceptive (OCP) use, and cessation of OCPs may be adequate to allow regression of the lesion if smaller than 4 cm. However, for lesions greater than 4 cm in size, surgical resection is advocated. Other indications for resection include failure to regress with cessation of OCPs or inability to stop taking OCPs and desire to become pregnant. Lesions greater than 4 cm in size have an increased risk of rupture with hemorrhage, which may in fact be the initial clinical presentation.

326. The answer is a. *(Brunicardi, pp 1160–1161.)* Focal nodular hyperplasia (FNH) is rarely symptomatic and unlike a hepatic adenoma does not carry an associated risk of malignant degeneration or rupture with hemorrhage. Therefore, surgical resection for FNH is indicated only if the lesion is symptomatic. If FNH cannot be distinguished from a hepatic adenoma on CT scan, a nuclear medicine scan can be obtained that may demonstrate a "hot" lesion in the setting of FNH and a "cold" lesion in the setting of hepatic adenoma.

327. The answer is d. *(Brunicardi, p 1260.)* Splenectomy is indicated for acute hemorrhage secondary to left-sided, or sinistrial, portal hypertension, which is characterized by gastric varices in the setting of splenic or portal vein thrombosis in the absence of cirrhosis. Patients who have either had an episode of acute or have chronic pancreatitis can develop either splenic or portal venous thrombosis. In the absence of bleeding complications, surgery is indicated only if other surgical procedures are planned.

328. The answer is b. *(Brunicardi, pp 1076–1081, 1127.)* Patients with regional enteritis usually have a chronic and slowly progressive course with intermittent symptom-free periods. The usual symptoms are anorexia, abdominal pain, diarrhea, fever, and weight loss. Extraintestinal syndromes that may be seen include ankylosing spondylitis, polyarthritis, erythema nodosum, pyoderma gangrenosum, gallstones, hepatic fatty infiltration, and fibrosis of the biliary tract, pancreas, and retroperitoneum. However, in about 10% of patients, especially those who are young, the onset of the disease is abrupt and may be mistaken for acute appendicitis. Appendectomy is indicated in such patients as long as the cecum at the base of the appendix is not involved; otherwise, the risk of fecal fistula must be considered. Interestingly, about 90% of patients who present with the acute appendicitis-like form of regional enteritis will not progress to development of the full-blown chronic disease. Thus, resection or bypass of the involved areas is not indicated at this time.

329. The answer is c. *(Brunicardi, pp 1211–1213.)* This scenario is typical for a patient with iatrogenic injury of the common bile duct. These injuries commonly occur in the proximal portion of the extrahepatic biliary system. The transhepatic cholangiogram documents a biliary stricture, which in this clinical setting is best dealt with surgically. Choledochoduodenostomy generally cannot be performed because of the proximal location of the stricture. The best results are achieved with end-to-side choledochojejunostomy (Roux-en-Y) performed over a stent. Percutaneous transhepatic dilatation has been attempted in select cases, but follow-up is too short to make an adequate assessment of this technique. Primary repair of the common bile duct may result in recurrent stricture.

330. The answer is e. *(Greenfield, pp 1097–1098.)* The term *carcinoma in situ* refers to the presence of malignant cells in the mucosal layer only. Endoscopic polypectomy is adequate treatment when malignant cells are identified in a colonic polyp, even if an invasive component is identified, if: (1) no vascular or lymphatic invasion is present, (2) there is an adequate negative margin (2mm), and the cancer is not poorly differentiated.

331. The answer is b. *(Brunicardi, pp 1042–1043.)* The effects of radiation on the intestine depend on a variety of factors, which include the age of the patient, temperature, degree of oxygenation, and metabolic activity. Acute intestinal radiation injury is manifested in the bowel by the cessation of viable cell production and is seen clinically as diarrhea or gastrointestinal bleeding. Progressive vasculitis and fibrosis are seen in the latter stages of radiation injury and may result in malabsorption, ulceration, fistulization, or perforation. Intussusception is generally not associated with radiation injury.

332. The answer is d. (*Greenfield, pp 741–744, 797–798.*) Drugs, hormones, or emotional states (e.g., fear) that stimulate or simulate sympathetic activity inhibit intestinal motility. Those factors that arouse parasympathetic activity (acetylcholine) stimulate motility. Gastrin has specific delaying effects on gastric emptying. Secretin and cholecystokinin are potent regulators of intestinal and digestive activities but probably have no effect on motility per se.

333. The answer is d. (*Greenfield, pp 696–713.*) Carcinoma of the esophagus occurs primarily in the sixth and seventh decades of life in a male-to-female ratio of 3:1. Although the cause is unknown, alcohol, tobacco, and dietary factors have been implicated as causative agents. A high incidence is reported in patients with corrosive esophagitis. Malignant tumors arising in the esophagus are usually squamous cell carcinomas, except those involving the esophagogastric junction, which are usually adenocarcinomas. Because the prognosis is poor for patients with esophageal carcinoma, multimodality therapy has been utilized in attempts to improve mortality. Neoadjuvant (preoperative) chemoradiation appears to result in improved local and regional control and to improve survival in patients with both squamous cell and adenocarcinoma. However, the standard of care is still esophageal resection. Radiation therapy alone has been used for palliation in patients with squamous cell carcinoma of the esophagus.

334. The answer is b. (*Greenfield, pp 905–907.*) This patient has a gastrin level suggestive of but not diagnostic of Zollinger-Ellison Syndrome (ZES). Given that there are multiple etiologies for hypergastrinemia (including acid suppression therapy with a proton pump inhibitor), a secretin stimulation test can be performed to diagnose ZES. A secretin stimulation test will cause a significant rise in serum gastrin levels greater than 200 pg/mL above baseline in patients with ZES.

335. The answer is c. (*Greenfield, p 906.*) Ninety percent of gastrinomas are located within the gastrinoma triangle—the three corners of the triangle are defined by the junction of the second and third portions of the duodenum, the junction of the neck and body of the pancreas, and the junction of the cystic and common bile duct.

336. The answer is b. *(Brunicardi, pp 1236–1237.)* The patient has acute gallstone pancreatitis. Ranson's criteria consist of 5 criteria on admission and 6 during the first 48 h that predict mortality: less than 2 criteria associated with 0% mortality, 3 to 5 criteria with 10 to 20% mortality, and 6 or more with greater than 50% mortality. All 11 criteria must be assessed; the first 5 criteria assess age, white blood cell count, LDH, AST, and glucose. The second set of criteria assesses hematocrit fall, BUN elevation, serum calcium, base deficit, and estimated fluid sequestration. Amylase is not one of the criteria, and in fact, amylase does not correlate with the severity of disease. The criteria are slightly different for gallstone pancreatitis and non–gallstone pancreatitis.

337. The answer is b. *(Greenfield, pp 903–905.)* Tumors arising from the pancreatic β cells give rise to hyperinsulinism. Seventy-five percent of these tumors are benign adenomas, and in fifteen percent of affected patients the adenomas are multiple. Symptoms relate to a rapidly falling blood glucose level and are due to epinephrine release triggered by hypoglycemia (sweating, weakness, tachycardia). Cerebral symptoms of headache, confusion, visual disturbances, convulsions, and coma are due to glucose deprivation of the brain. Whipple's triad summarizes the clinical findings in patients with insulinomas: (1) attacks precipitated by fasting or exertion, (2) fasting blood glucose concentrations below 50 mg/dL, and (3) symptoms relieved by oral or intravenous glucose administration. These tumors are treated surgically, and simple excision of an adenoma is curative in the majority of cases.

338. The answer is e. *(Greenfield, pp 1131–1136.)* Epidermoid cancers of the anal canal metastasize to inguinal nodes as well as to the perirectal and mesenteric nodes. The results of local radical surgery have been disappointing. Combined external radiation with synchronous chemotherapy (fluorouracil and mitomycin), also known as the Nigro protocol, has been used as the standard treatment of the disease, whereas radical surgical approaches are now generally reserved for treatment failures and recurrences.

339. The answer is c. *(Greenfield, pp 798–809.)* A markedly distended colon could have many causes in this 80-year-old man. The contrast study, however, reveals a classic apple core lesion appropriate prior to relief of this large-bowel obstruction. After medical preparation (e.g., hydration, normalization of electrolytes), this patient should undergo prompt surgical management of his mechanical obstruction; conservative management by resection and proximal colostomy would generally be preferred in this elderly patient with an obstructed, unprepared bowel.

340. The answer is c. *(Greenfield, pp 824–826.)* Surgical treatment of Crohn's disease is aimed at correcting complications that are causing symptoms. Intestinal obstruction is usually partial and secondary to a fixed stricture that is not responsive to anti-inflammatory agents. When the obstruction causes symptoms that compromise nutritional status, surgery is warranted. Fistula formation in itself is not an indication for surgery. Fistulas between the intestine and the bladder and the intestine and the vagina, however, generally cause significant symptoms and warrant surgical intervention, while an ileum–ascending colon fistula is very common yet rarely symptomatic. Perforation of bowel into the free abdominal cavity is obviously a surgical emergency.

341. The answer is e. *(Brunicardi, pp 1097–1098.)* The film shows a markedly distended colon. The differential diagnosis includes tumor, foreign body, and colitis, but far more likely is either cecal or sigmoid volvulus. Sigmoid volvulus may be ruled out quickly by proctosigmoidoscopy, which is preferable to barium enema, since sigmoid volvulus may be treated successfully by rectal tube decompression via the sigmoidoscope. If sigmoidoscopy is negative, the working diagnosis, based on this classic film, must be cecal volvulus; barium enema would clinch the diagnosis, but the colon might rupture in the intervening 1 to 2 h. Emergency celiotomy should be done.

342. The answer is c. *(Greenfield, pp 751–752, 763, 776.)* Helicobacter pylori is a spiral-shaped, gram-negative bacterium that is found in the viscous gastric mucus layer and has an affinity for epithelial cells. It was originally classified as a form of *Campylobacter*, but its genomic and phenotypic characteristics were subsequently found to be unique and it was given a new genus name. Urease and other peptides released by H. pylori may be toxic and cause direct gastroduodenal injury. Evidence is strong that H. pylori plays a role in the etiology of ulcer disease. There is an almost

100% association between gastric *H. pylori* infection and duodenal ulcer disease, and about 70% of patients with gastric ulcers are also infected with *H. pylori*. Furthermore, colonization with *H. pylori* increases the risk of developing a duodenal ulcer by up to twentyfold. Eradication of *H. pylori* from the stomach markedly decreases the rate of ulcer recurrence. This generally requires triple therapy with colloidal bismuth (Pepto-Bismol), an antibiotic (amoxicillin or ampicillin), and a nitroimidazole such as metronidazole. Recent studies have also demonstrated a possible association between *H. pylori* infection and gastric carcinoma.

343. The answer is e. *(Brunicardi, pp 1098–1099.)* The history, x-ray, and clinical findings are typical of a postoperative cecal volvulus, a condition in which the cecum is twisted on its mesentery (often, after aneurysm resection, a neomesentery) and becomes acutely obstructed. At 12 cm, the cecum is in imminent danger of perforation. Particularly in the presence of a prosthetic graft, cecal perforation is a catastrophe. Urgent decompression is needed. To attempt colonoscopic decompression would necessitate insufflation of additional air and increase the stress on the already compromised cecal wall. A transverse colostomy "decompression" would not decompress the cecum, nor would it provide detorsion of the cecal mesentery to allow restoration of adequate blood supply to the right colon. While untwisting the cecum and fixing it to the lateral abdominal wall (to inhibit recurrence) by a decompressing cecostomy might be advocated in some settings, the risk of contaminating the aortic graft would be excessive. Resection of the offending organ with ileotransverse colostomy would be the procedure of choice.

344. The answer is d. *(Greenfield, pp 945–946.)* Hydatid cysts secondary to echinococcal infection are most common in the liver in adults. Up to 20 to 30% of patients with hepatic cysts also have cysts in their lungs. In general, serologic tests are more likely to be positive the longer the lesion has been present, but false negativity occurs with sufficient frequency that results should not influence the decision to treat hepatic hydatid cysts. Spontaneous rupture of the cyst or leakage of cyst fluid during diagnostic or therapeutic aspiration may cause anaphylactic reactions or peritoneal dissemination of the disease. Classically, definitive treatment required surgical resection, enucleation, or evacuation of the cysts. As long as there is no evidence of biliary communication with the cyst, agents such as 0.5%

silver nitrate or hypertonic saline are introduced into the cyst at the time of surgery, and efforts are made to avoid spillage and contamination of the peritoneal cavity. Treatment of patients with liver cysts with mebendazole or albendazole combined with percutaneous drainage has been demonstrated to have comparable outcomes to surgical cystectomy and should be considered in these patients.

345. The answer is a. (*Mahmoodian, pp 19–24.*) Appendicitis complicates approximately 1 in 1700 pregnancies at an incidence comparable with that in nonpregnant women matched for age. It is the most prevalent extrauterine indication for laparotomy in pregnancy. The duration of gestation does not influence the severity of the disease, but the diagnosis does become more difficult as the pregnancy progresses. By the twentieth week of gestation, the appendix often lies at the level of the umbilicus and more lateral than usual. Pregnancy should not delay surgery if appendicitis is suspected; appendiceal perforation greatly increases the chance of premature labor and fetal mortality (approximately 20% for each). In contrast, negative laparotomy under general anesthesia and nonperforated appendicitis are associated with very low risk to both the fetus and the mother (less than 1% and 5%, respectively).

346. The answer is b. (*Greenfield, pp 726–728; Brunicardi, pp 911–918.*) Normal respiration creates negative pressure in the thoracic cavity. As a result of the pressure gradient, blood enters the chest via the venae cavae and air via the trachea; both are life-sustaining results of this pressure gradient. The pathophysiologic consequence of a hole in the diaphragm is that eventually abdominal viscera will be aspirated into the thorax. The sliding hernia, contained in the lower mediastinum by intact pleura, may rarely cause symptoms of reflux that would justify surgical attention, but such patients are in no danger of vascular compromise or of obstructive displacement of hollow viscera. The paraesophageal hernia, on the other hand, leaves the patient at substantial risk for both strangulation and obstruction. Either result would be a surgical catastrophe; with rare exceptions, paraesophageal hernias should be surgically repaired whenever diagnosed. A traction diverticulum is usually caused by inflammatory contraction around mediastinal nodes, is rarely of any symptomatic consequence, and need not be repaired. Neither the Schatzki's ring nor the esophageal web justifies esophageal surgery. They can be ignored or dilated as symptoms demand.

347. The answer is d. (*Greenfield, pp 810–811.*) Ogilvie syndrome describes the condition in which massive cecal and colonic dilation is seen in the absence of mechanical obstruction. Other terms used to describe this condition are acute colonic pseudo-obstruction, colonic ileus, and functional colonic obstruction. It tends to occur in elderly patients in the setting of cardiopulmonary insufficiency, in other systemic disorders that require prolonged bed rest, and in the postoperative state. The diagnosis of Ogilvie syndrome cannot be confirmed until mechanical obstruction of the distal colon is excluded by colonoscopy or contrast enema. Anticholinergic agents and narcotics need to be discontinued, but any delay in decompressing the dilated cecum is inappropriate since colonic ischemia and perforation become a distinct hazard as the cecum reaches this degree of dilation (>10 to 12 cm). In patients with less than 10 cm of dilation and no evidence of ischemic bowel, management consists of bowel rest, nasogastric suctioning if vomiting, correction of metabolic abnormalities, and discontinuation of medications that diminish gastrointestinal motility. In patients with persistent distention or a dilated cecum greater than 10 cm, cautious endoscopic colonic decompression can be performed, or a sympatholytic agent such as neostigmine can be administered, with appropriate hemodynamic monitoring. Surgery is indicated in all patients in whom perforation or ischemic bowel is suspected.

348. The answer is c. (*Greenfield, pp 724–726.*) Zenker's diverticulum is an acquired abnormality. Premature contraction of the cricopharyngeus muscle on swallowing, which leads to partial obstruction, is believed to be the cause of this pulsion-type diverticulum of the pharyngoesophageal junction. High intraluminal pressure results in an outpouching of mucosa through the oblique fibers of the pharyngeal constrictors. Dysphagia is common and is the usual presenting symptom. Because the diverticulum is located above the superior esophageal sphincter, no mechanism exists to prevent aspiration of the contents of the diverticulum, and patients can present with regurgitation and recurrent aspiration pneumonias; pulmonary complications are common. The diagnosis is established by barium swallow. Treatment is surgical: diverticulectomy with cricopharyngeal myotomy.

349. The answer is a. (*Merrell, pp 621–625.*) The classic Quincke triad of abdominal pain in the right upper quadrant, jaundice, and gastrointestinal bleeding is present in 30 to 40% of patients with hemobilia. With more frequent use of percutaneous liver procedures (e.g., transhepatic cholangiogram, transhepatic catheter drainage), iatrogenic injury has replaced other trauma as the most common cause of bloody bile. Other causes include spontaneous bleeding during anticoagulation, gallstones, parasitic infections/abscesses, and neoplastic lesions. Angiography and endoscopy are useful diagnostic studies, and intrahepatic bleeding can be controlled by angiographic embolization in up to 95% of cases. Surgical treatment is advocated for bleeding from extrahepatic bile ducts or the gallbladder or in cases of penetrating trauma in which associated injuries might need attention.

350. The answer is d. *(Podolosky, pp 928–937.)* The patient depicted in this question has Crohn's disease of the colon (Crohn's colitis). Crohn's colitis is characterized by linear mucosal ulcerations, discontinuous (skip) lesions, a transmural inflammatory process, and noncaseating granulomas in up to 50% of patients. Because their clinical features and management differ, Crohn's colitis must be distinguished from ulcerative colitis. Ulcerative colitis is usually found in the rectum, although in rare cases the rectum is spared involvement. The entire colon, from cecum to rectum, may be involved (pancolitis). Ulcerative colitis typically presents as a grossly continuous inflammatory process (without skip lesions) that microscopically is confined to the mucosa and submucosa of the colon. In addition, crypt abscesses and superficial ulcerations are common in ulcerative colitis.

351. The answer is c. *(Podolosky, pp 928–937.)* Patients with Crohn's disease can develop fistulas between the colon and other segments of intestine, the bladder, the urethra, the vagina, the skin, or the prostate. Intestinal perforation can occur in about 5% of patients. Toxic megacolon can occur in patients with Crohn's disease, ulcerative colitis, or any severe inflammatory process of the large intestine. Extraintestinal manifestations are usually associated with active disease. Finally, patients with Crohn's colitis have a 5.6-fold increased risk of colon cancer relative to an age-matched population.

352. The answer is c. *(Brunicardi, pp 911–918.)* The condition demonstrated is a paraesophageal hernia. It is encountered much less frequently (approximately 5%) than is the sliding hiatal hernia, and it has completely different therapeutic implications. Paraesophageal hernias are acquired, rarely present before middle age, and are most common in patients in their seventh decade. The position of the gastroesophageal junction distinguishes the different types of hernias, which occur near the esophageal hiatus of the diaphragm. In the more common sliding hernia, the gastroesophageal junction protrudes above the diaphragm (type I paraesophageal hernia). In the type II paraesophageal hernia, the anatomic junction between the esophagus and the stomach is anchored in its normal position below the diaphragm; the gastric cardia or fundus and occasionally other viscera herniate into the thorax within a true peritoneal sac alongside the gastroesophageal junction. In the type III paraesophageal hernia, the gastroesophageal junction and the gastric cardia or fundus are displaced above the level of the diaphragm. Surgical repair is indicated in patients with type II paraesophageal hernias as soon as the patient can be properly prepared for the procedure, as bleeding, ulceration, obstruction, necrosis of the stomach wall, and perforation are common.

353. The answer is b. (*Townsend, pp 1281–1288.*) The vast majority of pancreatic carcinomas are located in the head of the gland. Patients may present with painless jaundice by virtue of the carcinoma's obstruction of the intrapancreatic portion of the common bile duct. Approximately 10 to 15% of patients are candidates for resection. There is a very strong association with diabetes mellitus (but not diabetes insipidus), but the nature of this relationship is not known. Prognosis is poor; five-year survival after pancreaticoduodenectomy is about 10 to 15%.

354. The answer is d. (*Townsend, pp 1260–1262.*) The patient most likely has bleeding from the small bowel, given the findings on endoscopy, and the most common cause of small intestinal bleeding in patients under the age of 30 is a Meckel's diverticula. Because Meckel's diverticula can contain ectopic gastric mucosa, acid secretion can cause small-bowel ulcerations. Small-bowel enteroclysis is a contrast study that can sometimes identify masses or lesions in the small bowel. While enteroclysis, small-bowel endoscopy, angiography, and CT scanning can all be useful adjuncts in the workup of GI bleeding, the patient in this scenario should have a ^{99m}Tc pertechnate scan, which is diagnostic for a Meckel's diverticula.

355. The answer is d. (*Brunicardi, p 1134.*) Carcinoid tumors arise from the neuroectoderm and are a type of apudoma. The most common site of carcinoid tumors is the small bowel, although appendiceal carcinoids are also common. Carcinoid syndrome, which is characterized by flushing, diarrhea, and cardiac valvular disease, occurs in a small percentage of patients with carcinoid tumors; it is rarely seen with appendiceal carcinoids. It occurs when serotonin is released into the systemic circulation and thus avoids breakdown by the liver. The appropriate therapy for a small carcinoid (less than 2 cm) of the appendix is simple appendectomy.

356. The answer is b. *(Brunicardi, pp 1356–1357.)* Direct inguinal hernias occur medial to the inferior epigastric vessels and are best repaired by reapproximating the transversalis fascia to Cooper's ligament and thus reconstructing the floor of the inguinal canal or by a tension-free Lichtenstein-type repair. The hernia sac is opened and ligated routinely during indirect hernia repair but not during direct hernia repair. The most common inguinal hernia in women is an indirect hernia. Direct hernias rarely present with a scrotal component and are less likely to present with incarceration than indirect hernias.

357. The answer is b. *(Cosentino, pp 740–748.)* Choledochal cysts are congenital cystic dilations of the extrahepatic biliary ducts. Intrahepatic cystic dilation can coexist (Caroli's disease), but it represents a distinct problem and is managed differently. Patients may present with symptoms at any age, but the classic triad of epigastric pain, abdominal mass, and jaundice is not frequently seen. Rather, most patients present with other conditions such as cholecystitis, cholangitis, or pancreatitis. Ultrasonography or endoscopic retrograde cholangiopancreatography (ERCP) is helpful in demonstrating cysts. Nonsurgical treatment of these cysts results in high morbidity and mortality, and therefore surgery is advised in all cases. The present recommendation is for complete resection of the cyst and Roux-en-Y choledochojejunostomy. Since malignant changes in choledochal cysts have been frequently described, complete resection rather than the performance of an internal drainage procedure is preferred whenever the resection can be done safely.

358. The answer is d. *(Townsend, pp 1253–1254.)* Stress ulceration refers to acute gastric or duodenal erosive lesions that occur following shock, sepsis, major surgery, trauma, or burns. These lesions tend to be superficial and can involve multiple sites. McClelland and associates showed that patients subjected to trauma and subsequent hemorrhagic shock do not have increased gastric secretion, but rather show decreased splanchnic blood flow. Ischemic damage to the mucosa may therefore play a role. Unlike chronic benign gastric ulcers, which are generally found along the lesser curvature and in the antrum, acute erosive lesions usually involve the body and fundus and spare the antrum.

359. The answer is b. *(Brunicardi, p 1203.)* Cholangitis is suggested by the presence of the Charcot triad: fever, jaundice, and pain in the right upper quadrant. These symptoms are usually caused by choledocholithiasis, but they can also occur in association with obstructing neoplasms and choledochal cysts. The disease occurs primarily in the elderly. Therapy is aimed at decompression of the common bile duct. In patients with suppurative cholangitis who fail to respond to intravenous antibiotics and fluid resuscitation, the nonoperative approach is the preferred intervention via either percutaneous or endoscopic drainage of the obstructed common bile duct. If the nonoperative approach fails, surgery is indicated. This is usually best accomplished by surgical placement of a T tube into the duct. Percutaneous transhepatic catheter drainage is an acceptable alternative in select patients. This procedure can often provide effective decompression during the acute septic phase of the disease. Cholecystostomy will be effective only if there is free flow of bile into the gallbladder via the cystic duct and in general should not be depended on to secure drainage of the common bile duct.

360. The answer is a. *(Brunicardi, p 1200.)* High-risk, critically ill patients with multisystem disease and cholecystitis experience a significant increase in morbidity and mortality following operative intervention. Tube cholecystostomy can be performed under local anesthesia in the operating room or via a percutaneous approach in the radiology suite. Open or laparoscopic procedures would carry the same general anesthetic risk whether done urgently or in a delayed (elective) fashion. Lithotripsy has no role in the treatment of acute cholecystitis.

361. The answer is a. *(Townsend, pp 1658–1660.)* Pancreatic pseudocysts can develop in the setting of acute and chronic pancreatitis. They are cystic collections that do not have an epithelial lining and therefore have no malignant potential. Most pseudocysts spontaneously resolve. Therapy should not be considered for six weeks to allow for the possibility of spontaneous resolution as well as to allow for maturation of the cyst wall if the cyst persists. Complications of pseudocysts include gastric outlet and extrahepatic biliary obstructions as well as spontaneous rupture and hemorrhage. Pseudocysts can be excised, externally drained, or internally drained into the gastrointestinal tract (most commonly the stomach or a Roux-en-Y limb of jejunum).

362. The answer is d. *(Reilly, pp 1702–1707.)* Recently, Dieulafoy's lesion has been identified more frequently as a source of gastrointestinal bleeding. It is characteristically located within 6 cm distal to the gastroesophageal junction. Dieulafoy's lesion typically consists of an abnormally large submucosal artery that protrudes through a small, solitary mucosal defect. For unclear reasons, the lesions may bleed spontaneously and massively, in which case they require emergency intervention. Upper endoscopy is usually successful in localizing the lesion, and permanent hemostasis can be obtained endoscopically in most cases with injection sclerotherapy, electrocoagulation, or heater probe. If surgery is required, a gastrotomy and simple ligation or wedge resection of the lesion may be adequate. No large series have yet established the optimal surgical treatment for Dieulafoy's lesion; however, acid-reducing procedures have not been successful in preventing further bleeding.

363. The answer is b. *(Brunicardi, p 1134.)* Carcinoid tumors arise from enterochromaffin cells in the crypts of Lieberkühn. When they are encountered in the appendix and are less than 2 cm in size, simple appendectomy is the procedure of choice. When the tumors are larger than 2 cm, a right hemicolectomy should be performed. Carcinoid syndrome (hepatomegaly, diarrhea, cutaneous flushing, right heart valvular disease, and asthma) usually occurs in the presence of liver metastases but can also be seen when there are metastases to sites drained by systemic (as opposed to portal) veins or from primary carcinoids outside the portal system. Carcinoid syndrome is rare in patients with carcinoid of the appendix because the tumors are usually discovered before metastases occur.

364. The answer is d. *(Brunicardi, pp 1094–1095.)* Rectal carcinoids are slowly growing tumors, but they can be locally invasive and metastasize in up to 15% of patients. Patients manifest systemic signs of the carcinoid syndrome only in the rare circumstance where hepatic metastases have occurred. The malignant potential is low in carcinoid tumors when they are less than 2 cm in diameter, as is typically the case when diagnosed. The tumors are curable by wide local transanal resection that includes the muscle layer. Endoscopic treatment leaves tumor cells near the margin of resection and is felt to increase the risk of recurrence. Whether more aggressive resection (abdominoperineal or low anterior resection) improves the prognosis in larger tumors remains controversial. The prognosis is excellent for patients with local disease.

365. The answer is b. (*Reilly, pp 1702–1707.*) Polypoid lesions of the gallbladder are found most often in the third through fifth decades of life and are increasingly being detected by ultrasonography. These are generally small lesions that typically do not show a shadow on ultrasound. Ninety percent are benign lesions, such as cholesterol polyps (pseudotumors). True adenomas, which constitute about 10% of these benign lesions, can undergo malignant transformation. The indications for operative intervention remain controversial. Recent reviews suggest that the vast majority of malignant polypoid lesions are solitary, larger than 1.0 cm, and much more common in patients more than 50 years of age. There is also an increased incidence of malignancy if the lesions are associated with gallstones. Symptomatic lesions should be removed regardless of their size. Asymptomatic small lesions can probably be safely followed by ultrasonography.

366. The answer is a. (*Blumgart, p 1085.*) The metabolic consequences of total pancreatectomy are manifold. They include weight loss, malabsorption attended by hypocalcemia and hypophosphatemia, diabetes mellitus, diarrhea, and both iron deficiency and pernicious anemia. In theory, total pancreatectomy should provide good surgical treatment for pancreatic carcinoma; in reality, the severe metabolic problems that result from total removal of the pancreas make partial pancreaticoduodenectomy a frequently preferred treatment for most cases of pancreatic carcinoma that are resectable.

367. The answer is d. (*Brunicardi, p 1084.*) Cecal diverticula must be differentiated from the more common variety of diverticula that are usually found in the left colon. Cecal diverticula are thought to be congenital. The cecal diverticulum is often solitary and involves all layers of the bowel wall;

therefore, cecal diverticula are true diverticula. Diverticula elsewhere in the colon are almost always multiple and are thought to be an acquired disorder. These acquired diverticula are really herniations of mucosa through weakened areas of the muscularis propria of the colon wall. The preoperative diagnosis in the case of cecal diverticulitis is acute appendicitis about 80% of the time. If there is extensive inflammation involving much of the cecum, an ileocolectomy is indicated. If the inflammation is well localized to the area of the diverticulum, a simple diverticulectomy with closure of the defect is the procedure of choice. To avoid diagnostic confusion in the future, the appendix should be removed whenever an incision is made in the right lower quadrant, unless operatively contraindicated.

368. The answer is c. (*Brunicardi, pp 1161–1162.*) Hepatic hemangiomas are the most common of all liver tumors. The infantile forms are highly vascular and occasionally cause hepatomegaly or congestive cardiac failure that requires angiographic or surgical interruption. The diagnostic incidence of incidental cavernous hemangiomas in adults has increased in this era of noninvasive imaging of organs with MRI, ultrasonography, and CT. When this lesion is suspected, the diagnosis can be confirmed with sensitive and more specific imaging techniques such as labeled red blood cell scanning (not liver-spleen scans). The mean age of presentation in adults is about 50 years, and the vast majority of these lesions are asymptomatic. There is no evidence that they undergo malignant transformation. They may enlarge and become symptomatic more readily in women after multiple pregnancies or during the use of estrogen or oral contraceptives. The risk of rupture and severe hemorrhage into or from hemangiomas is extremely low; when it does occur, it is usually iatrogenic (following attempted biopsy). Given the typically benign and static nature of these lesions, management by angiographic embolization or resection should be reserved for the rare patient with symptomatic or complicated hemangioma.

369. The answer is d. (*Brunicardi, p 273.*) CEA is a nonspecific tumor marker that is elevated in only about one-half of patients with colorectal tumors and is often elevated in patients with lung, pancreatic, gastric, or gynecologic malignancies. CEA is also elevated in cigarette smokers. Patients in whom the primary colon tumor produced CEA and in whom the level falls below 2 to 3 ng/mL after resection have an excellent prognosis for disease control. In such patients, a subsequent rise in CEA has been demonstrated to be a very sensitive marker of the presence and extent of recurrent disease. Many surgeons follow CEA levels and perform second-look operations to resect local disease or possibly isolated metastatic disease if the levels become elevated postoperatively. Some surgeons recommend exploration in that circumstance even in the absence of other evidence (CT scan, colonoscopy) of recurrence. In some patients, the long-term survival seems to be improved following this aggressive approach. However, very high elevations of CEA suggest extensive liver disease or peritoneal spread, which is unresectable.

370. The answer is e. (*Brunicardi, p 985.*) Patients with Mallory-Weiss syndrome typically present with a massive, painless hematemesis after severe vomiting or retching. The majority of tears occur just below the gastroesophageal junction. These tears occur more commonly in cirrhotics than in the normal population. Most of the time (90%), bleeding will stop without any intervention. When bleeding persists, balloon tamponade, endoscopic control of the bleeding, and surgical intervention with gastrotomy and oversewing of the tear have all been successful. Both intravenous and intraarterial infusion of vasopressin are also useful in controlling bleeding but are contraindicated in patients with coronary artery disease.

371–373. The answers are 371-b, 372-d, 373-c, 374-a. (*Townsend, pp 1279, 1289–1295.*) Gastric ulcers have been classified as type I (incisura or most inferior portion of lesser curvature), type II (gastric and duodenal), type III (pyloric and prepyloric), and type IV (juxtacardial). Indications for surgery are intractability, perforation, obstruction, and bleeding. A patient with an intractable type I ulcer can be treated with an antrectomy alone or with a proximal gastric vagotomy. If done properly, antrectomy offers slightly lower recurrence rates and a higher incidence of postoperative sequelae as compared with proximal gastric vagotomy. However, significant scarring along the lesser curvature makes a proximal gastric vagotomy technically unfeasible. Gastric outlet obstruction and severe inflammation around the pylorus and duodenum make resection a difficult and dangerous option. Similarly, pyloroplasty is often not adequate to provide adequate drainage in the setting of gastric outlet obstruction. Vagotomy and gastrojejunostomy, although associated with the highest recurrence rate, offer the best choice in this setting. In an elderly patient with a bleeding duodenal ulcer, recurrence rates are less of a consideration and thus the simplest and most expedient operation offers the best surgical outcome. Vagotomy and pyloroplasty with oversewing of the ulcer are the best choice in this setting. In a young patient with intractable type III ulcers, antrectomy with vagotomy offers the best long-term outcome.

375–378. The answers are 375-d, 376-b, 377-b, 378-c. *(Townsend, pp 1431–1439; Brunicardi, pp 1076–1097.)* The definitive operation of choice for patients with ulcerative colitis is total proctocolectomy with either end ileostomy or ileoanal j-pouch anastomosis. Indications for operation in UC include high-grade dysplasia or carcinoma, toxic megacolon, and intractability to medical therapy. Patients with either UC or Crohn's can develop toxic megacolon, which is manifested by fever, abdominal pain, and marked dilation of the large bowel. Treatment consists of a subtotal colectomy with end ileostomy. For patients with UC and toxic megacolon, completion proctectomy can be performed at a later date.

For squamous cell carcinoma of the anus, the mainstay of therapy is chemoradiation with the Nigro protocol. However, recurrent or persistent disease after chemoradiation requires surgery—abdominal-perineal resection (APR) involves removing the rectum and anus with formation of a permanent end colostomy. APR is also the procedure of choice for distal rectal cancers that involve the sphincters or are too close to obtain an adequate margin (2 cm) and in patients for whom sphincter-sparing surgery is contraindicated because of fecal incontinence. Preoperative or neoadjuvant chemoradiation can sometimes cause distal rectal tumors to shrink in size such that a sphincter-sparing operation can be performed. For proximal and midrectal cancers, low anterior resection (LAR) is the procedure of choice. LAR involves the removal of the rectum to below the peritoneal reflection through an abdominal approach.

379–380. The answers are 379-b, 380-g. *(Townsend, pp 1226–1227, 1422–1424.)* A radiolucency under the right hemidiaphragm demonstrates pneumoperitoneum. Only a perforated viscus can produce this radiographic appearance in conjunction with diffuse peritonitis. A perforated diverticulum, perforated gastric ulcer, perforated transverse colon carcinoma, or strangulated hernia with necrotic bowel are all included in the differential diagnosis. A sigmoid volvulus appears radiographically on plain film of the abdomen as an upside-down U or bent inner tube. Acute sigmoid volvulus presents in the elderly with nausea, vomiting, abdominal distention, colicky abdominal pain, and obstipation. The first diagnostic and often therapeutic maneuver should be a sigmoidoscopy. Patients with evidence of necrosis or perforation should undergo emergent exploratory laparotomy. Recurrent sigmoid volvulus should be treated with sigmoid resection.

Cardiothoracic Problems

Questions

DIRECTIONS: Each item below contains a question followed by suggested responses. Select the **one best** response to each question.

381. A 42-year-old homeless man presents with a three-week history of shortness of breath, fevers, and pleuritic chest pain. CXR reveals a large left pleural effusion. Thoracentesis reveals thick purulent-appearing fluid, which is found to have a glucose less than 40 mg/dL and a pH of 6.5. A chest tube is placed, but the pleural effusion persists. Which of the following is the most appropriate management of this patient?

a. Placement of a second chest tube at the bedside and antibiotic therapy
b. Infusion of antibiotics via the chest tube
c. Intravenous antibiotics for six weeks
d. Thoracotomy with instillation of antibiotics into the pleural space
e. Thoracotomy with decortication and antibiotic therapy

382. A 63-year-old man is seen because of facial swelling and cyanosis, especially when he bends over. There are large, dilated subcutaneous veins on his upper chest. His jugular veins are prominent even while he is upright. Which of the following conditions is the most likely cause of these findings?

a. Histoplasmosis (sclerosing mediastinitis)
b. Substernal thyroid
c. Thoracic aortic aneurysm
d. Constrictive pericarditis
e. Bronchogenic carcinoma

383. During endoscopic biopsy of a distal esophageal cancer, perforation of the esophagus is suspected when the patient complains of significant new substernal pain. An immediate chest film reveals air in the mediastinum. Which of the following is the most appropriate management of this patient?

a. Placement of a nasogastric tube to the level of perforation, antibiotics, and close observation
b. Spit fistula (cervical pharyngostomy) and gastrostomy
c. Left thoracotomy, pleural patch oversewing of the perforation, and drainage of the mediastinum
d. Left thoracotomy with esophagectomy
e. Thoracotomy with chest tube drainage and esophageal exclusion

384. A 63-year-old woman with COPD presents with a several-week history of fever, night sweats, weight loss, and cough. On chest x-ray, she is noted to have a density in the left upper lobe with a relatively thin-walled cavity. Bronchoscopy and CT scan are suggestive of a lung abscess rather than a malignant process. Which of the following is the most appropriate initial management of this patient?

a. Percutaneous drainage of the lung abscess
b. Systemic antibiotics directed against the causative agent
c. Tube thoracostomy
d. Left upper lobectomy
e. Surgical drainage of the abscess

385. A 45-year-old man with poorly controlled hypertension presents with severe chest pain radiating to his back. An ECG demonstrates no significant abnormalities. A CT scan of the chest and abdomen is obtained, which demonstrates a descending thoracic aortic dissection extending from distal to the left subclavian takeoff down to above the iliac bifurcation. A Foley catheter is placed, and urine output is 30 to 40 cc/h. His feet are warm, with less than 2-s capillary refill. Which of the following is the most appropriate initial management?

a. Emergent operation for repair of the aortic dissection
b. Angiography to confirm the diagnosis of aortic dissection
c. Echocardiography to rule out cardiac complications
d. Initiation of a beta blocker
e. Initiation of a vasodilator such as nitroprusside

386. A stockbroker in his mid-40s presents with complaints of episodes of severe, often incapacitating chest pain on swallowing. Diagnostic studies on the esophagus yield the following results: endoscopic examination and biopsy—mild inflammation distally; manometry—prolonged high-amplitude contractions from the arch of the aorta distally, lower esophageal sphincter (LES) pressure 20 mmHg with relaxation on swallowing; barium swallow—2-cm epiphrenic diverticulum. Which of the following is the best management option for this patient?

a. Myotomy along the length of the manometric abnormality
b. Diverticulectomy, myotomy from the level of the aortic arch to the fundus, fundoplication
c. Diverticulectomy, cardiomyotomy of the distal 3 cm of esophagus and proximal 2 cm of stomach with antireflux fundoplication
d. A trial of calcium channel blockers
e. Pneumatic dilatation of the LES

387. A 4-year-old boy is seen 1 h after ingestion of a lye drain cleaner. No oropharyngeal burns are noted. Chest x-ray is normal, but the patient continues to complain of significant chest pain. Which of the following is the most appropriate next step in his management?

a. Parenteral steroids and antibiotics
b. Esophagogram with water soluble contrast
c. Administration of an oral neutralizing agent
d. Induction of vomiting
e. Rapid administration of a quart of water to clear remaining lye from the esophagus and dilute material in the stomach

388. A previously healthy 20-year-old male is admitted to the hospital with acute onset of left-sided chest pain. Electrocardiographic findings are normal, but chest x-ray shows a 40% left pneumothorax. Appropriate treatment consists of which of the following procedures?

a. Observation
b. Barium swallow
c. Thoracotomy
d. Tube thoracostomy
e. Thoracostomy and intubation

389. A 50-year-old salesman is on a yacht with a client when he has a severe vomiting and retching spell punctuated by a sharp substernal pain. He arrives in your emergency room 4 h later and has a chest film in which the left descending aorta is outlined by air density. Which of the following is the most appropriate next step in his workup?

a. Upper GI with water-soluble contrast
b. Echocardiogram
c. Flexible bronchoscopy
d. Flexible esophagogastroscopy
e. Aortography

390. A 26-year-old man is brought to the emergency room after being extricated from the driver's seat of a car involved in a head-on collision in which the patient was not wearing his seat belt. An echocardiogram (shown here) demonstrates wall motion abnormalities suggestive of a myocardial contusion. Which of the following is true regarding the diagnosis of and outcome after a traumatic myocardial contusion?

a. Significant pump failure occurs in less than 5% of patients with major chest trauma
b. ST and T wave abnormalities on EKG are diagnostic
c. An elevation in the CK-MB fraction of greater than 5% of total is predictive of increased mortality
d. Cardiac enzymes are the most sensitive test for diagnosing myocardial contusion
e. Patients should be placed on antiarrhythmics regardless of EKG findings for at least 24 h postinjury

391. A 63-year-old man underwent a three-vessel CABG 5 h ago. Initially, his mediastinal chest tube output was 300 mL blood per hour, but an hour ago, there was no further evidence of bleeding from the tube. His mean arterial pressure has fallen, and several fluid boluses were administered. His central venous pressure is elevated to 20 mmHg, and he has required the addition of inotropes. Which of the following is the best management strategy?

a. Addition of vasopressors along with the inotropes
b. Transfusion of packed red blood cells
c. Return to the operating room for exploration of the mediastinum
d. Placement of an intraaortic balloon pump
e. Infusion of streptokinase into the mediastinal chest tube

392. Several days following esophagectomy, a patient complains of dyspnea and chest tightness. A large pleural effusion is noted on chest radiograph, and thoracentesis yields milky fluid consistent with chyle. Which of the following is the most appropriate initial management of this patient?

a. Immediate operation to repair the thoracic duct
b. Immediate operation to ligate the thoracic duct
c. Tube thoracostomy and low-fat diet
d. Observation and low-fat diet
e. Observation and antibiotics

393. A 56-year-old woman presents for evaluation of a murmur suggestive of mitral stenosis and is noted on echocardiography to have a lesion attached to the fossa ovalis of the left atrial septum. The mass is causing obstruction of the mitral valve. Which of the following is the most likely diagnosis?

a. Endocarditis
b. Lymphoma
c. Cardiac sarcoma
d. Cardiac myxoma
e. Metastatic cancer to the heart

394. A 56-year-old woman has been treated for three years for wheezing on exertion, which was diagnosed as asthma. Chest radiograph, shown here, reveals a midline mass compressing the trachea. Which of the following is the most likely diagnosis?

a. Lymphoma
b. Neurogenic tumor
c. Lung carcinoma
d. Goiter
e. Pericardial cyst

395. A 59-year-old man is found to have a 6-cm thoracic aortic aneurysm for which he desires repair, but he is concerned about the risk of paralysis postoperatively. Which of the following maneuvers has not been demonstrated to decrease the risk of paraplegia after repair?

a. Infusion of a bolus of steroids immediately postoperatively with a continuous infusion for 24 h
b. Minimization of cross-clamping time
c. Reattachment of segmental intercostal and lumbar arteries
d. Cerebrospinal fluid drainage
e. Left heart bypass

396. An 89-year-old man has lost 30 lb over the past two years. He reports that food frequently sticks when he swallows. He also complains of a chronic cough. Pulmonary function tests show a vital capacity of 60% of expected values, and forced expiratory volume is 50% of predicted values. Barium swallow is shown here. Which of the following statements is true?

a. Radiation therapy and stenting can be expected to produce the same long-term survival as would surgery
b. Esophagoscopy and biopsy should be performed to confirm the x-ray findings
c. This patient is atypical in that the lesion usually appears in the second or third decade of life
d. The patient should be treated with antituberculous medications before any surgical intervention is considered
e. The carotid bifurcation lies adjacent to the lesion

397. A 70-year-old woman is seeking a surgical opinion following her heart catheterization, which was performed because of exertional chest pain. Her pain is worsening. Which of the following statements is true concerning aortocoronary bypass grafting?

a. It is indicated for crescendo (preinfarction) angina
b. It is indicated for congestive heart failure
c. It is not indicated for chronic disabling angina
d. It is associated with a 10% operative mortality in low-risk patients
e. It is indicated only if significant triple vessel disease is documented angiographically

398. A 27-year-old woman seeks your advice regarding pain and numbness in the right arm and hand. She reports that it is exacerbated by raising her arm over her head. A provisional diagnosis is made. Which of the following statements is true regarding this condition?

a. It is associated with cervical spine disk disease
b. It is reliably diagnosed by positional obliteration of the radial pulse
c. If conservative measures fail, it is best treated by surgical decompression of the brachial plexus
d. It most commonly affects the median nerve
e. It can be reliably ruled out by angiography

399. A 35-year-old man presents with a history of four days of severe substernal pain and fever to 38.89°C (102°F). He has a past medical history of peptic ulcer disease that resulted in a Billroth II procedure five years earlier. On admission, the chest film shown here is obtained. A true statement regarding this patient's case is which of the following?

a. Pericardial effusion is present
b. The condition may be managed with antibiotics and close observation if the patient remains hemodynamically stable
c. The condition could have resulted from recurrent peptic ulcer disease
d. The condition could have resulted from a myocardial infarction
e. The previous Billroth II procedure effectively rules out peptic ulcer as the cause of the condition

400. A 65-year-old woman has had pain in her right shoulder and has been treated with analgesics without relief. Chest x-ray reveals a mass in the apex of the right chest. A transthoracic needle biopsy documents carcinoma. Superior pulmonary sulcus carcinomas (Pancoast tumors) are bronchogenic carcinomas that typically produce which of the following clinical features?

a. Atelectasis of the involved apical segment
b. Horner's syndrome
c. Pain in the T_4 and T_5 dermatomes
d. Nonproductive cough
e. Hemoptysis

401. A 63-year-old man has a chylothorax that after two weeks of conservative therapy appears to be persistent. The chest tube output is approximately 600 mL/d. Appropriate management at this time includes which of the following procedures?

a. Neck exploration and ligation of the thoracic duct
b. Subdiaphragmatic ligation of the thoracic duct
c. Thoracotomy and repair of the thoracic duct
d. Thoracotomy and ligation of the thoracic duct
e. Thoracotomy and abrasion of the pleural space

402. A 32-year-old woman has a screening chest x-ray, and a 1.5-cm mass is noted in the right lower lobe. She is a nonsmoker. Bronchoscopy shows a mass in the right lower lobe orifice, covered with mucosa. Biopsy indicates this is compatible with a carcinoid tumor. Which of the following statements is true regarding carcinoids in the lung?

a. They frequently metastasize
b. They most commonly arise in peripheral terminal bronchioles
c. They rarely produce the carcinoid syndrome
d. They are radiosensitive
e. Five-year survival rate is less than 50%

403. Six months ago at the time of lumpectomy for breast cancer, a 60-year-old female attorney quit a 30-year smoking habit of two packs per day. She had the chest radiograph shown here as part of her routine follow-up examination. True statements about the lesion visualized on the film include which of the following?

a. It is more apt to be metastatic breast carcinoma than primary lung carcinoma
b. There is a 90% chance that this mass is malignant
c. Since the diagnosis can be established with certainty only by a tissue diagnosis, the mass should be biopsied
d. If the mass is malignant, the possibility for cure with excision is remote
e. The mass is most likely benign

404. A 42-year-old man presents with a solitary lung lesion. At the time of operation on this patient, a firm, rubbery lesion in the periphery of the lung is discovered. It is sectioned in the operating room to reveal tissue that looks like cartilage and smooth muscle. Which of the following is the most likely diagnosis?

a. Fibroma
b. Chondroma
c. Osteochondroma
d. Hamartoma
e. Aspergilloma

405. The condition shown in these x-rays is most compatible with which of the following manifestations?

a. Difficulty swallowing solids but not liquids
b. Higher than normal incidence of esophageal carcinoma
c. Failure of the upper esophageal sphincter to relax in response to swallowing
d. Normal pressure in the body of the esophagus
e. Normal esophageal motility

DIRECTIONS: Each group of questions below consists of lettered options followed by a set of numbered items. For each numbered item, select the **one** lettered option with which it is **most** closely associated. Each lettered option may be used once, more than once, or not at all.

Questions 406–410

For each physical finding or group of findings, select the cardiovascular disorder with which it is most likely to be associated.

a. Massive tricuspid regurgitation
b. Aortic regurgitation
c. Coarctation of the aorta
d. Thoracic aortic aneurysm
e. Myocarditis

406. An elderly man with abnormal pupillary responses (Argyll Robertson pupil)

407. A 24-year-old drug addict with jugular venous distention and exophthalmos

408. A patient with flushing and paling of the nail beds (Quincke pulse) and a bounding radial pulse

409. A patient with conjunctivitis, urethral discharge, and arthralgia

410. A patient with short stature, webbed neck, low-set ears, and epicanthal folds

Questions 411–415

For each clinical scenario, select the mediastinal tumor with which it is most likely to be associated.

a. Thymoma
b. Hodgkin's disease
c. Pheochromocytoma
d. Parathyroid adenoma
e. Cystic teratoma

411. A 23-year-old patient with hypertension and increased urinary catecholamine levels.

412. A 21-year-old woman presents with generalized weakness and double vision. During her workup, she is noted to have a widened mediastinum on chest x-ray prompting a CT scan, which demonstrates an anterior mediastinal mass.

413. A 63-year-old woman with vague symptoms of fatigue and depression who presents with hematuria. CT scan of the abdomen and pelvis reveals a stone at the ureteropelvic junction.

414. A 35-year-old woman with fever and weight loss. CT scan revealed a mediastinal mass, which was biopsied and revealed Reed-Sternberg cells.

415. A 33-year-old woman presents with cough and chest pain for two months. More recently, she complains of coughing up hair. Chest x-ray reveals a mediastinal mass.

Questions 416–420

Match the appropriate pharmacologic agent with each description.
a. Epinephrine
b. Norepinephrine
c. Isoproterenol
d. Dobutamine
e. Milrinone
f. Digitalis
g. Nitroprusside
h. Nitroglycerin

416. A patient requires lowering of systolic blood pressure and central venous pressure (balanced arterial and venous dilation).

417. A patient has a high systemic vascular resistance and low cardiac output (action as an inotrope and vasodilator by inhibiting endogenous phosphodiesterase).

418. A patient requires a dramatic increase in cardiac output due to profound bradycardia; an external pacemaker is nonfunctional (pure α agonist with profound chronotropic properties).

419. Endogenous catecholamine that is secreted into the circulation under normal conditions.

420. A patient requires augmented contractility and antiarrhythmic properties to treat supraventricular tachycardia with rapid ventricular response (inotropic and antiarrhythmic properties).

Cardiothoracic Problems

Answers

381. The answer is e. (*Way, pp 360–366.*) The patient has an empyema or the accumulation of pus in the pleural cavity. Based on the history (three weeks of symptoms) and the fluid analysis demonstrating a glucose level less than 40 mg/dL and a pH less than 7.0 and its thick consistency, the patient's empyema is in the most advanced stage or the chronic organizing phase. In this phase, the fluid collection is loculated and depositions of fibrin create a thick pleural rind, which prevents apposition of the lung to the parietal pleura. Reexpansion of the lung requires thoracotomy with decortication to remove the purulent fluid and the pleural rind. Antibiotic therapy tailored to the organism(s) identified is necessary but not sufficient to treat an empyema.

382. The answer is e. (*Greenfield, pp 1431–1432.*) Superior vena cava obstruction (SVC syndrome) is almost always due to malignancy (90% of cases) and in three out of four cases, results from invasion of the vena cava by bronchogenic carcinoma. Lymphomas are the second most common cause of the superior vena cava syndrome. Fibrosing mediastinitis as a complication of histoplasmosis or ingestion of methysergide may occur but is rare. Rarely, a substernal thyroid or thoracic aortic aneurysm may be responsible for the obstruction. SVC syndrome can be caused iatrogenically secondary to indwelling catheters. Although constrictive pericarditis may decrease venous return to the heart, it does not produce obstruction of the superior vena cava. Whatever the cause of the superior vena cava syndrome, the resultant increased venous pressure produces edema of the upper body, cyanosis, dilated subcutaneous collateral vessels in the chest, and headache. Cervical lymphadenopathy may also be present as a result of either stasis or metastatic involvement. Initial management of superior vena cava syndrome consists of diuresis, and for malignancies, the treatment consists of radiation and chemotherapy if applicable. Occasionally, surgical intervention or thrombolysis may be indicated for severe life-threatening complications.

383. The answer is d. (*Greenfield, pp 717–722.*) Perforation of the esophagus in the chest is a surgical catastrophe that requires aggressive intervention in virtually all circumstances. In a patient with no underlying esophageal disorder, surgical intervention is directed at primary repair of the perforation and drainage of the mediastinum. In patients with an underlying motility disorder, stricture, or malignancy, surgical intervention must address both the perforation and the esophageal abnormality. For patients with a distal esophageal carcinoma, treatment usually requires esophagectomy. Esophageal exclusion or proximal diversion (with a cervical esophagostomy or "spit fistula") are typically reserved for patients in whom a late diagnosis of esophageal perforation was made.

384. The answer is b. (*Brunicardi, pp 573–575.*) Initial treatment of a lung abscess, once the diagnosis has been made, is systemic antibiotics directed against the causative agent. The duration of therapy is dependent on the severity of the underlying pneumonia that resulted in the abscess and can last up to 12 weeks. Often, the abscess drains spontaneously via the tracheobronchial tree, but if it fails to resolve with medical therapy, intervention may be required, ranging from percutaneous to surgical drainage of the abscess or resectional therapy.

385. The answer is d. (*Brunicardi, pp 707–709.*) The initial treatment for a descending aortic dissection is reduction in the change in blood pressure over the change in time (dP/dT), which is achieved with beta blockade. Nitroprusside may be added after beta blockade has been achieved. Indications for operative intervention for a descending aortic dissection are end-organ failure (renal failure, lower extremity ischemia, intestinal ischemia), inadequate pain relief despite optimal medical therapy, and rupture or signs of impending rupture (increasing diameter or periaortic fluid).

386. The answer is a. (*Brunicardi, pp 878–880.*) The finding of prolonged high-amplitude contractions in the body of the esophagus in a highly symptomatic patient is diagnostic of diffuse esophageal spasm (DES). None of the findings revealed by the diagnostic studies listed (minimal reflux esophagitis, normal LES relaxation and pressure, and an incidental small epiphrenic diverticulum) justifies treatment and none explains the patient's symptoms. The cause of the hypermotility disorder known as DES is unknown, but its symptoms can be disabling. The recommended treatment for this relatively rare disorder is a long myotomy guided by the manometric evidence. More than 90% of patients treated in this fashion will experience acceptable relief of symptoms if the myotomy is performed correctly.

387. The answer is b. (*Greenfield, pp 713–717.*) Corrosive injuries of the esophagus most frequently occur in young children due to accidental ingestion of strong alkaline cleaning agents. Signs of airway injury or imminent obstruction warrant close observation and possibly tracheostomy. An initial esophagogram with water-soluble contrast (Gastrografin) is performed if a perforation is suspected or for localization of a perforation prior to surgical intervention. Vomiting should be avoided, if possible, to prevent further corrosive injury and possible aspiration. Administration of oral antidotes is ineffective unless given within moments of ingestion; even then, the additional damage potentially caused by the chemical reactions of neutralization often makes use of them unwise. Attempted dilution of the caustic agent is not recommended, given that most of the damage has already occurred, and increasing the gastric volume may induce nausea and vomiting. Based on lack of evidence of efficacy in preventing strictures and potential deleterious side effects, steroids are not recommended. Parenteral antibiotics are indicated in cases with significant esophageal injury. It is probably wise to avoid all oral intake until the full extent of injury is ascertained.

388. The answer is d. (*Greenfield, pp 1420–1425.*) Spontaneous pneumothorax usually results from the rupture of subpleural blebs in young men (age 20 to 40), which is often signaled by a sudden onset of chest and shoulder pain. Large pneumothoraxes require placement of a chest tube; thoracotomy with bleb excision and pleural abrasion is generally recommended if spontaneous pneumothorax is recurrent. Small pneumothoraxes in patients with minimal symptoms usually resolve and therefore can simply be observed. A spontaneous perforation of the esophagus (Boerhaave's syndrome) can result in hydropneumothorax as well as the more usual pneumomediastinum, but would not present with an isolated 40% pneumothorax. Gastrografin swallow followed by a barium study are appropriate diagnostic tests for evaluation of a suspected leaking esophagus.

389. The answer is a. (*Way, pp 490–491.*) The presence of air in the mediastinum after an episode of vomiting and retching is virtually pathognomonic of spontaneous rupture of the esophagus (Boerhaave's syndrome). Radiographic studies, performed in a timely fashion, are indicated to confirm the diagnosis and define the location of the perforation. Esophagogram with water-soluble contrast is the initial test of choice. CT scanning may be useful if a small, contained leak is suspected. If the leak is contained and the patient does not have any evidence of sepsis, then the leak can be managed with antibiotics and expectant management. For leaks associated with systemic signs, patients should undergo prompt surgical therapy. The operation of choice is dependent on the time to diagnosis. Leaks that are less than 24 h old in patients without an underlying esophageal disorder may be managed with thoracotomy, repair, and drainage. Leaks older than 24 h typically require more extensive surgery.

390. The answer is a. (*Greenfield, p 331; Brunicardi, p 134.*) Significant pump failure occurs in less than 5% of patients with major chest trauma. There are no universally accepted criteria for the diagnosis of myocardial contusion, but an ECG may demonstrate ST or T-wave changes (which are not specific for a myocardial contusion), arrhythmias, or bundle branch blocks. Similarly, cardiac enzymes may be elevated, including the CK-MB fraction, but are neither sensitive nor specific for a myocardial contusion. Echocardiography may demonstrate wall motion abnormalities, valvular disruption, or a pericardial effusion with or without tamponade. Antiarrhythmics are not indicated prophylactically in a patient with a myocardial contusion, but should be used to treat any rhythm disturbances. Supportive therapy for myocardial contusion is directed at inotropic support of the ventricle; the coronary arteries are usually intact after the injury, so there is little role for coronary vasodilators and less for coronary artery bypass grafting.

391. The answer is c. (*Townsend, pp 1864–1865.*) Cardiac tamponade is a life-threatening complication that can occur after coronary artery bypass grafting. If the patient has bleeding postoperatively, the patient's coagulopathy should be corrected. Clotting of the mediastinal chest tube followed by hemodynamic decompensation with decreased mean arterial pressures (MAPs) and cardiac output with increasing filling pressures is suggestive of tamponade. Equalization of pressures across the four chambers on Swan-Ganz catheter monitoring or collapse of the right atrium on echocardiography are diagnostic of tamponade. The patient should return to the operating room for exploration and drainage of the mediastinal hematoma.

392. The answer is c. *(Greenfield, pp 1417–1419.)* Chylothorax may occur after intrathoracic surgery, or it may follow malignant invasion or compression of the thoracic duct. Intraoperative recognition of a thoracic duct injury is managed by ligation of the duct. Direct repair is impractical owing to the extreme friability of the thoracic duct. Injuries not recognized until several days after intrathoracic surgery frequently heal following the institution of a low-fat diet and either repeated thoracentesis or tube thoracostomy drainage. A low-fat, medium-chain triglyceride diet often reduces the flow of chyle.

393. The answer is d. *(Brunicardi, pp 679–680.)* The most common benign cardiac tumor is a myxoma. Symptoms can include valvular obstruction (mitral or tricuspid valve) or embolization systemically. They are often attached by a pedicle to the fossa ovalis of the left atrial septum. Treatment is resection.

394. The answer is d. *(Greenfield, pp 1425–1431.)* The boundaries of the mediastinum are the thoracic inlet, the diaphragm, the sternum, the vertebral column, and the pleura bilaterally. The mediastinum itself is divided into three portions delineated by the pericardial sac: the anterosuperior and posterosuperior regions are in front of and behind the sac, respectively, while the middle region designates the contents of the pericardium. In adults, mediastinal masses occur most frequently in the anterosuperior region and less often in the posterosuperior and middle regions. Cysts (pericardial, bronchogenic, or enteric) are the most common tumors of the middle region; neurogenic tumors are the most common of the primary tumors of the posterior mediastinum. The primary neoplasms of the mediastinum in the anteroposterior region (in order of descending frequency) are thymomas, lymphomas, and germ cell tumors. More commonly, though, a mass in this area represents the substernal extension of a benign substernal goiter. Diagnosis may be made by visualization of an enhancing structure on CT; radioactive iodine scanning is useful in management because it may make the diagnosis if the mediastinal tissue is functional and will also document the presence of functioning cervical thyroid tissue to prevent removal of all functional thyroid tissue during mediastinal excision.

395. The answer is a. *(Brunicardi, pp 691–701.)* Operative intervention is usually recommended for thoracic aortic aneurysms greater than 5 or 6 cm in diameter or those that are increasing in size. Spinal cord ischemia can result in paraplegia with a risk of 5 to 15%, depending on the extent of the repair. Various strategies that have been employed to prevent spinal cord ischemia include minimizing cross-clamp time, hypothermia, moderate systemic heparinization, left heart bypass, and cerebrospinal fluid drainage (using a lumbar drain). The rationale for CSF drainage is that it decreases the pressure on the blood supply to the spinal cord and therefore improves perfusion. Postoperative steroids do not reduce the risk of paraplegia.

396. The answer is e. (*Greenfield, pp 724–726.*) Pharyngoesophageal (Zenker's) diverticulum is an outpouching of mucosa between the lower pharyngeal constrictor and the cricopharyngeus muscles. It is thought to result from an incoordination of cricopharyngeal relaxation with swallowing. These diverticula occur in elderly patients and more commonly on the left. The typical patient presents with complaints of dysphagia, weight loss, and choking. Other patients present symptoms such as repeated aspiration, pneumonia, or chronic cough. A mass is sometimes palpable, and a gurgle may be heard. Surgical treatment is excision of the diverticulum and division of the cricopharyngeus muscle (cricopharyngeal myotomy), which can be done under local anesthesia in a cooperative patient. Esophagoscopy should be performed cautiously because the blind pouch is easily perforated; diagnosis is made with a barium swallow. Even though the pouch may extend down into the mediastinum, the origin of the diverticulum is at the cricopharyngeus muscle near the level of the bifurcation of the carotid artery.

397. The answer is a. (*Greenfield, pp 1495–1503.*) Coronary artery bypass surgery was developed in the late 1960s and is now being regularly performed. Indications for surgery include chronic disabling angina and crescendo (or preinfarction) angina. Cardiac catheterization with selective coronary angiography defines the extent of disease, which generally is localized to the proximal segments of the vessels. Operative mortality depends on the presence of risk factors such as age, other comorbidities, and preoperative ventricular function; mortality is approximately 3% in lower-risk, younger patients. Relief of angina is obtained in most affected patients. Patients with left main coronary artery disease as well as those with triple vessel disease and ventricular dysfunction have an increased longevity following successful bypass. Data regarding extension of life in other groups is conflicting. Coronary artery bypass is not indicated for congestive heart failure unless this condition is ischemic in origin and angiography identifies disease amenable to surgical revascularization.

398. The answer is c. (*Greenfield, pp 1413–1414.*) The thoracic outlet syndrome designates a symptom complex whose precise cause is unknown. It is felt to result from compression of the brachial plexus or subclavian vessels, or both, in the anatomic space bounded by the first rib, the clavicle, and the scalene muscles. Carpal tunnel syndrome (compression of the median nerve as it passes through the carpal tunnel of the wrist) and cervical disk disease are the two entities most commonly confused with the thoracic outlet syndrome, whose symptoms and signs include pain, paresthesias, edema, venous congestion, and digital vasospastic changes. Positional dampening or obliteration of the radial pulse is an unreliable finding, since it is present in up to 70% of the normal population. Plain films may diagnose bony abnormalities, and MRI can be useful in detecting cervical disease. Neurologic abnormalities may be documented by nerve conduction studies. Angiographic studies are often negative. Conservative management, which generally should precede surgery, consists of an exercise program to strengthen shoulder girdle muscles and decrease shoulder droop. Operative treatment includes division of the scalenus anticus and medius muscles, first rib resection, cervical rib resection, or a combination of all three.

399. The answer is c. (*Cummings, pp 511–518.*) This x-ray demonstrates an air-fluid level in the pericardium. Pneumopericardium can result from penetrating or blunt chest trauma, spontaneous formation of gas from anaerobic bacteria, iatrogenic causes, or direct extension into the pericardium by diseased adjacent organs. In this case, a patient with a high gastrojejunostomy developed a recurrent ulcer that eroded through the diaphragm and into the pericardium and thus caused a pneumopyopericardium. Often these patients have an unrecognized gastrinoma (Zollinger-Ellison syndrome) and therefore continue to have peptic ulcer disease despite aggressive surgical therapy. The presence of pneumopyopericardium as seen in this chest film should be treated as a surgical emergency in this setting. Inability to demonstrate a fistula on radiographic investigation should not preclude the diagnosis of this entity. If the cause of the pericardial fluid is not clearly diagnosed by available means, then a pericardial window should be performed for diagnostic as well as therapeutic reasons.

The pericardial sac should be irrigated, and adequate continuing drainage should be ensured. Although myocardial infarction may result in pericardial effusion or (rarely) tamponade, it does not cause pneumopericardium.

400. The answer is b. (*Greenfield, p 1411.*) Pancoast tumors are peripheral bronchogenic carcinomas that produce symptoms by involvement of extrapulmonary structures adjacent to the cupula. These structures include the nerve roots of C8 and T1, as well as the sympathetic trunk. Interruption of the cervical sympathetic trunk leads to miosis, ptosis, and anhidrosis, the triad of signs that constitutes Horner's syndrome. Involvement of the nerve roots causes pain along the corresponding dermatomes. The peripheral location of the neoplasm makes pulmonary signs, such as atelectasis, cough, and hemoptysis, unlikely.

401. The answer is d. (*Brunicardi, pp 602–603.*) The initial treatment for a chylothorax consists of nonoperative therapy: drainage of the chest cavity, bowel rest, and total parenteral nutrition. However, if chyle drainage continues to be greater than 500 mL/d, then operative ligation of the thoracic duct should be performed. The best approach is from a right thoracotomy.

402. The answer is c. (*Greenfield, pp 1389–1390.*) Bronchial carcinoid tumors rarely produce the carcinoid syndrome. They are slow-growing, infrequently metastatic tumors that histologically resemble carcinoid tumors of the small intestine. Over 80% arise in the major proximal bronchi, and their intraluminal growth is responsible for the frequent presentation of bronchial obstruction. The only therapy for this lesion is operative resection, because neither the primary tumor nor the infrequent lymph node metastasis is radiosensitive. The low malignant potential for this lesion is reflected by a long-term survival rate that approaches 90%.

403. The answer is c. (*Brunicardi, pp 556–557.*) Coin lesions have been defined as densities within the lung field of up to 3 cm, usually round, and free of signs of infections such as cavitation or surrounding infiltrates. Malignant solitary lesions may contain flecks of calcification, but heavy calcification or concentric rings of calcium generally suggest a benign etiology. The differential diagnosis for coin lesions includes primary pulmonary carcinomas, metastatic carcinomas to the lung, benign lung neoplasms such as chondromas, other benign lung processes such as granulomas, or vascular abnormalities such as arteriovenous malformations. Coin lesions should be biopsied to rule out malignancy. Transthoracic fine-needle aspiration (FNA) can be used for diagnosis, with an accuracy of 95% for peripheral pulmonary lesions, but is associated with a high rate of complications. Thoracoscopic resection can be used for peripheral nodules not amenable to FNA. If the patient has had a previous malignancy of tissue other than lung, the likelihood that the lesion represents a metastatic lesion depends on the tissue of origin of the previous malignancy. If all patients with a history of prior cancer are considered together, a lung nodule will be a new lung primary in 60%, a metastatic lesion in 25%, and a benign process in 15% of cases. However, 80% of solitary lesions in patients with melanoma represent metastatic disease, while only 40% of lesions in patients with breast cancer represent metastasis, and solitary lesions in patients with colon carcinoma are equally likely to be metastatic or primary lung cancers.

404. The answer is d. (*Greenfield, p 1397.*) The term *hamartoma* denotes a tumor that arises from the disorganized arrangement of tissues normally found in an organ. Pulmonary hamartomas are solitary lesions of the pulmonary parenchyma and generally appear as asymptomatic peripheral nodules; they represent the most common benign epithelial and mesodermal elements. Pulmonary chondromas consist of mesodermal elements alone and arise centrally in major bronchi, where they produce signs and symptoms of bronchial obstruction. Fibromas are the most common benign mesodermal tumors found in the lung; they may occur either within the lung parenchyma or, more commonly, within the tracheobronchial tree. Osteochondromas are lesions of bone and are not found in the lung. Aspergillomas are due to infection with the fungus *Aspergillus* and most commonly appear in the upper lobes as oval, friable, necrotic gray or yellow masses often surrounded by evidence of preexisting parenchymal lung disease.

405. The answer is b. (*Brunicardi, pp 877–878.*) The x-rays are consistent with a diagnosis of achalasia, a motility disorder of the esophagus that usually affects persons between 30 and 50 years of age. The x-rays show a classic beaklike narrowing of the distal esophagus and a large, dilated esophagus proximal to the narrowing. The diagnosis of achalasia is generally suspected on the basis of barium studies, but, because other esophageal disorders may mimic the condition, an esophageal motility study is usually required to confirm the diagnosis. The characteristic findings on a motility study are small-amplitude, repetitive, simultaneous postdeglutition contractions in the body of the esophagus, failure of the lower esophageal sphincter to relax after deglutition, and a higher than normal pressure in the body of the esophagus. Carcinoma of the esophagus is approximately seven times more frequent in persons who have achalasia than in the general population. Patients usually describe difficulty in swallowing solids and liquids.

406–410. The answers are 406-d, 407-a, 408-b, 409-e, 410-c. (*Greenfield, pp 1468–1478.*) The Argyll Robertson pupil (a pupil that constricts with accommodation but not in response to light) is characteristic of central nervous system syphilis and is associated with vascular system manifestations of that disease. *Treponema pallidum* invades the vasa vasorum and causes an obliterative endarteritis and necrosis. The resulting aortitis gradually weakens the aortic wall and predisposes it to aneurysm formation. Once an aneurysm has formed, the prognosis is grave. Massive isolated tricuspid regurgitation produces a markedly elevated venous pressure, usually manifested by a severely engorged (often pulsating) liver. If the venous pressure is sufficiently elevated, exophthalmos may result. Tricuspid regurgitation of rheumatic origin is almost never an isolated lesion, and the major symptoms of patients who have rheumatic heart disease are usually attributable to concurrent left heart lesions. Bacterial endocarditis from intravenous drug abuse is becoming an increasingly important cause of isolated tricuspid regurgitation. A Quincke pulse, which consists of alternate flushing and paling of the skin or nail beds, is associated with aortic regurgitation. Other characteristic features of the peripheral pulse in aortic regurgitation include the waterhammer pulse (Corrigan pulse, caused by a rapid systolic upstroke) and pulsus bisferiens, which describes a double systolic hump in the pulse contour. The finding of a wide pulse pressure provides an additional diagnostic clue to aortic regurgitation. Myocarditis, aortitis, and pericarditis have all been described in association with Reiter's syndrome; the original description included conjunctivitis, urethritis, and arthralgias. Although its cause is unknown, Reiter's syndrome is associated with HLA-B27 antigen, as are aortic regurgitation, pericarditis, and ankylosing spondylitis. Short stature, webbed neck, low-set ears, and epicanthal folds are the classic features of patients who have Turner's syndrome. Persons affected by the syndrome, which is commonly linked with aortic coarctation, are genotypically XO. However, females and males have been described with normal sex chromosome constitutions

(XX, XY) but with the phenotypic abnormalities of Turner's syndrome. Additional cardiac lesions associated with Turner's syndrome include septal defects, valvular stenosis, and anomalies of the great vessels.

411–415. The answers are 411-c, 412-a, 413-d, 414-b, 415-e. (*Greenfield, pp 1427–1431.*) Mediastinal pheochromocytomas comprise less than 2% of all pheochromocytomas. Their presentation is consistent with overproduction of catecholamines resulting in paroxysmal or sustained hypertension. Diagnosis is by measurement of urinary catecholamines and their metabolites. Thymomas are associated with myasthenia gravis, agammaglobulinemia, and red blood cell aplasia. These tumors are typically cystic and occur in the anterior mediastinum. Most thymic lesions associated with myasthenia gravis are hyperplastic rather than neoplastic. Renal stones occur in about half the cases of hyperparathyroidism. Other disorders sometimes associated with hyperparathyroidism include peptic ulcers, pancreatitis, and bone disease; central nervous system symptoms may also arise in connection with hyperparathyroidism. Occasionally, parathyroid adenomas occur in conjunction with neoplasms of other endocrine organs, a condition known as multiple endocrine adenomatosis. Persons afflicted with Hodgkin's disease have impaired cell-mediated immunity and are particularly susceptible to mycotic infections and tuberculosis. The severity of the immune deficiency correlates with the extent of the disease. The nodular sclerosing variant of primary mediastinal Hodgkin's disease is the most common type. Histology reveals Reed-Sternberg cells. Cystic teratomas, or dermoid cysts, include endodermal, ectodermal, and mesodermal elements. They are characteristically cystic and contain poorly pigmented hair, sebaceous material, and, occasionally, teeth. If there is a connection between the teratoma and the tracheobronchial tree, the patient may present with symptoms of coughing up hair or sebaceous material. Dermoid cysts occur in the gonads and central nervous system, as well as in the mediastinum. With rare exceptions, these lesions are benign.

416–420. The answers are 416-g; 417-e; 418-c; 419-a; 420-f. (*Greenfield, pp 212–213.*) Epinephrine is a circulating endogenous catecholamine, released mainly from the adrenal medulla, whose effects are mediated by binding of free circulating hormone to β_1 and β_2 receptors, with lesser effects on α adrenoreceptors. Norepinephrine is also endogenously produced, but acts locally through release at nerve synapses. Isoproterenol is a synthetic sympathomimetic that acts as a pure β agonist, resulting in profound vasodilator and chronotropic effects. Dopamine (not listed) is an endogenous catecholamine that is released into the circulation and acts by binding to α_1 receptors as well as to specific dopamine receptors in the renal, mesenteric, coronary, and intracerebral vascular beds, causing vasodilation. Dobutamine is a synthetic sympathomimetic structurally related to dopamine and is a potent inotrope but possesses only small chronotropic properties. Milrinone and amrinone (not listed) are bipyridine derivatives that induce vasodilation and inotropy via inhibition of phosphodiesterase, thereby enhancing intracellular concentrations of cyclic AMP. Digitalis exerts positive inotropic effects by inhibition of Na,K-activated ATPase, resulting in increased intracellular sodium concentrations, which lead to increased intracellular calcium concentrations. Digitalis is also used in the management of arrhythmias, most commonly atrial fibrillation. Nitroprusside and nitroglycerin (not listed) are systemic vasodilators. While nitroprusside causes balanced arterial and venous dilation, the effects of nitroglycerin are less pronounced in the arterial than in the venous system, often resulting in venous pooling.

Peripheral Vascular Problems

Questions

DIRECTIONS: Each item below contains a question followed by suggested responses. Select the **one best** response to each question.

421. A 64-year-old woman complains of calf pain and swelling following an uncomplicated left hemicolectomy for colon cancer. An ultrasound confirms the presence of deep vein thrombosis of the calf. Which of the following statements is true?

a. The patient can expect asymptomatic recovery if treated promptly with anticoagulants
b. This condition may be effectively treated with low-dose heparin
c. This condition may be effectively treated with pneumatic compression stockings
d. This condition may be effectively treated with acetylsalicylic acid
e. The patient is at risk for significant pulmonary embolism

422. For the first 6 h following surgical repair of a leaking abdominal aortic aneurysm in a 70-year-old man, oliguria (total urinary output of 25 mL since the operation) has become a concern. Which of the following is the most appropriate diagnostic test?

a. Renal scan
b. Aortogram
c. Left heart preload pressures
d. Urinary sodium concentration
e. Creatinine clearance

423. A 72-year-old man undergoes an aortobifemoral graft for symptomatic aortoiliac occlusive disease. The inferior mesenteric artery is ligated at its aortic attachment. Which of the following is the most reliable way to assess colonic viability postoperatively?

a. Intraoperative measurement of inferior mesenteric artery stump pressure
b. Intraoperative Doppler arterial signal in the sigmoid mesentery
c. Intraoperative observation of bowel peristalsis
d. Postoperative sigmoidoscopy
e. Postoperative barium enema

424. A 25-year-old woman presents to the emergency room complaining of redness and pain in her right foot up to the level of the midcalf. She reports that her right leg has been swollen for at least 15 years, but her left leg has been normal. On physical examination, she has a temperature of 39°C (102.2°F). The left leg is normal. The right leg is not tender, but it is swollen from the inguinal ligament down, and there is an obvious cellulitis of the right foot. Which of the following is the patient's most likely underlying problem?

a. Popliteal entrapment syndrome
b. Acute arterial insufficiency
c. Primary lymphedema
d. Deep-venous thrombosis
e. None of the above

425. A 76-year-old woman is admitted with back pain and hypotension. A CT scan (shown here) is obtained, and the patient is taken to the operating room. Three days after resection of a ruptured abdominal aortic aneurysm, she complains of severe, dull left flank pain and passes bloody mucus per rectum. Which of the following is the most likely diagnosis?

a. Staphylococcal enterocolitis
b. Diverticulitis
c. Bleeding AV malformation
d. Ischemia of the left colon
e. Bleeding colonic carcinoma

426. A 65-year-old man presents with symptoms of claudication and undergoes a lower extremity arteriogram (shown here). Based on the angiographic findings, which of the following risk factors does the patient most likely have?

a. Cigarette smoking
b. Alcoholism
c. Hypertension
d. Diabetes
e. Type I hyperlipoproteinemia

427. An 80-year-old man is found to have an asymptomatic abdominal mass. An arteriogram is obtained and is pictured here. Which of the following treatment recommendations is most appropriate?

a. Surgery should be performed, but a 20% chance of mortality is to be anticipated
b. Surgery should be performed only if symptoms develop
c. Surgery will improve his chance of five-year survival
d. Surgery this extensive should not be performed in a patient of his age
e. Surgery should be performed only if follow-up ultrasound demonstrates increasing size

428. A 75-year-old man is found by his internist to have an asymptomatic carotid bruit. Which of the following is the most appropriate next test?
a. Transcranial Doppler studies
b. Doppler ultrasonography (duplex)
c. Spiral CT angiography
d. Arch aortogram with selective carotid artery injections
e. Magnetic resonance arteriogram (MRA)

429. A 69-year-old man with mild hypertension and COPD presents with transient ischemic attacks and the angiogram shown here. Which of the following is the most appropriate treatment recommendation?

a. Medical therapy with aspirin 325 mg/d and medical risk factor management
b. Medical therapy with warfarin
c. Angioplasty of the carotid lesion followed by carotid endarterectomy if the angioplasty is unsuccessful
d. Carotid endarterectomy
e. Medical risk factor management and carotid endarterectomy if neurologic symptoms develop

430. A 55-year-old man with recent onset of atrial fibrillation presents with a cold, pulseless left lower extremity. He complains of left leg paresthesia and is unable to dorsiflex his toes. Following a successful popliteal embolectomy, with restoration of palpable pedal pulses, the patient is still unable to dorsiflex his toes. Which of the following is the most appropriate next step in management?

a. Electromyography (EMG)
b. Measurement of anterior compartment pressure
c. Elevation of the left leg
d. Immediate fasciotomy
e. Application of a posterior splint

431. Changes consistent with peripheral vascular insufficiency are found on an examination for complaints of calf pain on walking more than half a block. Distal pulses are absent, and the ankle-brachial index on the right is 0.5. Conservative management rather than reconstructive arterial surgery is generally recommended for patients with which of the following symptoms or signs of arterial insufficiency?

a. Ischemic ulceration
b. Ischemic neuropathy
c. Claudication
d. Nocturnal foot pain
e. Toe gangrene

432. A 64-year-old man with a history of a triple coronary bypass two years ago now has calf claudication. His only medication is a thiazide diuretic. You are considering administration of antiplatelet therapy. Which of the following statements concerning antiplatelet therapy is correct?

a. Aspirin has been shown to be an effective antiplatelet agent
b. Most antiplatelet agents work by enhancing prostaglandin synthesis
c. Antiplatelet agents have not been shown to increase patency rates of coronary artery bypass grafts
d. Aspirin can be used to treat deep-venous thrombophlebitis
e. The antiplatelet effect of aspirin will last for the life of the platelet, which is generally 20 to 25 days

433. A patient who has had angina as well as claudication reports feeling light-headed on exertion, especially when lifting and working with his arms. The subclavian steal syndrome is associated with which of the following hemodynamic abnormalities?

a. Antegrade flow through a vertebral artery
b. Venous congestion of the upper extremities
c. Occlusion of the carotid artery
d. Occlusion of the vertebral artery
e. Occlusion of the subclavian artery

434. You are reviewing the angiogram of a patient to be referred to you for a surgical opinion. Almost total occlusion of the aorta has occurred at the aortoiliac bifurcation. You would expect which of the following symptoms when you interview and examine the patient?

a. Claudication of the buttock and thigh
b. Causalgia of the lower leg
c. Retrograde ejaculation
d. Gangrene of the feet
e. Dependent rubor of the feet

435. A 66-year-old woman with a history of smoking has a slowly enlarging abdominal aortic aneurysm. Surgery is considered, but her hypertension, smoking, and diabetes put her at risk for associated coronary heart disease. What test is most predictive of postoperative ischemic cardiac events following peripheral vascular surgery?

a. Exercise stress testing
b. Gated blood pool studies that demonstrate an ejection fraction of 50% or less
c. Coronary angiography
d. Dipyridamole-thallium imaging
e. Transesophageal echocardiography

436. Fourteen months after a femoropopliteal bypass graft procedure, a 64-year-old man is admitted with a cold foot and no graft pulse. Urokinase infusion is begun. Which of the following statements regarding management is true?

a. Clot lysis is accomplished in 25% of patients
b. After successful clot lysis, surgical revision of the opened graft should be considered only if early reocclusion occurs
c. With optimal treatment, a 20% reocclusion rate is expected within one year
d. Urokinase is less successful in lysing acute thromboses of prosthetic grafts than those of vein grafts
e. Streptokinase is the preferred thrombolytic agent when treating graft occlusions

437. A 60-year-old man is admitted to the coronary care unit with a large anterior wall myocardial infarction. On his second hospital day, he begins to complain of the sudden onset of numbness in his right foot and an inability to move his right foot. On physical examination, the right femoral, popliteal, and pedal pulses are no longer palpable. Vascular consultation is obtained. Diagnosis of acute arterial embolus is made. Which of the following statements concerning this condition is true?

a. Appropriate management is embolectomy of the right femoral artery under general anesthesia
b. Noninvasive hemodynamic testing is required
c. Prophylactic exploration of the contralateral femoral artery should be done despite the presence of a normal pulse
d. The source of the embolus is most likely the left ventricle
e. Arteriography is mandatory prior to operative intervention

438. Which of the following statements concerning the condition depicted on the arteriogram shown here is true?

a. Surgery should be performed only if the patient is symptomatic
b. Limb loss is a definite risk in the untreated patient
c. The contralateral limb is affected in a similar fashion in over 85% of cases
d. Embolization is unlikely
e. Bleeding into the leg is the most common presentation

439. A 65-year-old male cigarette smoker reports onset of claudication of his right lower extremity approximately three weeks previously. His walking radius is limited to three blocks before the onset of claudication. Physical examination reveals palpable pulses in the entire left lower extremity, but no pulses are palpable below the right groin level. Noninvasive flow studies are obtained and are pictured here. Which of the following statements regarding this patient's condition is true?

a. Femoropopliteal bypass is indicated on a relatively urgent basis in order to salvage the right leg
b. The occlusive process is in the right superficial femoral artery, with flow to the right foot supplied by the profunda femoris artery
c. About half of patients with similar symptoms will ultimately require amputation
d. The occlusive process is most likely caused by embolic disease
e. The noninvasive studies suggest iliac as well as superficial femoral occlusive disease on the right side

440. Indications for placement of the device pictured in the abdominal x-ray shown here include which one of the following?

a. Recurrent pulmonary embolus despite adequate anticoagulation therapy
b. Axillary vein thrombosis
c. Pulmonary embolus in a patient with a perforated duodenal ulcer
d. Pulmonary embolus due to deep vein thrombosis of the lower extremity that occurs two weeks postoperatively
e. Pulmonary embolus in a patient with metastatic pancreatic carcinoma

441. Two days after admission to the hospital for a myocardial infarction, a 65-year-old man complains of severe, unremitting midabdominal pain. His cardiac index is 1.6. Physical examination is remarkable for an absence of peritoneal irritation or distention despite the patient's persistent complaint of severe pain. Serum lactate is 9 (normal is less than 3). Which of the following is the most appropriate next step in this patient's management?

a. Perform computed tomography
b. Perform mesenteric angiography
c. Perform laparoscopy
d. Perform flexible sigmoidoscopy to assess the distal colon and rectum
e. Defer decision to explore the abdomen until the arterial lactate is greater than 10

442. During evaluation for the repair of an expanding abdominal aortic aneurysm, a patient is discovered to have a horseshoe kidney. Which of the following is the optimal surgical approach?

a. Midline abdominal incision, preservation of the renal isthmus
b. Midline abdominal incision, division of the renal isthmus
c. Retroperitoneal approach, implantation of anomalous renal arteries
d. Nephrectomy, repair of aneurysm, chronic dialysis
e. Repair of aneurysm after autotransplantation of the kidney into the iliac fossa

443. A postoperative patient with swelling and pain in his right calf is suspected of having a deep-venous thrombosis. Prior to initiating treatment with anticoagulants, he requires a confirmatory examination. Both venography and Doppler ultrasound are available. Which of the following statements regarding contrast venography is true?

a. It is more accurate than Doppler analysis and B-mode ultrasound (duplex scan) at detecting thrombi in the deep veins responsible for pulmonary emboli
b. It identifies incompetent deep, superficial, and perforating veins
c. It is totally noninvasive, painless, and safe
d. It is easily performed in a vascular laboratory or radiology suite or at the bedside
e. It is particularly sensitive in identifying the proximal extent of an iliofemoral thrombus

444. A 52-year-old man with HIV and a history of intravenous drug use presents with a new heart murmur and a fever. He also complains of severe back pain and on further evaluation is found to have an enlarged, saccular-appearing abdominal aorta below the renal arteries. Which of the following statements is correct regarding his diagnosis and treatment options?

a. The most likely organisms involved are staphylococcus and salmonella
b. The mainstay of therapy should consist of antifungal antibiotics for three to six months
c. Surgical intervention is indicated only if he remains febrile after six weeks of intravenous antibiotics
d. The treatment of choice is aortic replacement with a synthetic graft and perioperative antibiotics only
e. The treatment of choice is six weeks of intravenous antibiotics followed by aortic replacement with a synthetic graft.

445. A 72-year-old woman with severe COPD that requires home oxygen is unable to ambulate inside her home without experiencing severe left hip pain. She was hospitalized one year ago for a viral pneumonia and was ventilator-dependent at that time for six weeks. On examination, her blood pressure is 165/80. She has weakly palpable bilateral femoral pulses. An angiogram demonstrates severe aortoiliac disease involving bilateral iliac vessels. Which of the following is the most appropriate vascular procedure for this patient?

a. Femorofemoral bypass
b. Axillofemoral bypass
c. Femoropopliteal bypass
d. Aortobifemoral bypass
e. Common femoral and profunda femoral endarterectomies

Peripheral Vascular Problems

Answers

421. The answer is e. (*Greenfield, pp 1883–1886.*) Both low-dose heparin and pneumatic compression stockings are acceptable prophylactic measures in patients at moderate risk for deep vein thrombosis; however, they are not effective against established thrombosis, the initial treatment for which is therapeutic heparinization (either with intravenous heparin or low-molecular-weight heparin administered subcutaneously). Salicylate has not been convincingly shown to have either a prophylactic or a therapeutic role in the treatment of deep vein thrombosis. Even following prompt, aggressive treatment of deep vein thrombosis of the calf, as many as half of affected patients will develop symptoms of chronic venous hypertension, and a larger number will have abnormal venous hemodynamic findings. Untreated vein thrombosis of the calf may propagate into the larger popliteal veins and cause life-threatening pulmonary embolism.

422. The answer is c. (*Greenfield, pp 208–215, 1818.*) By far the most likely cause of the oliguria observed in this patient is hypovolemia. Volume status would be best assessed by floating a Swan-Ganz catheter to measure the preload pressures in the left atrium (by inference from the pulmonary capillary wedge pressures). Patients who have had a leaking aneurysm and then a long, usually difficult operation with large surgical fields that collect third-space fluids may be intravascularly depleted despite large volumes of intravenous fluid and blood replacement. The proper management usually involves titrating the cardiac output by providing as much fluid as necessary to keep the wedge pressures near 15 mmHg. The other studies listed might become useful if urinary flow remains depressed after optimal cardiac output has been achieved, but in view of the probability of hypovolemia, they are not indicated as first diagnostic studies.

423. The answer is d. (*Schroeder, pp 299–303; Brunicardi, p 948.*) Viability of the colon can be evaluated intraoperatively by Doppler auscultation of the bowel mesentery and serosa, observation of bowel peristalsis, and measurement of the IMA stump pressure. A strong, pulsatile Doppler signal in the mesentery, active sigmoid peristalsis, a chronically occluded IMA, or a patent IMA with stump pressure greater than 40 mmHg presage viability of the sigmoid colon postoperatively. However, none of these observations excludes the possibility of late sigmoid ischemia. Serial postoperative sigmoidoscopic examination is the best predictor of ischemic colitis and in experienced hands allows assessment of the depth of ischemic injury before frank perforation has occurred. Barium enema is not as accurate as sigmoidoscopy in determining depth of injury and carries grave risks of contamination by barium and feces if perforation occurs.

424. The answer is c. *(Greenfield, pp 1897–1900.)* This patient is at high risk for developing cellulitis of her right foot because her underlying problem is unilateral primary lymphedema. Hypoplasia of the lymphatic system of the lower extremity accounts for more than 90% of cases of primary lymphedema. If edema is present at birth, it is referred to as congenital; if it starts early in life (as in this woman), it is called praecox; if it appears after age 35, it is tarda. The inadequacy of the lymphatic system accounts for the repeated episodes of cellulitis that these patients experience. Swelling is not seen with acute arterial insufficiency or with popliteal entrapment syndrome. Deep-venous thrombophlebitis will result in tenderness and is generally not a predisposing factor for cellulitis of the foot.

425. The answer is d. *(Brewster, pp 447–454, 1991.)* The CT scan reveals a fractured ring of calcification in the abdominal aorta with significant density in the paraaortic area. The inferior mesenteric artery (IMA) is always at risk in patients with the changes in the vessel wall characteristic of abdominal aneurysms, but particularly so in the presence of rupture and retroperitoneal dissection of blood under systemic arterial pressures. The incidence of ischemic colitis following abdominal aortic resection is about 2%. Blood flow to the left colon normally derives from the IMA with collateral flow from the middle and inferior hemorrhoidal vessels. The superior mesenteric artery (SMA) may also contribute via the marginal artery of Drummond. If the SMA is stenotic or occluded, flow to the left colon will be primarily dependent on an intact IMA. The IMA is usually ligated at the time of aneurysmorrhaphy. Patients at highest risk for diminished flow through collateral vessels are those with a history of visceral angina, those found to have a patent IMA at the time of operation, those who have suffered an episode of hypotension following rupture of an aneurysm, those in whom preoperative angiograms reveal occlusion of the SMA, and those in whom Doppler flow signals along the mesenteric border cease following occlusion of the IMA. Bowel ischemia recognized at the time of operation should be treated by reimplantation of the IMA into the graft to restore flow.

426. The answer is a. (*Greenfield, p 1740.*) The angiogram demonstrates an isolated segment of atherosclerotic occlusion of the superficial femoral artery. Patients who have isolated femoropopliteal disease tend to be smokers, whereas those who have isolated tibioperoneal disease frequently are diabetic. Hypertension and hyperlipidemia predispose to accelerated atherosclerosis. However, type I hyperlipoproteinemia (hyperchylomicronemia), which is associated with dramatic levels of plasma triglyceride and formation of xanthomas, does not cause accelerated vascular disease.

427. The answer is c. (*Greenfield, pp 1807–1819.*) Most abdominal aortic aneurysms (AAAs) are asymptomatic and are discovered on palpation by a physician. A radiograph of the abdomen is useful in demonstrating the aneurysm if there is calcification in the walls. Ultrasound is generally the first diagnostic procedure in confirming the presence of an aneurysm, with arteriography being performed if the aneurysm is considered large enough to require resection (typically greater than 4 to 5 cm in diameter). CT scan is also useful as a preoperative study in patients suspected of having aneurysms. All symptomatic AAAs should be repaired; the minimum size for asymptomatic AAAs before surgery should be entertained is controversial. For good surgical candidates (young, low operative risks), repair is advocated for aneurysms more than 4 cm in size. With leaking or ruptured aneurysms, the operative mortality associated with this emergency situation is significantly increased, with 50% of patients never reaching the hospital. The patient's age is not a contraindication to surgery, because several studies have demonstrated a low mortality rate (less than 5%) and satisfactory long-term survival and quality of life in elderly, even octogenarian, patients.

428. The answer is b. (*Greenfield, pp 1676–1677.*) Doppler ultrasonography (duplex) is the best initial test for screening patients with carotid disease. It has become a highly accurate test, often obviating the need for carotid arteriography prior to carotid endarterectomy. Carotid arteriography remains the gold standard when quantifying the degree of carotid stenosis, but it is usually performed after noninvasive testing suggests significant stenosis. Spiral CT angiography is a noninvasive modality that has been used to evaluate many segments of the vascular tree, but as yet its accuracy does not approach that of standard arteriography and it would certainly not be used in the initial evaluation of a patient with an asymptomatic bruit. Magnetic resonance arteriography (MRA) is also a modality that has enjoyed success in the investigation of carotid disease. Although not quite as accurate as standard arteriography, it has been used in conjunction with the duplex as a complementary study. Once again, because of its cost, MRA would not be used as the primary screening modality. Transcranial Doppler studies are used to assess the intracranial vasculature.

429. The answer is d. (*Executive Committee, pp 1421–1428.*) In a prospective, randomized, multicenter trial involving 1662 patients in a study known as the Asymptomatic Carotid Atherosclerosis Study, patients with asymptomatic carotid artery stenosis causing 60% or greater reduction in diameter and whose general health made them good candidates for elective surgery were found to have a significant reduction in the five-year risk for ipsilateral stroke with surgery compared with medically treated cohorts (5.1 versus 11.0%). Medically treated patients were treated with aspirin on a daily basis. Warfarin has not been shown to be effective in the management of patients with carotid disease. Angioplasty of carotid stenoses is being performed in some institutions but to date has not replaced surgery as the treatment for high-grade carotid stenoses.

430. The answer is d. (*Greenfield, pp 2093–2094.*) This case illustrates two (among many) conditions that lead to the anterior compartment syndrome, namely, acute arterial occlusion without collateral inflow and rapid reperfusion of ischemic muscle. Treatment for a compartment syndrome is prompt fasciotomy. Assessing a compartment syndrome and proceeding with fasciotomy are generally based on clinical judgment. Inability to dorsiflex the toes is a grave sign of anterior compartment ischemia. EMG studies and compartment pressure measurements would probably be abnormal, but are unnecessary in view of the known findings and would delay treatment. Mere elevation of the leg would be an ineffective means of relieving compartment pressure, although elevation should accompany fasciotomy. Application of a splint has no role in the acute management of this problem.

431. The answer is c. (*Brunicardi, pp 767–770.*) The major threat to patients with arterial occlusive disease is limb loss. Ischemic ulceration, neuropathy, rest pain, and gangrene represent advanced stages of arterial insufficiency and warrant reconstructive surgery whenever clinically feasible. Claudication, in most cases, reflects mild ischemia; the majority of affected patients are successfully managed without surgery. Most will stabilize or improve with development of increased collateral blood flow following institution of a program of daily exercise, cessation of smoking, and weight loss. Vasodilator drugs have been shown to have little benefit in the conservative management of intermittent claudication.

432. The answer is a. (*Willerson, pp 12A–18A.*) Aspirin exerts an antiplatelet effect that will last for the life of the platelet (approximately 7 to 10 days). Patients who take aspirin will experience its effect for 7 to 10 days after stopping the medication. Aspirin interferes with platelet function by inhibiting the synthesis of thromboxane A2 and the subsequent production of prostaglandins. The platelet does not have a nucleus and thus cannot remanufacture the prostaglandins necessary for its functioning. Antiplatelet agents are generally used to prevent thrombotic and embolic events on the arterial side of the circulation. The Canadian Cooperative Study has shown antiplatelet therapy to be effective in preventing strokes in men with carotid artery disease, but it is not used to treat thrombophlebitis in the deep-venous system. Antiplatelet therapy has been shown to increase graft patency rates following coronary artery bypass grafting if the medication is started preoperatively and continued postoperatively.

433. The answer is e. (*Brunicardi, pp 796–797.*) Atherosclerotic occlusion of the subclavian artery proximal to the vertebral artery is the anatomic situation that results in the subclavian steal syndrome. On being subjected to exercise, the involved extremity (usually the left) develops relative ischemia, which gives rise to reversal of flow through the vertebral artery with consequent diminished flow to the brain. The upper extremity symptom is intermittent claudication. Venous occlusive disease is not a feature of the syndrome. The operative procedure for treating the subclavian steal syndrome consists of delivering blood to the extremity by creating either a carotid-subclavian bypass or a subclavian-carotid transposition. Dilatation and stenting of the artery by endovascular techniques is effective as well.

434. The answer is a. (*Greenfield, pp 1725–1737.*) The slow progression of aortoiliac atherosclerotic occlusive disease is usually associated with the development of collateral flow through the lumbar branches of the aorta, anastomosing via retroperitoneal branches of the gluteal arteries with the profunda femoris arteries in the legs. This network of collateral vessels provides sufficient blood flow to nourish the extremities at rest but cannot prevent claudication of the upper and lower muscle groups of the leg during exercise. Sexual impotence, also part of Leriche's syndrome, is believed to be a result of bilateral stenosis or occlusion of the hypogastric (internal iliac) arteries. Retrograde ejaculation can occur after disruption of the sympathetic chain overlying the distal aorta and left iliac and can occur after dissection around these vessels during vascular reconstructions. Gangrene of the feet or toes is rarely seen unless distal embolization of atherosclerotic material from the aorta occludes the pedal or digital arteries. Dependent rubor is usually a sign of significant ischemia resulting from lower extremity occlusive and not aortoiliac disease. Causalgia or reflex sympathetic dystrophy is a disorder of the sympathetic nervous system that can affect the upper or lower extremities.

435. The answer is d. (*Boucher, pp 389–394; Pasternack, pp 13–17.*) The occurrence of perioperative ischemic cardiac events among patients undergoing peripheral vascular reconstruction has been found to correlate with gated blood pool ejection fractions of 35% or less and with reversible perfusion defects (thallium redistribution) on dipyridamole-thallium imaging. Ischemic rest pain or early onset of claudication after minimal exercise limits the effectiveness of stress testing as a screening procedure for occult coronary artery disease in this group of patients. Screening coronary angiography, followed by angioplasty or bypass of asymptomatic lesions, had an adverse effect on patient survival in a large prospective study of patients who had peripheral vascular surgery. Transesophageal echocardiography has no role in the preoperative screening of peripheral vascular patients.

436. The answer is c. (*Belkin, pp 769–773; Eisbud, pp 160–165.*) Management of acute graft occlusion must include both reestablishment of peripheral perfusion and correction of any underlying hemodynamic problem. Urokinase is associated with fewer allergic reactions than streptokinase and is the preferred thrombolytic agent. Treatment results in total clot lysis in 75% of patients. However, high reocclusion rates are observed (20% within one year) even if angioplasty or anastomotic revision is performed after successful lysis. Without surgical revision following clot lysis, a 50% reocclusion rate is expected within three months. Urokinase has proved equally successful in opening both vein and prosthetic graft thromboses.

437. The answer is d. (*Greenfield, pp 1568–1577.*) The heart is the most common source of arterial emboli and accounts for 90% of cases. Within the heart, sources include diseased valves, endocarditis, the left atrium in patients with unstable atrial arrhythmias, and mural thrombus on the wall of the left ventricle in patients with myocardial infarction. The diagnosis in this patient is clear, and therefore neither noninvasive testing nor arteriography is indicated. In fact, arteriography may prove too stressful for a patient undergoing an acute myocardial infarction. Embolectomy of the femoral artery can be performed under local anesthesia with minimal risk to the patient. Emboli typically lodge in one femoral artery; contralateral exploration is not indicated in the absence of signs or symptoms. The contralateral groin should always be prepared in case flow is not restored via simple thrombectomy, and femoral-femoral bypass is needed to provide inflow to the affected limb.

438. The answer is b. (*Greenfield, pp 1856–1859.*) Popliteal aneurysms are usually due to atherosclerosis, are bilateral 60 to 70% of the time, and are associated with extrapopliteal aneurysms 55% of the time (aortic, femoral). Many patients are asymptomatic when diagnosed (40%), but can develop embolization (25%) or thrombosis (40%) with resultant gangrene. Rupture of the aneurysm (less than 5%) can occur but is an uncommon presentation compared with embolization. All symptomatic popliteal aneurysms should be treated, usually with exclusion of the aneurysm (which is ligated and left in situ) combined with surgical bypass. Because of the risk of complications, in good surgical candidates, treatment of small asymptomatic popliteal aneurysms is recommended as well.

439. The answer is b. (*Greenfield, pp 1743–1747.*) This patient has occlusion of the right superficial femoral artery caused by atherosclerosis, and this is confirmed by both the physical examination and the flow study findings, which indicate a sharp decrease in the blood pressure below the level of the common femoral artery. Fewer than 10% of patients with claudication progress to gangrene and the need for amputation. Operative therapy would not be suggested at this time because it is quite likely that, with cessation of cigarette smoking and adherence to an exercise program, the patient could markedly improve his walking radius as collateral vessels enlarge to deliver more blood to the affected tissues. Operative therapy (femoropopliteal bypass) would be indicated at this time in this patient only if symptoms of rest pain or ischemic ulceration were present. Physical examination and flow studies indicate disease distal to the aortoiliac distribution.

440. The answer is a. *(Greenfield, pp 1884–1885.)* The Greenfield filter pictured on the x-ray is used to interrupt migration of emboli to the lungs from the veins below the level of the filter. It is indicated in patients who sustain a recurrent pulmonary embolus despite adequate anticoagulant therapy or in patients with pulmonary emboli who cannot receive anticoagulants because of a contraindication (e.g., bleeding ulcer, intracranial hemorrhage). The filter is not used in patients who sustain a single pulmonary embolus. It is placed in the inferior vena cava just below the renal veins and therefore would not be effective for emboli that arise cephalad to its position. Despite the hypercoagulable state seen in some patients with metastatic pancreatic cancer, anticoagulation can still be used as a first-line defense.

441. The answer is b. *(Greenfield, pp 1698–1702.)* Abdominal pain out of proportion to findings on physical examination is characteristic of intestinal ischemia. The etiology of ischemia may be embolic or thrombotic occlusion of the mesenteric vessels or nonocclusive ischemia due to a low cardiac index or mesenteric vasospasm. Differentiation among these etiologies is best made by mesenteric angiography. While not without serious risks, angiography also offers the possibility of direct infusion of vasodilators into the mesenteric vasculature in the setting of nonocclusive ischemia. This patient, with a recent myocardial infarction and a low cardiac index, is at risk for embolism of clot from a left ventricle mural thrombus as well as low-flow mesenteric ischemia. If embolism or thrombosis is found angiographically (usually involving the superior mesenteric artery), thrombolytic therapy can be attempted in the absence of suspicion of ischemic bowel. Otherwise, operative embolectomy or vascular bypass is indicated to restore flow. If occlusive disease cannot be demonstrated, efforts should be made to simultaneously increase cardiac output with inotropic agents and dilate the mesenteric vascular bed by angiographic instillation of papaverine, nitrates, or calcium channel blockers. Computed tomography is not helpful in delineating the cause of intestinal ischemia because it does not provide a sufficiently detailed image of the mesenteric vessels. Laparoscopy and/or laparotomy would be useful if ischemic bowel were suspected, although laparoscopy would not allow for adequate assessment of the visceral vessels. Flexible sigmoidoscopy, while useful in patients with ischemic colitis, has no role in the workup of mesenteric ischemia, which involves primarily the small intestine and right colon. Serum lactate is helpful in raising the suspicion of intestinal ischemia, but no absolute level should be used to decide whether or not to explore a patient.

442. The answer is c. (*O'Hara, pp 940–947.*) A horseshoe kidney is a fused kidney that occupies space on both sides of the vertebral column. The fusion is ordinarily at the lower poles, with the isthmus anterior to the aorta. The ureters run anterior to the isthmus, and the kidney frequently has an anomalous blood supply. The arterial supply to the kidney is highly variable, with vessels arising not only from the normal position in the aorta but also from a variable number of accessory segmental end arteries from the lower aorta and iliac arteries. Most cases of abdominal aortic aneurysm associated with a horseshoe kidney can be successfully resected, but these anomalies make the repair challenging. When the horseshoe kidney is recognized preoperatively, an arteriogram helps to define the vascular anatomy. The preferred operative approach is then via a retroperitoneal dissection. This allows the kidney and its collecting system to be swept anteromedially and provides relatively unobstructed access to the aneurysm. All anomalous renal arteries should be implanted into the graft after the aneurysm sac is opened, since the proportionate contribution from each may be hard to determine. The renal isthmus and collecting system restrict access to the aneurysm and make the anterior approach less desirable. Though division of the isthmus can be accomplished, there is high risk of calyceal or ureteral injury. Given the numerous arterial, venous, and collecting system anomalies, autotransplantation of the kidney is not a good option. The presence of the fresh intravascular foreign body (aortic graft) contraindicates dialysis because of the excessive risk of infecting the graft.

443. The answer is b. (*Greenfield, pp 1882–1883.*) Doppler analysis and B-mode ultrasonography (duplex scan) is the diagnostic test of choice in the evaluation of deep-venous thrombosis. The duplex scanning device is portable, and therefore the study is easily performed at the bedside, in a vascular laboratory, or in a radiology suite. It is completely noninvasive, painless, and safe. Venography must be performed in a radiology suite and requires the use of an intravenous contrast medium that is painful on injection and is itself thrombogenic. Incompetent deep, superficial, and perforating veins can be accurately identified by either venography or duplex scan. Both venography and duplex scan are highly accurate in diagnosing deep-venous thrombi that may result in pulmonary embolism. Significantly, however, contrast venography does not provide information regarding the proximal extent of an iliofemoral thrombus when it fails to fill the deep femoral system due to total occlusion by blood clot.

444. The answer is a. (*Brunicardi, pp 742–744.*) The patient has a mycotic aortic aneurysm, which is a sequela of infection, most commonly with either staphylococcus or salmonella. Treatment for infrarenal mycotic aortic aneurysms has traditionally been that an axillofemoral bypass is performed and then the involved intraabdominal aorta is excised. If the aorta is debrided and replaced, autogenous graft material is used (e.g., superficial femoral vein). Antibiotic therapy is also administered for three to six months.

445. The answer is b. (*Greenfield, pp 1731–1738.*) Given her comorbidities, the patient should undergo axillofemoral bypass grafting. In a patient with severe symptoms of claudication that are interfering with his or her lifestyle, intervention is indicated. In a young, healthy patient with unilateral iliac artery occlusive disease, when angioplasty is not a treatment option, an aortofemoral bypass offers excellent long-term relief. Aortobifemoral bypass, while clearly the most risky of the treatment options offered, provides the best long-term patency. In elderly patients with severe comorbidities who are considered at high risk for complications, extraanatomic bypasses (femorofemoral or axillofemoral bypasses) offer fair long-term patencies while not subjecting the patient to the risks of general anesthesia. Femorofemoral bypass offers the additional benefit of not disturbing sexual function; however, femorofemoral bypass is not an option in a patient with bilateral iliac artery disease. Axillofemoral bypass grafts are an alternative to aortofemoral procedures, but have a lower five-year patency rate and should be reserved for high-risk patients with bilateral iliac disease or an infected aortic aneurysm or graft.

Urology

Questions

DIRECTIONS: Each item below contains a question followed by suggested responses. Select the **one best** response to each question.

446. A 65-year-old woman complains of urinary incontinence and desires a surgical consultation regarding treatment options. Which of the following statements about incontinence is correct?

a. Pelvic floor exercises improve symptoms in patients with mild urge incontinence
b. Continuous urinary incontinence suggests the presence of a vesicovaginal or vesicocutaneous fistula
c. Anticholinergic medications may improve symptoms in patients with mild stress incontinence
d. Spinal cord injuries at the level of the cauda equina can result in urge incontinence
e. Urge incontinence never improves after a urethral sling procedure

447. A 26-year-old man is seen in the emergency ward because of symptoms of urinary burning, frequency, and urgency. Urinalysis shows bacteriuria. His meatus is inferiorly displaced on the glans. Which of the following statements regarding hypospadias is correct?

a. It is often associated with chordee (ventral curvature of the penis)
b. It is associated with undescended testes in more than 50% of cases
c. It is a rare fusion defect of the posterior male urethra
d. It occurs sporadically, without evidence of familial inheritance
e. The most common location is penoscrotal

448. A 60-year-old man sees a urologist for what he describes as bloody urine. A urine sample is positive for cytologic evidence of malignancy. Cystoscopy confirms the presence of superficial transitional cell carcinoma. Which of the following is the recommended treatment for stage A (superficial and submucosal) transitional cell carcinoma of the bladder?

a. Local excision
b. Radical cystectomy
c. Radiation therapy
d. Topical (intravesicular) chemotherapy
e. Systemic chemotherapy

449. A 36-year-old man presents to the emergency room with renal colic. A radiograph reveals a 1.5-cm stone. Which of the following statements regarding this disorder is correct?

a. Conservative treatment including hydration and analgesics will not result in a satisfactory outcome
b. Serial kidney-ureter-bladder (KUB) radiographs should be used to follow this patient
c. Urinalysis will nearly always reveal microhematuria
d. When the acute event is correctly treated, this disease seldom recurs
e. Elevated BUN and creatinine are expected

450. An eight-month-old boy is seen by a pediatrician for the first time. The physician notes that there are no testes in the scrotum. Which of the following is the optimal management of bilateral undescended testicles in an infant?

a. Immediate surgical placement into the scrotum
b. Chorionic gonadotropin therapy for one month; operative placement into the scrotum before age one if descent has not occurred
c. Observation until the child is two years old because delayed descent is common
d. Observation until age five; if no descent by then, plastic surgical scrotal prostheses before the child enters school
e. No therapy; reassurance of the parent that full masculinization and normal spermatogenesis are likely even if the testicle does not fully descend

451. A 32-year-old medical student notes an asymptomatic mass in his right testicle. On examination, the mass cannot be transilluminated. The urologist suspects seminoma. Seminoma is accurately described by which of the following statements?

a. It is the most common type of testicular cancer
b. Metastases to liver and bone are frequently found
c. It does not respond to radiation
d. The five-year survival rate approaches 50%
e. Common presentation is that of a painful lump that transilluminates

452. A 10-year-old boy presents to the emergency room with testicular pain of 5 h duration. The pain was of acute onset and woke the patient from sleep. On physical examination, he is noted to have a high-riding, indurated, and markedly tender left testis. Pain is not diminished by elevation. Urinalysis is unremarkable. Which of the following statements regarding the patient's diagnosis and treatment is true?

a. There is a strong likelihood that this patient's father or brother has had or will have a similar event
b. Operation should be delayed until a technetium scan clarifies the diagnosis
c. The majority of testicles that have undergone torsion can be salvaged if surgery is performed within 24 h
d. If torsion is found, both testes should undergo orchiopexy
e. The differential diagnosis includes spermatocele

453. A patient is noted incidentally on an ultrasound to have a right renal mass. Which of the following statements is true regarding further workup and treatment of a renal mass?

a. Presence of a simple cyst requires follow-up imaging in a year
b. Diagnosis of an angiomyolipoma of the kidney requires surgical resection
c. Presence of a 3-cm lesion suspicious for renal cell carcinoma can be treated with a partial nephrectomy
d. CT scanning is diagnostic for oncocytomas
e. Presence of a solid, enhancing lesion in the right kidney should always be biopsied percutaneously

454. A 48-year-old African American man undergoes a screening exam. His prostate-specific antigen (PSA) is found to be high. A rectal exam confirms a mass in the prostate, and the biopsy is read as carcinoma. Which of the following statements regarding carcinoma of the prostate is true?

a. It has a higher incidence among American blacks than among other American ethnic groups
b. A single microscopic focus of prostate cancer discovered on transurethral resection of the prostate (TURP) is an indication for radical prostatectomy
c. It arises initially in the gland's central portion
d. It commonly produces osteoclastic bony metastases
e. Screening for PSA, although easily done, offers no advantage over simple rectal examination in the detection of the disease

455. A 60-year-old man seeks medical attention because of increasing difficulty in urination (decreased flow, straining, hesitancy). A prostate biopsy proves benign. Which of the following statements regarding benign prostatic hyperplasia (BPH) is true?

a. Initial management of BPH is transurethral resection of the prostate
b. Low bladder pressures and low flow rates are suggestive of outflow obstruction
c. All patients with BPH should be treated to prevent renal failure due to outflow obstruction
d. Indications for surgery include urinary retention refractory to medical therapy and recurrent urinary tract infections (UTIs)
e. Hypernatremia is a complication of transurethral resection of the prostate for BPH

456. During the course of an operation on an unstable, critically ill patient, the left ureter is lacerated through 50% of its circumference. If the patient's condition is felt to be too serious to allow time for definitive repair, which of the following would be an appropriate damage control procedure?

a. Placement of an external stent through the proximal ureteral stump with delayed reconstruction
b. Ipsilateral nephrectomy
c. Placement of a catheter from the distal ureter through an abdominal wall stab wound
d. Placement of a suction drain adjacent to the injury without further manipulation that might convert the partial laceration into a complete disruption
e. Bringing the proximal ureter up to the skin as a ureterostomy

457. A pedestrian is hit by a speeding car. Radiologic studies obtained in the emergency room, including a retrograde urethrogram, are consistent with a pelvic fracture with a rupture of the urethra superior to the urogenital diaphragm. Which of the following is the most appropriate next step in this patient's management?

a. Immediate percutaneous nephrostomy
b. Immediate placement of a Foley catheter through the urethra into the bladder to align and stent the injured portions
c. Immediate reconstruction of the ruptured urethra after initial stabilization of the patient
d. Immediate exploration of the pelvis for control of hemorrhage from pelvic fracture and drainage of pelvic hematoma
e. Immediate placement of a suprapubic cystostomy tube

Urology

Answers

446. The answer is b. (*Brunicardi, pp 1543–1544.*) There are several types of urinary incontinence: stress, urge, overflow, and total. Stress incontinence in women is associated with previous birth trauma, aging, and neurologic injuries. Nonoperative treatment includes estrogen therapy, pelvic floor exercises, and timed voiding. Surgical therapy in women consists of a urethral sling procedure. Urge incontinence can be treated symptomatically with anticholinergic medications, biofeedback, and timed voiding. If there is a contributory component from stress incontinence, urge incontinence may improve with a urethral sling procedure. A spinal cord injury above the level of the sacrum results in a hyperreflexic bladder and urge incontinence. Overflow incontinence may result from bladder outlet obstruction. Total incontinence, or continuous leakage of urine, suggests the presence of a fistula and typically requires surgical intervention.

447. The answer is a. (*Brunicardi, pp 1555–1556.*) Hypospadias is a common congenital anomaly of the penis resulting from incomplete development of the anterior urethra. It occurs in about 1 in 300 live births and is believed to have a multifactorial genetic mode of inheritance. Of those with hypospadias, about 7% have a father with the disorder, 14% a brother, and 20% a second family member. Hypospadias occurs in the corona in about 75% of cases, where it is often accompanied by chordee. Undescended testes occur in about 10% of cases of hypospadias, as do inguinal hernias. Hypospadias in the scrotal area is associated with bilateral undescended testes and infertility and must be differentiated from pseudohermaphroditism and adrenogenital syndrome.

448. The answer is d. (*Greenfield, pp 2186–2188.*) Bladder cancer represents 2% of all cancers, and 90% of bladder cancers are of transitional cell origin. It is most prevalent among men with a history of heavy smoking and is usually multifocal and superficial, even when recurrent. When the disease is still superficial, transurethral resection of visible lesions and intravesicular chemotherapy are most often recommended. More radical surgical resection is reserved for advanced stages of the disease.

449. The answer is a. (*Greenfield, pp 2181–2186.*) Initial management of kidney stones should include hydration and analgesics. However, as this patient's stone is larger than 1 cm, it is unlikely to pass spontaneously, though stones smaller than 0.5 cm usually do pass spontaneously. The size of the stone also makes a high-grade obstruction more likely; therefore, an intravenous pyelogram (IVP) must be urgently performed. A high-grade obstruction will require nephrostomy or the passage of a ureteral stent. If the stone is completely occluding the lumen of the ureter, urinalysis may not show microhematuria and thus may be misleading. Approximately 50% of patients may have a recurrence within 5 to 10 years. Elevated BUN and creatinine are expected only in the setting of an obstructed single functioning kidney.

450. The answer is b. (*Greenfield, p 2052.*) Surgical intervention consisting of inguinal orchiopexy, should be performed before one year of age. By the second year, a testicle not in the cooler environment of the scrotal sac will begin to undergo histologic changes characterized by reduced spermatogonia. Testicles left longer in the undescended state not only have a higher incidence of malignant degeneration, but are inaccessible for examination. If a malignancy should occur, diagnosis will be delayed. There is also a substantial psychological burden when children reach school age or are otherwise subjected to exposure of their deformed genitalia. Gel-filled prostheses are generally inserted when a testicle cannot be placed in the scrotum. Close follow-up by a physician until the late teens is indicated in all patients who have had an undescended testicle. Since these patients may be at increased risk for malignancy throughout life, careful training should be given in self-examination.

451. The answer is a. (*Greenfield, pp 2194–2195.*) Seminomas tend to grow slowly and metastasize late. They usually present as a nonpainful lump that does not transilluminate. They represent about 40% of malignant testicular tumors; embryonal cell carcinoma and teratocarcinoma each represent about 25%. Because most tumors have mixed elements, they are usually classified according to the most malignant cell type encountered, whatever the predominant cell type. When metastases occur, they are usually along the regional lymphatic drainage pathways to the iliac, aortic, and renal lymph nodes. Because of their slow growth and radiosensitivity, seminomas are associated with a 90% five-year survival rate. Therapy generally consists of removing the affected testis and sampling the lymph nodes (usually external iliac) for evidence of metastasis. If metastases are present, radiation therapy is given locally to areas of known involvement. Radiation therapy is highly effective in seminoma, and metastatic disease may be palliated for extended periods.

452. The answer is d. (*Greenfield, pp 2052–2053.*) Testicular torsion occurs commonly in adolescents. The underlying pathology is secondary to an abnormally narrowed testicular mesentery with tunica vaginalis surrounding the testis and epididymis in a bell clapper deformity. As the testis twists, it comes to lie in a higher position within the scrotum. Urinalysis is usually negative. Elevation will not provide a decrease in pain (negative Prehn sign); a positive Prehn sign might indicate epididymitis. A ^{99m}Tc pertechnetate scan or Doppler ultrasound may be helpful in making the diagnosis if clinical suspicion of torsion is low; however, operation should not be delayed in order to maximize testicular salvage. This patient's presentation warrants immediate operation. Both the affected and the unaffected testes should undergo orchiopexy. The differential diagnosis between torsion of the testicle and epididymitis is sometimes quite difficult. On occasion, the physician has to explore a patient with epididymitis just to rule out a torsion of the testicle.

Epididymitis usually occurs in sexually active males. Urinalysis is usually positive for inflammatory cells, and urethral discharge is often present.

Spermatocele is a cyst of an efferent ductule of the rete testis. It presents as a painless, transilluminable cystic mass that is separate from the testes.

453. The answer is c. (*Brunicardi, pp 1531–1532.*) Lesions that are solid and enhancing on CT scan should raise the suspicion for a renal cell carcinoma. Because of a high false-negative rate, suspicious lesions should not routinely be biopsied. For renal cell cancers less than 4 cm, a partial nephrectomy can be performed, but for larger lesions, a radical nephrectomy (which includes the kidney, ipsilateral adrenal gland, and perirenal fat) is indicated. Benign kidney lesions include simple cysts, angiomyolipomas, and oncocytomas. Simple cysts do not require further follow-up, but multiple septations or calcifications should increase suspicion for malignancy. Angiomyolipomas can be diagnosed based on appearance on CT scan and do not require removal; larger lesions are at increased risk for hemorrhagic complications. Oncocytomas can be diagnosed only on pathology.

454. The answer is a. (Brunicardi, pp 1535–1538; Greenfield, pp 2191–2195.) Prostate cancer is one of the most frequent causes of male cancer deaths; it is common, affecting one in every six men in the United States during their lifetime. Family history, African American race, and diet have all been implicated as risk factors. Prostate cancer (adenocarcinoma) arises initially in the periphery of the gland. Therefore, one of the best screening tests is careful rectal examination (DRE). Screening for prostate cancer with prostate-specific antigen (PSA), which is increased not only in prostate cancer but in benign conditions such as benign prostatic hypertrophy (BPH) as well, and DRE increases the detection rate. However, routine PSA screening is controversial because of the low positive predictive value. Spread of prostate cancer is by direct local extension and via lymphatic and vascular channels. The most common locations of distant metastases are in the axial skeleton with osteoblastic bony lesions. A single focus of disease discovered on TURP or simple prostatectomy is considered stage T_1 by the TNM classification system; management of these lesions is dependent on the patient's life expectancy—for example, expectant management in patients older than 65 years of age. More locally advanced disease is treated with radiation or surgical prostatectomy.

455. The answer is d. (Brunicardi, pp 1529–1531.) Indications for surgery in patients with BPH include urinary retention refractory to medical therapy, upper tract dilation, renal insufficiency secondary to outflow obstruction, and bladder stones. Recurrent urinary tract infections are also an indication for surgical intervention. BPH increases in incidence with age, and is almost universal in men in their 90s. Treatment should be directed at alleviating symptoms; initial management consists of alpha blockade. Outflow obstruction is characterized by high bladder pressures and low flow rates. Low bladder pressures and low flow rates are present when the bladder muscles are poorly contractile due to overdistention and persistent obstruction. Although persistent outflow obstruction can ultimately lead to renal failure, BPH does not always progress to this stage. Surgical treatment for BPH consists of transurethral resection of the prostate (TURP). Because of the use of large volumes of hypotonic fluid during TURP, patients should be monitored postoperatively for hyponatremia due to hemodilution secondary to absorption of the irrigation solution.

456. The answer is a. (*Greenfield, pp 360–361; Moore, pp 835–837.*) If time and the patient's condition permit, primary ureteral reconstruction should be carried out. In the middle third of the ureter, this will usually consist of ureteroureterostomy (primary anastamosis) using absorbable sutures over a stent. If the injury involves the upper third, ureteropyeloplasty may be necessary. In the lower third, ureteral implantation into the bladder using a tunneling technique is preferred. If time does not permit definitive repair, suction drainage adjacent to the injured segment alone is inadequate; placement of a catheter into the proximal ureter is an acceptable alternative that would allow reconstruction to be performed later. The creation of a watertight seal is difficult and nephrectomy may be required if the injury occurs during a procedure in which a vascular prosthesis is being implanted (e.g., an aortic reconstructive procedure) and contamination of the foreign body by urine must be avoided.

457. The answer is e. (*Brunicardi, pp 1545–1546.*) If a rupture of the urethra is suspected, a retrograde urethrogram (RUG) should be obtained before any attempts are made to place a Foley catheter, as efforts to do so may result in the creation of multiple false passages or conversion of a partial laceration into complete rupture. If there is incomplete disruption of the urethra, a transurethral Foley catheter can be cautiously placed across the injury. However, if there is complete disruption, a suprapubic catheter is placed temporarily and definitive repair is delayed four to six months, at which time the hematoma will have resolved and the prostate will have descended into the proximity of the urogenital diaphragm. Percutaneous nephrostomy has no role in the management of this problem.

Orthopedics

Questions

DIRECTIONS: Each item below contains a question followed by suggested responses. Select the **one best** response to each question.

458. An 18-year-old football player is seen in the emergency ward with severe knee pain incurred after being hit by a tackler while running. Physical exam is consistent with tearing of a meniscus. Meniscal tears usually result from which of the following circumstances?

a. Hyperextension
b. Flexion and rotation
c. Simple hyperflexion
d. Compression
e. Femoral condylar fracture

459. A patient has severe pain, pallor, and paresthesias distal to an extremity injury. There is concern regarding the dressing/cast associated with this injury. Which of the following is associated with a Volkmann's ischemic contracture?

a. Intertrochanteric femoral fracture
b. Supracondylar fracture of the humerus
c. Posterior dislocation of the knee
d. Traumatic shoulder separation
e. Colles (silver fork) fracture

460. While playing with his children, a 44-year-old man falls and lands on his right shoulder. There is immediate pain and deformity. In an uncomplicated dislocation of the glenohumeral joint, the humeral head usually dislocates primarily in which of the following directions?

a. Anteriorly
b. Superiorly
c. Posteriorly
d. Laterally
e. Medially

461. A 10-year-old girl falls and fractures her femur. You try to explain what, if any, growth disturbances might be expected in the future because of the location of the fracture. The most severe epiphyseal growth disturbance is likely to result from which of the following types of fracture?

a. Fracture dislocation of a joint adjacent to an epiphysis
b. Fracture through the articular cartilage extending into the epiphysis
c. Transverse fracture of the bone shaft on the metaphyseal side of the epiphysis
d. Separation of the epiphysis at the diaphyseal side of the growth plate
e. Crushing injury compressing the growth plate

462. EMS calls to notify you that they are bringing a young man to your ER with multiple injuries incurred subsequent to a fall down a very steep hill. Which of the following fractures is most commonly seen in healthy bones subjected to violent falls?

a. Colles fracture
b. Femoral neck fracture
c. Intertrochanteric fracture
d. Clavicular fracture
e. Vertebral compression fracture

463. A 29-year-old construction worker fell 15 feet from a roof and broke his right humerus, as depicted in the accompanying radiograph. Given his injury, which of the following nerves is most at risk?

a. Median nerve
b. Radial nerve
c. Posterior interosseous nerve
d. Ulnar nerve
e. Ascending circumflex brachial nerve

464. In a failed suicide gesture, a depressed student severs her radial nerve at the wrist. Which of the following is her expected disability?

a. Loss of ability to extend the wrist
b. Loss of ability to flex the wrist
c. Wasting of the intrinsic muscles of the hand
d. Sensory loss over the thenar pad and the thumb web
e. Palmar insensitivity

465. After being injured by a bull on his mother's farm, a young man is placed in a cast for a supracondylar fracture of his humerus. He begins to experience intense pain and weakness in the ipsilateral hand. Compartment pressures are measured and are markedly elevated. Which of the following statements regarding compartment syndromes following orthopedic injuries is true?

a. The first sign is usually loss of pulse in the extremity
b. Passive flexion of the extremity proximal to the involved compartment will aggravate the pain
c. Surgical decompression (fasciotomy) is necessary only as a last resort
d. These syndromes are most commonly associated with supracondylar fractures of the humerus and tibial shaft
e. The syndrome is often painless

466. Your son falls and breaks his tibia while ice skating. The orthopedic surgeon suggests an operation to reduce and fixate the fracture. You recall from your medical school reading that there is controversy regarding open versus closed treatment of fractures. In contrast to closed reduction, which of the following is true regarding the open reduction of a fracture?

a. Produces a shorter healing time
b. Decreases trauma to the fracture site
c. Produces a higher incidence of nonunion
d. Reduces the risk of infection
e. Requires longer periods of immobilization

DIRECTIONS: Each group of questions below consists of lettered options followed by a set of numbered items. For each numbered item, select the **one** lettered option with which it is **most** closely associated. Each lettered option may be used once, more than once, or not at all.

Questions 467–470

For each description, select the type of fracture or dislocation with which it is most likely to be associated.

a. Navicular (scaphoid) fracture
b. Monteggia's deformity
c. Greenstick fracture
d. Spiral fracture
e. Posterior shoulder dislocation

467. A patient has a seizure with gross tonic-clonic movements.

468. A patient experiences prolonged pain and radiologic evidence of nonhealing after an injury.

469. A 30-year-old cyclist falls and injures her forearm. The radial head is dislocated and the proximal third of the ulna is fractured.

470. A patient has tenderness in the anatomical snuffbox.

Questions 471–474

For each description, select the type of bone disease with which it is most likely to be associated.
a. Osteogenesis imperfecta
b. Osteopetrosis
c. Osteitis fibrosa cystica
d. Osteomalacia
e. Osteitis deformans

471. Your patient has renal stones and needs an operation in the neck. Parathyroid hormone levels are elevated.

472. Your patient is taking high doses of vitamin D to supplement a defect in the mineralization of adult bone due to abnormalities in vitamin D metabolism.

473. A genetically determined disorder in the structure or processing of type I collagen may require your patient to wear various orthoses to protect himself.

474. A patient has bossing of his frontal bones and an abnormal skull radiograph. (Synonym for Paget's disease.)

Questions 475–477

For each description, select the type of bone lesion with which it is most likely to be associated.

a. Osteoma
b. Osteoid osteoma
c. Osteoblastoma
d. Osteosarcoma
e. Paget's disease
f. Ewing's sarcoma

475. An 11-year-old boy presents with pain in his right leg. A radiograph shows a sunburst appearance with bone destruction, soft tissue mass, new bone formation, and sclerosis limited to the metaphysis of the lower femur.

476. A 25-year-old man presents with severe pain in the left femur. The pain is relieved by aspirin. On plain film, a 0.5-cm lucent lesion, which is surrounded by marked reactive sclerosis, is seen.

477. A 12-year-old boy complains of pain in his left leg that is worse at night. He has been experiencing fevers and also has a 9-lb weight loss. X-ray demonstrates an aggressive lesion with a permeative pattern of bone lysis and periosteal reaction. There is an associated large soft tissue mass as well. Pathology demonstrates the tumor to be of the round cell type.

Orthopedics

Answers

458. The answer is b. (*Brunicardi, p 1711.*) Most meniscal tears are produced by flexion and rapid rotation. A classic example (football knee) involves a player who is hit while running. The knee, supporting all the player's weight, usually is slightly flexed, and the foot is anchored to the ground by cleats. Impact from an opposing player usually causes rotation almost entirely restricted to the knee. The injury involves rapid rotation of the flexed femoral condyles about the tibial plateau, which most frequently tears the medial meniscus. (Less frequently, the lateral meniscus is torn.) A tear in the inner free border of the cartilage is also common whenever excessive rotation without flexion or extension occurs. Early surgical removal of the displaced menisci is usually recommended to prevent further damage to the cartilage or ligaments.

459. The answer is b. (*Brunicardi, p 349.*) Compromise of blood supply to the muscles of the forearm can lead to a compartment syndrome and permanent serious functional deformity of the arm. Any patient with a compressive dressing or cast of the upper extremity can experience this potential catastrophe. Whenever a patient has increasing pain in the presence of a circular dressing around the arm or forearm, the dressing should be removed immediately. If there is tenderness on either the ulnar or the dorsal aspect of the forearm, a fasciotomy should be considered.

460. The answer is a. (*Brunicardi, pp 1694–1696.*) The glenohumeral joint is bounded posteriorly by the teres minor and infraspinatus muscles and partially by the long head of the triceps. It is bounded laterally by the powerful deltoid muscle; superiorly, the acromion process precludes upward dislocation. However, anteriorly and inferiorly the pectoralis major and the long head of the biceps do not completely stabilize the glenohumeral joint; in this region the articular ligaments and joint capsule provide the major structural support. Thus, the joint is not strongly supported in its anteroinferior aspect, and consequently anterior (or anteroinferior) dislocations are the most common glenohumeral dislocations. The humeral head is driven anteriorly, which tears the shoulder capsule, detaches the labrum from the glenoid, and produces a compression fracture of the humeral head. Most glenohumeral dislocations result from a posteriorly directed force on an arm that is partially abducted. Posterior dislocation is much rarer and should raise the possibility of a seizure as the precipitating cause.

461. The answer is e. *(Brunicardi, pp 1654–1655.)* Longitudinal growth of bone follows ossification of cartilage that forms at the epiphyseal plate. Fractures that involve separation of the growth plate (type I; almost always on the diaphyseal side) may be realigned; normal growth usually follows epiphyseal separation because the proliferative cells are still attached to their blood supply in the bone epiphysis. Fractures that extend perpendicular to and through the epiphysis (types II, III, IV) may result in the formation of bony bridges across the epiphysis that can disrupt later growth. Though all the fractures listed place the epiphyseal growth plate in some jeopardy, crushing injuries to the epiphysis (type V) have the worst prognosis; numerous bony bridges may form and prevent longitudinal growth.

462. The answer is d. *(Brunicardi, p 1655.)* Postmenopausal osteoporosis is responsible for a large number of fractures in elderly women. Though bone mineralization is normal in osteoporosis, total bone mass and trabecular volume are decreased. Common fracture sites are the vertebrae, distal radius, and hip. Vertebral compression fractures are often sustained by elderly men and women even without trauma. A minor fall on an outstretched hand can lead to a Colles fracture when the distal radius is weakened by osteoporosis. Similarly, either a femoral neck fracture or an intertrochanteric fracture can follow a fall on the hip. Clavicular fractures are less likely to result from osteoporosis. While these fractures occur in both children and adults, they are common in healthy children and young adults after violent falls onto an outstretched hand.

463. The answer is b. *(Brunicardi, p 1696.)* The radiograph demonstrates a transverse fracture of the distal half of the humeral shaft. The radial nerve runs in a groove on the posterior aspect of the humerus as it courses into the forearm compartment and is therefore at high risk of injury. If the nerve injury is apparent before any manipulation has been done, the fracture should be reduced; the nerve injury should be observed, since the nerve function will likely improve with time. If the nerve injury is present only after reduction, immediate surgical exploration is warranted because the nerve might be trapped in the fracture site. At this level of the arm, the ulnar and median nerves are well protected by muscle. The posterior interosseous nerve is a distal branch of the radial nerve and may be injured in fractures near the radial head, but it is in no danger from injuries at the level seen in this radiograph. There is no ascending circumflex brachial nerve.

464. The answer is d. *(Brunicardi, p 1771.)* An injury to the radial nerve at the wrist would cause primarily sensory abnormalities. The dorsum of the hand from the radial aspect of the fourth digit over the thumb, including the thenar pad and thumb web, becomes insensate after severance of the radial nerve at the wrist. Radial injuries more proximally would impair extension of the wrist and digits as well as forearm supination.

465. The answer is d. *(Brunicardi, p 349.)* Compartment syndromes result from increasing pressures in the fascial compartments of the arm or leg. When the pressure in the muscles is greater than that of the capillaries, ischemia and necrosis of the muscles occur even though the arterial pressure is still high enough to produce pulses; pulselessness is an unreliable sign. Extreme pain (out of proportion to the injury), pain on passive extension of the fingers or toes, pallor of the extremity, motor paralysis, and paresthesias are all components of the syndrome. The patient will usually hold the injured part in a position of flexion to maximally relax the fascia and reduce the pain; passive extension will usually produce severe pain. The diagnosis can be confirmed by measuring intracompartmental pressures, but whenever physical findings or symptoms are suspicious, immediate surgical decompression by fasciectomy is indicated, since delay is likely to lead to irreversible damage.

466. The answer is c. *(Brunicardi, pp 1681–1686.)* Open reduction of a fracture involves the restoration of normal bone alignment under direct observation at surgery. In effect, open reduction converts a simple fracture into a compound (or open) fracture and thereby increases the risk of infection. Operative manipulation also increases trauma at the fracture site and may consequently add to the probability of infection. Hematomas at the site of fracture may be important for early healing; open reduction, which usually involves removing the clots in the field, could contribute to a delay in bone healing and to nonunion. The major advantage of open reduction is the shorter period of immobilization it allows, an advantage that often outweighs all the disadvantages previously mentioned, as in the open reduction of femoral neck fractures in the elderly. This allows these patients to get out of bed much sooner than if they were treated with several weeks of traction.

467–470. The answers are 467-e, 468-a, 469-b, 470-a. (*Brunicardi, pp 1694–1696, 1730–1736.*) Fractures of the navicular bone of the wrist should be suspected in anyone, particularly a young person, who falls on an outstretched hand. Although x-rays are mandatory, it is important to realize that the fracture may not be seen on the initial x-ray and that a presumptive diagnosis can and should be made on clinical grounds alone. Typically, there will be tenderness to palpation over the navicular tuberosity and limitation of wrist flexion and extension. Immobilization of the wrist for about 16 weeks and sometimes up to six months is required.

Nonunion or avascular necrosis is not uncommon and may require bone grafting for correction. Dislocation of the radial head with a fracture of the proximal third of the ulna is known as Monteggia's deformity. Usually, the radial head is dislocated anteriorly. The injury is usually caused by forced pronation. The injury can be treated by reduction and stabilization of the ulna followed by reduction of the radial head via supination and direct pressure.

Greenstick fractures are common in children. The bones of young children are able to bend to a greater degree than those of adults; the fracture may occur only at the site of maximal cortical stress but not at the opposite cortex, the site of maximal longitudinal compression. A spiral fracture, frequently seen in the tibia in skiers, results from the application of torque to a long bone. Anterior shoulder dislocations occur more frequently than posterior dislocations. However, posterior dislocations are seen in special situations, such as during an epileptiform convulsion and during electroshock therapy. Closed reduction followed by immobilization is usually sufficient therapy.

471–474. The answers are 471-c, 472-d, 473-a, 474-e. (*Brunicardi, pp 231, 1655.*) Osteitis fibrosa cystica is commonly associated with hyperparathyroidism. Hemorrhagic cystic lesions (brown tumors) usually occur in the long bones. Treatment is parathyroidectomy. Osteomalacia is defined as a defect in mineralization of adult bone that results from abnormalities in vitamin D metabolism. Treatment generally involves vitamin D supplementation. Osteogenesis imperfecta is a genetically determined disorder in the structure or processing of type I collagen. Treatment is surgical and involves orthoses to prevent fractures and correction of deformities by multiple osteotomies. Osteitis deformans is also known as Paget's disease.

Osteopetrosis is a rare skeletal deformity associated with increased density of the bones.

475–477. The answers are 475-d, 476-b, 477-f. *(Brunicardi, pp 1664–1673.)* Osteosarcoma, or osteogenic sarcoma, usually is seen in patients between the ages of 10 and 25 years. The distal femur is the site most frequently involved. The radiograph has a blastic, or sunburst, appearance. The tumor is not sensitive to radiation but does respond well to combination chemotherapy followed by surgical resection or amputation.

An osteoid osteoma typically presents with severe pain that is characteristically relieved by aspirin. On radiograph, the lesion appears as a small lucency (usually <1.0 cm) within the bone that is surrounded by reactive sclerosis. These lesions gradually regress over 5 to 10 years, but most are excised to relieve symptoms. Surgical extirpation is usually curative.

Ewing's sarcoma is a round cell–type tumor. This is a highly malignant tumor that affects children (age range 5 to 15 years) and tends to occur in the diaphyses of long bones. The spine and pelvis can also be primary sites.

There is a permeative pattern of bone lysis and periosteal reaction often associated with a large soft tissue mass. Fever and weight loss are common. The pain is often more pronounced at night. Treatment usually involves a combination of radiation and systemic chemotherapy, with five-year survivals around 50%. Adjuvant surgery in combination with radiation and chemotherapy improves the five-year survival rate to about 75%.

Neurosurgery

Questions

DIRECTIONS: Each item below contains a question followed by suggested responses. Select the **one best** response to each question.

478. A severely traumatized woman is seen in the ER with a Glasgow coma scale of 5T. Her family asks what the significance of this measurement is. Which of the following statements regarding the Glasgow coma scale is true?

a. It serves to assess the long-term sequelae of head trauma
b. A high score correlates with a high mortality rate
c. It includes measurement of intracranial pressure
d. It includes measurement of pupillary reflexes
e. It includes measurement of verbal response

479. A 25-year-old unhelmeted man involved in a motorcycle collision has multiple cerebral contusions on head CT scan. He is agitated but hemodynamically stable, with a heart rate of 80 beats per minute and a mean arterial pressure of 90 mmHg. An intracranial pressure (ICP) monitor is placed, and the initial ICP reading is 30 mmHg. Which of the following is the most appropriate in the management of his traumatic brain injury?

a. Hyperventilation to maintain a cerebral P_{CO_2} of 25 to 30 mmgHg
b. Administration of neosynephrine to increase his mean arterial pressure and, consequently, his cerebral perfusion pressure
c. Administration of mannitol (1 g/kg) to reduce his intracranial pressure
d. Placement of the patient in Trendelenburg position to increase cerebral perfusion
e. Avoidance of all sedating drugs in the first 24 to 48 h in order to accurately assess his neurologic status

480. A 50-year-old woman complains of headaches and lateralizing weakness. A CT scan of the brain reveals an irregular mass in the right cerebral hemisphere. A biopsy documents that this is a glioblastoma. Which of the following statements regarding glioblastoma multiforme is true?

a. It is a neuronal cell tumor
b. It arises from the malignant degeneration of an astrocytoma
c. With aggressive treatment, most patients can live up to 10 years with this disease
d. It is the most common childhood intracranial neoplasm
e. With combined surgery, chemotherapy, and radiation therapy, cure rates now approach 50%

481. A 60-year-old woman presents to her physician with a three-week history of severe headaches. A contrast CT scan reveals a small, circular, hypodense lesion with ringlike contrast enhancement. Which of the following is the most likely diagnosis?

a. Brain abscess
b. High-grade astrocytoma
c. Parenchymal hemorrhage
d. Metastatic lesion
e. Toxoplasmosis

482. During the secondary survey of a trauma patient, it becomes apparent that there is a depressed skull fracture. You must decide if this changes the management plan for this patient in any way. Which of the following statements regarding skull fractures is true?

a. Depressed fractures are those in which the patient's level of consciousness is diminished or absent
b. Compound fractures are those in which the skull is fractured and the underlying brain is lacerated
c. Any bone fragment displaced more than 1 cm inward should be elevated surgically
d. Drainage of cerebrospinal fluid via the ear or nose requires prompt surgical treatment
e. Most skull fractures require surgical treatment

483. A 39-year-old man presents to his physician with the complaint of loss of peripheral vision. Which of the following findings are demonstrated by the subsequent magnetic resonance imaging (MRI) scan, shown here?

a. Cerebral atrophy
b. Pituitary adenoma
c. Optic glioma
d. Pontine hemorrhage
e. Multiple sclerosis plaque

484. An 18-year-old male is admitted to the emergency room following a motorcycle accident. He is alert and fully oriented, but witnesses to the accident report an interval of unresponsiveness following the injury. Skull films disclose a fracture of the left temporal bone. Following x-ray, the patient suddenly loses consciousness and dilation of the left pupil is noted. Which of the following is the most likely diagnosis?

a. A ruptured berry aneurysm
b. An acute subdural hematoma
c. An epidural hematoma
d. An intraabdominal hemorrhage
e. A ruptured arteriovenous malformation

485. A 42-year-old woman presents to the emergency room with the worst headache of her life. She undergoes a noncontrast CT scan, which demonstrates no intracerebral lesions and is negative for acute hemorrhage. She then undergoes a lumbar puncture, which appears bloody. All four tubes collected have red blood cell counts greater than 100,000/mL. Which of the following steps is the most appropriate management of this patient?

a. Repeat the head CT scan with intravenous contrast
b. Perform an angiogram of the aorta and lumbar branches for immediate embolization of the injured vessel
c. Perform a four-vessel cerebral angiogram
d. Administer a dose of mannitol
e. Consult neurosurgery for immediate ventriculostomy

486. A trauma patient with a closed head injury is being monitored in the neurosurgical ICU. His ICP measurement is seen to rise precipitously. An acute increase in intracranial pressure is characterized by which of the following clinical findings?

a. Respiratory irregularities
b. Decreased blood pressure
c. Tachycardia
d. Papilledema
e. Compression of the fifth cranial nerve

487. A 32-year-old nonsmoking housewife has a chest x-ray, which shows a posterior mass in the right upper chest. CT documents a pleural-based rounded mass in the posterior mediastinum. The clinical diagnosis is schwannoma of the intercostal nerve. Which of the following statements about schwannomas is true?

a. They represent central nerve tumors
b. Treatment is via excision
c. They arise most frequently in motor nerves
d. They often degenerate to malignancy
e. The most common presentation is a painful mass

488. An 18-year-old high school senior develops peripheral vision abnormalities. A CT of the brain reveals a cystic suprasellar mass with some calcification noted. Clinically, this is compatible with a craniopharyngioma. Which of the following statements about craniopharyngiomas is true?

a. The tumors are uniformly solid
b. The tumors are usually malignant
c. Children with these tumors often develop signs and symptoms of acromegaly
d. The tumors may cause compression of the optic tracts and visual symptoms
e. The primary mode of treatment is radiation therapy

489. Following significant head trauma, a 34-year-old woman receives a CT scan that demonstrates bilateral frontal lobe contusions of the brain. There is no midline shift. Which of the following statements regarding cerebral contusions is true?

a. They occur most frequently in the occipital lobes
b. They may occur opposite the point of skull impact
c. They are rarely accompanied by parenchymal bleeding
d. They may occur spontaneously in patients receiving anticoagulants
e. Anticonvulsants have no role in the early management of this disorder

490. A patient's left-sided weakness prompts a CT scan, which demonstrates a mass in the left hemisphere with well-circumscribed edges abutting the skull. The clinical diagnosis is meningioma. You are about to speak with the patient and her family regarding management recommendations and prognosis. Which of the following statements is true regarding meningiomas?

a. They are malignant in 50% of cases
b. They occur predominantly in men
c. They are treated primarily by surgical excision
d. They are cured, when properly treated, in nearly 95% of cases
e. They arise from the dura

DIRECTIONS: Each group of questions below consists of lettered options followed by a set of numbered items. For each numbered item, select the **one** lettered option with which it is **most** closely associated. Each lettered option may be used once, more than once, or not at all.

Questions 491–492

For each description, select the type of vascular event with which it is most likely to be associated.

a. Subdural hematoma
b. Epidural hematoma
c. Carotid dissection
d. Brain contusion
e. Ruptured intracranial aneurysm

491. While watching a golf tournament, a 37-year-old man is struck on the side of the head by a golf ball. He is conscious and talkative after the injury, but several days later he is noted to be increasingly lethargic, somewhat confused, and unable to move his right side.

492. A 42-year-old woman complains of the sudden onset of a severe headache, stiff neck, and photophobia. She loses consciousness. She is later noted to have a dilated pupil.

Neurosurgery

Answers

478. The answer is e. *(Townsend, pp 492–493.)* The Glasgow coma scale was developed to enable an initial assessment of the severity of head trauma. It is now also used to standardize serial neurologic examinations in the early postinjury period. It measures the level of consciousness using three parameters: verbal response (5 points), motor response (6 points), and eye opening (4 points); a "T" is used in lieu of a verbal score when the patient is intubated. The score is the sum of the highest number achieved in each category and ranges from 3 for a completely unresponsive patient to 15 for a fully oriented and alert patient. A score of 13 to 15 is considered a mild traumatic brain injury (TBI), 9 to 12 a moderate TBI, and 8 or less a severe TBI. The GCS score can be used to prognosticate outcome and likelihood of neurosurgical intervention.

479. The answer is c. *(Townsend, pp 2154–2155.)* The cerebral perfusion pressure (CPP) is calculated as the difference between the mean arterial pressure (MAP) and the intracranial pressure (ICP); optimally the CPP should be maintained at greater than 70 mmHg and the ICP at less than 20 mmHg. Methods for reducing ICP include elevation of the head of the bed (reverse Trendelenburg), administration of mannitol or other diuretics to improve cerebral blood flow, use of short-acting sedatives to decrease patient agitation (the drugs should be intermittently held to perform neurological examinations), prevention of hypovolemia and treatment of hypotension, and prevention of hypoventilation and hypercapnia. Hypoventilation and hypercapnia cause vasodilation of the cerebral vessels, which increases the intracranial volume and pressure. Currently, prolonged hyperventilation is not recommended. Use of pressors to maintain a CPP above 70 mmHg is controversial.

480. The answer is b. *(Townsend, p 2144.)* Glioblastoma multiforme is the most common form of primary intracranial neuroepithelial tumor. It is a heterogeneous glial cell tumor derived from the malignant degeneration of an astrocytoma or anaplastic astrocytoma. These tumors are most commonly found in the cerebral hemispheres during the fifth decade of life. CT and MRI scans typically reveal an irregular lesion with hypodense central necrosis, peripheral ring enhancement of the highly cellular tumor tissue, and surrounding edema and mass effect. Curative resections are rare. Therapy consists of surgical resection followed by external beam radiation. The course of the disease progresses rapidly after presentation, with median survival being one year.

481. The answer is d. *(Townsend, pp 2142, 2150.)* The CT findings are consistent with any of the suggested lesions. However, the most likely diagnosis is metastatic disease, which has an incidence of approximately 150,000 to 250,000 cases per year as compared to primary intracranial tumors, which have an incidence of 35,000 per year. Roughly 15 to 30% of cancer patients develop intracranial metastases during the course of their disease. The cancers that most frequently metastasize to the brain parenchyma include those of the lung, breast, kidney, GI tract, and melanomas. Leukemia shows a predilection for the leptomeninges. A large majority of these lesions become symptomatic owing to mass effect from white matter edema. Treatment is dependent on the number and size of the lesions and the physical condition of the patient, but may include a combination of surgery, radiosurgery, and whole-brain radiation therapy.

482. The answer is c. *(Brunicardi, pp 1615–1617.)* Most skull fractures do not require surgical treatment unless they are depressed or compound. A general rule is that all depressed skull fractures—defined as fractures in which the cranial vault is displaced inward—should be surgically elevated, especially if they are depressed more than 1 cm, if a fragment is over the motor strip, or if small, sharp fragments are seen on x-ray (as they may tear the underlying dura). Compound fractures, defined as fractures in which the bone and the overlying skin are broken, must be cleansed and debrided and the wound must be closed. When a skull fracture occurs in the area of the paranasal sinuses, the mastoid air cells, or the middle ear, a tear in the meninges may result in cerebrospinal fluid drainage from the ear or nose. The presence of rhinorrhea or otorrhea requires observation; although meningitis is a serious sequela, the role of prophylactic antibiotics is controversial. Otorrhea usually heals within a few days. Persistent cerebrospinal fluid from the nose or ear for more than 14 days requires surgical repair of the torn dura.

483. The answer is b. (*Brunicardi, p 1636.*) This T_1-weighted sagittal MRI scan reveals a dumbbell-shaped homogeneous mass involving the sella turcica and the suprasellar region. This lesion is most consistent with a pituitary adenoma, a benign tumor arising from the adenohypophysis. Pituitary adenomas are the most common sellar lesion and constitute 10 to 15% of all intracranial neoplasms. Macroadenomas are greater than 1 cm in size and microadenomas less than 1 cm. Pituitary adenomas may be functional, resulting in endocrinopathies from excessive hormone secretion, such as prolactin (amenorrhea or galactorrhea), growth hormone (gigantism or acromegaly), or ACTH (Cushing's syndrome). The tumor pictured is a macroadenoma; these larger tumors may cause symptoms secondary to mass effect; for example, a bitemporal visual field defect can result due to a compression of the optic chiasm. This tumor's dumbbell shape results from impingement on the adenoma by the diaphragm of the sella turcica. The suprasellar extension seen here makes a frontal craniotomy rather than the more commonly utilized transsphenoidal approach more appropriate.

484. The answer is c. (*Brunicardi, p 1619.*) Epidural hematomas are typically caused by a tear of the middle meningeal artery, and they may be associated with linear skull fractures, usually in the temporal region. The lesion appears as a hyperdense biconvex mass between the skull and the brain on CT scan. Clinical presentation is highly variable, and outcome depends largely on promptness of diagnosis and surgical evacuation. The typical history is one of head trauma followed by a momentary alteration in consciousness and then a lucid interval lasting for up to a few hours. This is followed by a loss of consciousness, dilation of the pupil on the side of the epidural hematoma, and then hemiparesis of the contralateral side. If treated promptly, outcome is favorable in 85 to 90% of cases. Treatment consists of temporal craniectomy, evaluation of the hemorrhage, and control of the bleeding vessel.

485. The answer is c. (*Townsend, pp 2135–2139.*) The patient's history of the "worst headache of her life" and initial exam findings are suggestive of a subarachnoid hemorrhage. As opposed to traumatic lumbar taps, the red blood cell count does not diminish between the first and last tubes collected when a subarachnoid hemorrhage is present; xanthochromia, due to bilirubin in the cerebrospinal fluid, causes the fluid to appear yellow.

Workup should proceed to a four-vessel cerebral angiogram to assess for a cerebral aneurysm. Given that only about 85% of cerebral aneurysms are identified on the initial study, a second angiogram should be performed within 7 to 10 days after the first study to completely rule out an aneurysm. Initial management consists of medical therapy to counteract vasospasm, blood pressure control, and anticonvulsant therapy. Although hydrocephalus can result from blockage of the arachnoidal channels, ventriculostomy is not the surgical management of choice. Surgical treatment should be initiated within the first 48 h and consists of craniotomy with clipping of the aneurysm.

486. The answer is a. (*Brunicardi, pp 1613–1614.*) The onset of irregular respirations, bradycardia, and, finally, increased blood pressure with increasing intracranial pressure (ICP) is termed the Cushing response. These physiologic alterations are caused by brainstem compression. Slow rises in ICP are, by contrast, autoregulated by the brain's compensatory mechanisms and lead to a late onset of neurologic sequelae. A mass lesion is more apt to compromise local cerebral blood flow and to increase cerebral edema and ICP. The vector of the mass effect may lead to herniation of brain parenchyma through the tentorial incisura or foramen magnum, with resultant brainstem compression. Herniation usually causes compression of the third cranial nerve and thus leads to a fixed and dilated pupil on that side. Papilledema is a finding with chronic increases in ICP.

487. The answer is b. (*Townsend, pp 2147–2149, 2151.*) Benign schwannomas, or peripheral nerve sheath tumors that arise from perineural fibroblasts (Schwann cells), are treated with surgical excision. Because schwannomas do not involve the motor roots, sacrifice of the involved nerve and affected nerve root are of no significant consequence. Malignant schwannomas, which are rare, are treated with radiation therapy if curative resection is not possible. Intracranial schwannomas most frequently originate in the vestibular branch of the eighth cranial nerve and represent 10% of all intracranial neoplasms. Symptoms include hearing loss, tinnitus, and vertigo. Bilateral vestibular schwannomas are associated with neurofibromatosis-2; patients with this disease also present with meningiomas and ependymomas. Neurofibromas are also Schwann cell tumors but are histologically distinguishable from schwannomas; patients with multiple neurofibromas typically have neurofibromatosis-1 or von Recklinghausen's disease. Other peripheral nerve tumors include ganglioneuromas, neuroblastomas, chemodectomas, and pheochromocytomas.

488. The answer is d. *(Brunicardi, p 1637.)* Craniopharyngiomas are cystic tumors with areas of calcification and originate in the epithelial remnants of Rathke's pouch. These usually benign tumors are found in the sellar and suprasellar region and lead to compression of the pituitary, optic tracts, and third ventricle. As a result, they show up on radiographic imaging as an area of sellar erosion with calcification within or above the sella. Craniopharyngiomas are most commonly found in children but may also present in adulthood. In children, they can cause growth retardation because of hypothalamic-pituitary dysfunction. Treatment consists of subfrontal or transsphenoidal excision with adjuvant radiotherapy if total removal is not possible.

489. The answer is b. *(Brunicardi, p 1618.)* Cerebral contusions are bruises of neural parenchyma that most commonly involve the convex surface of a gyrus. The most frequent sites of cerebral contusion are the orbital surfaces of the frontal lobes and the anterior portion of the temporal lobes. The etiology of the contusion is always traumatic. Injuries may be seen both at the site of impact (coup) and in parenchyma opposite the site (contrecoup). Patients deemed to have a substantial contusion should receive anticonvulsive medication to prevent seizures in the early posttraumatic period.

490. The answer is c. *(Townsend, p 2147.)* Meningiomas are relatively benign tumors that arise from the arachnoid layer of the meninges. They occur predominantly in women and are treated primarily by surgical excision. Even with a grossly complete resection, there is a 10% 10-year recurrence rate.

491–492. The answers are 491-a, 492-e. *(Townsend, pp 2135–2142, 2152–2157.)* Subdural hematomas usually arise from tears in the veins bridging from the cerebral cortex to the dura or venous sinuses, often after only minor head injuries. They can become apparent several days after the initial injury. Treatment is drainage of the hematoma through a burr hole; a formal craniotomy may be required if the fluid reaccumulates. Significant brain contusions due to blunt trauma are usually associated with at least transient loss of consciousness; similarly, epidural hematomas result in a period of unconsciousness, although a lucid interval may follow, during which neurologic findings are minimal.

Subarachnoid hemorrhage (SAH) in the absence of antecedent trauma most commonly arises from a ruptured intracranial aneurysm, which typically is found at the bifurcation of the major branches of the circle of Willis. Other, less frequent causes of SAH include hypertensive hemorrhage, trauma, and bleeding from an arteriovenous malformation. Patients typically present with the sudden onset of an excruciating headache. Complaints of a stiff neck and photophobia are common. Loss of consciousness may be transient or may evolve into frank coma. Cranial nerve palsies are seen as a consequence both of increased intracranial pressure due to hemorrhage and pressure of the aneurysm on adjacent cranial nerves. CT scans followed by cerebral arteriography help to confirm the diagnosis as well as to identify the location of the aneurysm. Treatment consists of surgical ligation of the aneurysm by placing a clip across its neck. Early surgical intervention (within 72 h of SAH) may prevent aneurysmal rebleeding and allow aggressive management of posthemorrhage vasospasm.

Otolaryngology

Questions

DIRECTIONS: Each item below contains a question followed by suggested responses. Select the **one best** response to each question.

493. A 14-year-old boy is brought to medical attention because of nasal fullness and bleeding. Inspection and biopsy confirm nasopharyngeal carcinoma. Which of the following statements concerning nasopharyngeal cancer is true?

a. It has an unusually high incidence among Chinese
b. It occurs primarily after the sixth decade of life
c. It undergoes early metastasis to the lungs
d. The treatment of choice is wide surgical excision of the primary tumor
e. Radiation therapy has little role in the treatment of nasopharyngeal cancer

494. A young motorcycle driver is thrown against a concrete bridge abutment and sustains severe trauma about the face, with marked deformity and bleeding. Regarding these injuries, which of the following statements is true?

a. Evaluation of the cervical spine should precede that of the facial injuries
b. Severe hemorrhage from the nasopharynx rarely occurs with LeFort fractures
c. Direct oral or nasotracheal intubation should be performed promptly to prevent airway obstruction
d. Standard facial x-ray series are preferable to computed tomography to assess facial fractures because they may be obtained in the emergency department, are performed faster, and are equally accurate
e. Definitive management of fractures of facial bones should not be delayed

495. A 48-year-old man with a strong history of cigarette use and heavy alcohol intake presents with an intraoral mass. Biopsy shows squamous cell cancer. Which of the following statements regarding squamous cell carcinoma of the head and neck is true?

a. Squamous cancers of the head and neck are caused by smoking tobacco rather than chewing tobacco
b. Chemotherapy rarely produces a response with pharyngeal carcinoma and is not employed
c. Squamous cancers of the nasopharynx are best treated by radiotherapy; surgery is reserved for lymph node metastases that have not responded to radiation
d. Squamous cancers of the oropharynx are best treated by radiotherapy; surgery is not recommended
e. For squamous cancers of the hypopharynx, radical neck dissection is performed only if lymph nodes are enlarged

496. Your patient presents with a complaint of small masses inside her lips, which have been slowly enlarging. Biopsy shows a pleomorphic adenoma. You must discuss this tumor with your patient in preparation for surgery. Pleomorphic adenomas (mixed tumors) of the salivary glands are characterized by which of the following?

a. They occur most commonly on the lips, tongue, and palate
b. They grow rapidly
c. They rarely recur if simply enucleated
d. They present as rock-hard masses
e. They have no malignant potential

497. A 5-year-old child presents with a small mass near the anterior border of the sternocleidomastoid muscle. Which of the following statements about branchial cleft anomalies is true?

a. A fistula that lies between the external auditory canal and the submandibular region originates from the second branchial cleft
b. The course of the first branchial cleft fistula is through the bifurcation of the carotid artery
c. Injury to the hypoglossal nerve may occur during excision of a second branchial cleft fistula
d. The internal opening of the second branchial cleft fistula is usually found in the maxillary sinus
e. The internal opening of the first branchial cleft cyst is just underneath the base of the tongue

498. A 21-year-old woman asks you to evaluate a small painless lump in the midline of her neck that moves with swallowing. You make the clinical diagnosis of thyroglossal duct cyst. Which of the following statements regarding symptomatic thyroglossal duct cysts is true?

a. Over 90% manifest themselves before age 12
b. Treatment includes resection of the hyoid bone
c. They usually present as a painful swelling in the lateral neck
d. Approximately 10 to 15% contain malignant elements
e. They rarely become infected

499. A 60-year-old smoker is seen because of an ulcerating mass on his tongue. Biopsy establishes that this is cancer. He declines surgical intervention. Which of the following statements regarding cancer of the tongue is true?

a. Carcinomas of the tongue are best treated by irradiation alone rather than surgery
b. Metastases to the preauricular lymph nodes is common
c. Cancer of the tongue most commonly occurs near the frenulum
d. Local invasion may result in hypoglossal or lingual nerve dysfunction
e. Elective neck dissection is not indicated in early-stage tumors

500. A dentist notices a shaggy white mass in the gingivobuccal recess in a 68-year-old man who chews tobacco. Carcinoma of the buccal mucosa is identified with which of the following characteristics?

a. It is not associated with tobacco chewing
b. Stage I and II tumors are best treated initially with chemotherapy
c. Surgery followed by radiation therapy is the treatment of choice for advanced buccal carcinomas
d. Involvement of the mandible or maxilla at presentation is rare
e. It rarely spreads to cervical lymph nodes

Otolaryngology

Answers

493. The answer is a. (*Greenfield, p 655.*) There is an unusually high incidence of carcinoma of the nasopharynx among Chinese, and it is associated with Epstein-Barr virus infections. The incidence of nasopharyngeal carcinoma has a bimodal distribution in the teen years and between ages 45 and 55. Most patients present with a neck mass, and up to 20% of patients may already have bilateral cervical nodal involvement at that time. Less than 5% of patients have distant metastases on presentation. Diagnosis of nasopharyngeal cancer, which tends to arise in relatively young people, should be made by biopsy of the primary tumor. Radiation therapy is the initial treatment of choice for the primary nasopharyngeal cancer.

494. The answer is a. (*Greenfield, pp 305–319.*) In patients with severe facial or mandibular trauma, airway difficulties may develop secondary to the effects of massive hemorrhage, tissue swelling, or associated laryngeal trauma. If oral or nasotracheal intubation cannot be performed easily, cricothyroidotomy or emergency tracheostomy should be performed. Evaluation of the cervical spine is a top priority and should be performed in any patient with head trauma prior to further facial studies. Although most facial fractures can be diagnosed easily with a standard radiographic facial series, computed tomography (CT) is more accurate and allows assessment of areas (e.g., intracerebral contents) that cannot be evaluated by conventional techniques. CT is the preferred method of evaluation for patients with severe maxillofacial trauma. Maxillary fractures are categorized by the LeFort classification, and, unlike other facial fractures, are frequently associated with severe nasal and nasopharyngeal hemorrhage. This may be treated with head elevation and ice compresses. Nasal packing also affords good control of hemorrhage, and in extreme cases ligation or embolization of the internal maxillary artery may be necessary. Definitive reduction and fixation of fractures may be delayed while other injuries and medical problems are addressed. In addition to control of hemorrhage, initial management of facial fractures may include temporary stabilization and wound closure.

495. The answer is c. *(Brunicardi, pp 515–536.)* Squamous cell cancers of the head and neck appear to arise as a response to tobacco in general (including chewing tobacco), rather than just to cigarette smoking, especially when used in combination with alcohol ingestion. Chemotherapy for squamous cell pharyngeal cancer has been used very successfully in childhood and adolescence, although its role in adult pharyngeal cancer is uncertain. Treatment of nasopharyngeal squamous cell carcinoma is by radiation, followed by radical neck dissection if lymph node metastases have not been controlled. Oropharyngeal cancers have responded equally well to surgery and radiation, and both treatments are routinely employed. In the hypopharynx, surgery is the optimal treatment, often supplemented by postoperative radiation therapy. Surgery for hypopharyngeal cancers includes radical neck dissection because lymph node metastases occur frequently and are not well controlled by radiation alone.

496. The answer is a. *(Brunicardi, pp 538–540.)* Pleomorphic adenomas (mixed tumors) can occur in either the major (submandibular, parotid, and sublingual) or minor salivary glands. These round tumors have a rubbery consistency and are slow-growing; all are potentially malignant. Unless adequately excised, they tend to recur locally in a high percentage of cases. The sites most commonly affected by pleomorphic adenomas of the salivary glands are the lips, tongue, and palate.

497. The answer is c. *(Greenfield, pp 1932–1935.)* Branchial cleft cysts, sinuses, and fistulas are remnants of the first and second branchial pouches. The internal opening of the first is the external auditory canal; for the second, it is the posterolateral pharynx below the tonsillar fossa. The facial nerve may be injured during dissection of the first fistula. The second fistula passes between the carotid bifurcation and adjacent to the hypoglossal nerve. In childhood, most branchial cleft anomalies present as a painless nodule along the lateral border of the sternocleidomastoid muscle. In adults, superinfection of the cyst or fistulous drainage via an orifice in the supraclavicular region may occur. Treatment is surgical excision.

498. The answer is b. *(Greenfield, pp 1935–1936.)* Thyroglossal duct cysts result from retention of an epithelial tract between the thyroid and its embryologic origin in the foramen cecum at the base of the tongue. This tract usually penetrates the hyoid bone. There is no sex predilection, and although these cysts are more frequently detected in children, they may not become symptomatic until adulthood. The most common presentation is a painless swelling in the midline of the neck that moves with protrusion of the tongue or swallowing. The cysts are prone to infection and progressive enlargement. Although rare (less than 1%), epidermoid or papillary carcinomas do occur within thyroglossal duct cysts. Surgical resection is the standard therapy. The Sistrunk procedure, which involves local resection of the cyst and the central portion of the hyoid bone, is the operation of choice. Simple excision of the cyst results in an unacceptably high recurrence rate.

499. The answer is d. *(Brunicardi, p 519; Greenfield, pp 653–654.)* Cancers of the tongue commonly present on the lateral or ventral surface of the tongue. Metastases to the submandibular or cervical nodes are common. Local invasion may result in tongue deviation due to involvement of the hypoglossal nerve or decreased sensation due to involvement of the lingual nerve. Treatment is surgical—wide local excision of the tumor and neck dissection as needed. In patients without nodal metastases, neck dissection is indicated for more invasive tumors.

500. The answer is c. *(Brunicardi, p 521; Greenfield, p 654.)* Buccal carcinoma is an uncommon oral cavity cancer, which tends to be locally aggressive. Because of the lack of symptoms, patients often present with involvement of the mandible or maxilla and up to half of patients present with cervical metastases. Predisposing risk factors include lichen planus and tobacco chewing. Wide excision is the best initial treatment for this neoplasm. Advanced tumors should be treated with surgery followed by postoperative radiation. Chemotherapy does not have a significant role in the treatment of buccal carcinomas.

Pediatric Surgery

Questions

DIRECTIONS: Each item below contains a question followed by suggested responses. Select the **one best** response to each question.

501. A neonate is examined in the nursery and found to have no anal orifice; only a small perineal fistulous opening is visualized. Decision as to the operative approach necessitates determining how high or low the anus has descended. Which of the following statements concerning imperforate anus is true?

a. Imperforate anus affects males more frequently than females
b. In females, a low imperforate anus often occurs with a persistent cloaca
c. The rectum usually ends in a blind pouch
d. The chance for eventual continence is greater when the rectum has descended to below the levator ani muscles
e. Immediate definitive repair of the anatomic defect is required to maximize the chance of eventual continence

502. A 2-month-old boy is examined because he has been straining while passing stool and has a distended abdomen. He is very low on the growth chart for age. A rectal examination and biopsy is performed. Which of the following statements concerning Hirschsprung's disease is true?

a. It is initially treated by colostomy
b. It is best diagnosed in the newborn period by barium enema
c. It is characterized by the absence of ganglion cells in the transverse colon
d. It is associated with a high incidence of genitourinary tract anomalies
e. It is the congenital disease that most commonly leads to subsequent fecal incontinence

503. A newborn has a midline defect in the anterior abdominal wall. The parents ask what, if anything, should be done. Spontaneous closure of which of the following congenital abnormalities of the abdominal wall generally occurs by the age of 4?

a. Umbilical hernia
b. Patent urachus
c. Patent omphalomesenteric duct
d. Omphalocele
e. Gastroschisis

504. A neonate is found to have an imperforate anus. As the pediatric surgeon consulting, you recommend studies to search for other anomalies because infants with anorectal anomalies tend to have other congenital anomalies. Associated abnormalities include which of the following?

a. Abnormalities of the cervical spine
b. Hydrocephalus
c. Duodenal atresia
d. Heart disease
e. Corneal opacities

505. A 36-h-old infant presents with bilious vomiting and an increasingly distended abdomen. At exploration, the segment pictured here is found as the point of obstruction. Which of the following statements regarding this finding is true?

a. Resection with primary anastomosis should not be performed
b. Gentle, persistent traction on the specimen usually corrects the defect and removes the need for a resection
c. The lesion is much more common in the jejunum than in the ileum in this age group
d. This problem is probably related to mesenteric vascular insufficiency
e. A properly monitored barium enema might have corrected this defect and removed the need for an operation

506. A 1-year-old child has repeated episodes of vomiting and abdominal distention. An x-ray shows obstruction at the second portion of the duodenum. Laparotomy is performed and an annular pancreas is discovered. For a symptomatic partial duodenal obstruction secondary to an annular pancreas, which of the following is the operative treatment of choice?

a. A Whipple procedure
b. Gastrojejunostomy
c. Vagotomy and gastrojejunostomy
d. Partial resection of the annular pancreas
e. Duodenoduodenostomy

507. Approximately two weeks after a viral respiratory illness, an 18-month-old child complains of abdominal pain and passes some bloody mucus per rectum. A long, thin mass is palpable in the right upper quadrant of the abdomen. Intussusception is suspected. Correct statements concerning intussusception in infants include which of the following?

a. Recurrence rates following treatment are high
b. It is frequently preceded by a gastrointestinal viral illness
c. A one- to two-week period of parenteral alimentation should precede surgical reduction when surgery is required
d. Hydrostatic reduction without surgery rarely provides successful treatment
e. The most common type occurs at the junction of the descending colon and the sigmoid colon

508. An 18-year-old female presents with abdominal pain, fever, and leukocytosis. With the presumptive diagnosis of appendicitis, a right lower quadrant (McBurney) incision is made and a lesion 60 cm proximal to the ileocecal valve is identified (see photo). Which of the following statements is true regarding this lesion?

a. Can best be diagnosed by preoperative angiogram, which should be done whenever the diagnosis is suspected
b. Should routinely be removed when incidentally discovered during celiotomy
c. Is embryologically derived from a persistent vitelline duct (omphalomesenteric duct)
d. Often contains ectopic adrenal tissue
e. Is frequently associated with cutaneous flushing and episodic tachycardia

509. A 17-year-old girl presents with an anterior neck mass. Her thyroid scan, shown here, is most consistent with which of the following disorders?

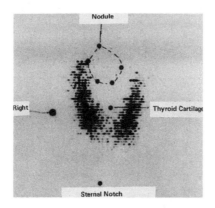

a. Hypersecreting adenoma
b. Parathyroid adenoma
c. Thyroglossal duct cyst
d. Graves' disease
e. Carcinoma

510. A full-term male newborn experiences respiratory distress immediately after birth. A prenatal sonogram was read as normal. An emergency radiograph is shown here. The patient is intubated and placed on 100% O_2. Arterial blood gases reveal pH 7.24, P_{O_2} 60 kPa, and P_{CO_2} 52 kPa. The baby has sternal retractions and a scaphoid abdomen. Which of the following statements correctly refers to this condition?

a. The most likely cause of this problem is in utero traumatic rupture of the diaphragm
b. The most important aspect in management is immediate exploration and repair of the defect
c. The size of the defect directly correlates with severity of the disease
d. The defect is usually anteromedial in location
e. Any abdominal organ can be involved

511. A 2-year-old asymptomatic child is noted to have a systolic murmur, hypertension, and diminished femoral pulses. Which of the following is true about this child's disorder?

a. Atrial septal defects (ASDs) are frequently associated
b. The child is unlikely to become normotensive even with surgical intervention
c. Rib notching is often seen on x-ray
d. Claudication is frequently noted
e. Older children with this disorder almost always have symptoms of heart failure

512. A 35-week term infant presents with cyanosis shortly after birth. His arterial oxygen saturation is only 30%. Which of the following is the most likely diagnosis?

a. Patent ductus arteriosus
b. Coarctation of the aorta
c. Atrial septal defect
d. Ventricular septal defect
e. Transposition of the great vessels

DIRECTIONS: Each group of questions below consists of lettered options followed by a set of numbered items. For each numbered item, select the **one** lettered option with which it is **most** closely associated. Each lettered option may be used once, more than once, or not at all.

Questions 513–514

For each patient, select the most likely congenital cardiac anomaly.

a. Tetralogy of Fallot
b. Ventricular septal defect
c. Tricuspid atresia
d. Transposition of the great vessels
e. Patent ductus arteriosus

513. A noncyanotic two-day-old child has a systolic murmur along the left sternal border; examination is otherwise normal. Chest x-ray and electrocardiogram are normal.

514. A 3-year-old child has congenital cyanosis.

Pediatric Surgery

Answers

501. The answer is d. (*Brunicardi, pp 1497–1499.*) Imperforate anus affects males and females with equal frequency, occurring in 1 in 5000 live births. It is due to failure of descent of the urorectal septum. Imperforate anus may be broadly classified into high or low, depending on whether the rectum ends above or below the level of the levator ani complex. The rectal fistula may end in the prostatic urethra or vagina in the high cases, while the low cases terminate in a perineal fistula. In females, high imperforate anus often occurs with a persistent cloaca. For the low cases, only a perineal operation may be required, and these children will be expected to be continent. A pull-through procedure will be required for the high imperforate anus, and the likelihood of continence is smaller. If there is doubt about the level or location of the termination of the rectum, it is better to perform a temporary colostomy than to compromise the ultimate chances of continence by an injudicious perineal approach.

502. The answer is a. (*Brunicardi, pp 1496–1497.*) Hirschsprung's disease, which is the congenital absence of ganglion cells in the rectum or rectosigmoid colon, is definitively diagnosed by rectal biopsy. The typical findings on barium enema—a distal narrow segment of bowel with markedly distended colon proximally—may not be seen early in life. Symptoms may go unrecognized in the newborn period, with consequent development of malnutrition or enterocolitis. Initial treatment is colostomy decompression. Definitive repair is best delayed until nutritional status is adequate and the chronically distended bowel has returned to normal size. Unlike the situation with imperforate anus, which is associated with a high incidence of genitourinary tract anomalies and risk of long-term fecal incontinence, in Hirschsprung's disease repair leads to satisfactory bowel function in most affected patients.

503. The answer is a. (*Brunicardi, pp 1501–1504.*) In most children, umbilical hernias close spontaneously by the age of 4 and need not be repaired unless incarcerated or symptomatic. Omphalocele and gastroschisis result in evisceration of bowel and require emergency surgical treatment to effect immediate or staged reduction and abdominal wall closure. Patent urachal or omphalomesenteric ducts result from incomplete closure of embryonic connections from the bladder and ileum, respectively, to the abdominal wall. They are appropriately treated by excision of the tracts and closure of the bladder or ileum.

504. The answer is d. (*Brunicardi, p 1498.*) Congenital anorectal anomalies are frequently associated with other congenital anomalies including heart disease, esophageal atresia, abnormalities of the lumbosacral spine, double urinary collecting systems, hydronephrosis, and communication between the rectum and the urinary tract, vagina, or perineum. Patients may present with a number of anomalies collectively known as the VACTERL syndrome: **V**ertebral anomalies, **A**nal atresia, **C**ardiac defect (e.g., ventricular septal defect), **T**racheo**E**sophageal fistula, **R**enal anomalies, and **L**imb defects (e.g., radial dysplasia). They occur in approximately 1 in 5000 live births. A variety of surgical procedures have been devised to treat the problem, depending on the type of anomaly (whether the rectum ends above or below the level of the levator ani complex). However, even when anatomic integrity is established, the prognosis for effective toilet training is poor. In 50% of cases, continence is never achieved. Cervical spine abnormalities, hydrocephalus, duodenal atresia, and corneal opacities have no significant association with congenital anorectal anomalies.

505. The answer is d. (*Brunicardi, p 1488.*) This is an example of an ileal atresia. Whether the atresia is jejunal or ileal does not affect treatment, and there is no predilection for one site over the other. The basis of jejunoileal atresia is probably a mesenteric vascular accident during intrauterine growth. Resection and primary anastomosis should be performed if possible, but the bowel should be exteriorized if there is a question of viability or a large size discrepancy between two segments. Plain films will reveal a small-bowel obstruction with no gas beyond the lesion. A carefully administered Gastrografin enema can help in the differential diagnosis. Midgut volvulus and meconium ileus can be apparent on an enema, which is important, as meconium ileus should be managed nonoperatively.

506. The answer is e. (*Brunicardi, pp 1487–1488.*) A bypass procedure is the operation of choice for obstruction secondary to an annular pancreas. A Whipple procedure (pancreaticoduodenectomy) is too radical a therapy for this benign condition, and a partial resection of the annular pancreas often is complicated by fistula. Duodenoduodenostomy is much more physiologic than gastrojejunostomy and does not require a vagotomy to prevent marginal ulceration; it is therefore the procedure of choice.

507. The answer is b. *(Brunicardi, pp 1493–1494.)* Intussusception is the result of invagination of a segment of bowel into distal bowel lumen. The most common type is ileocolic, which typically appears as a coiled spring on barium enema. Ileoileal and colocolic intussusceptions occur less commonly and are not easily diagnosed on barium enema. If bloody mucus, peritonitis, or systemic toxicity have not developed, hydrostatic reduction by barium enema is the appropriate initial treatment. Most patients are successfully managed this way and do not require surgical intervention. Immediate treatment should be instituted to avert the danger of bowel infarction. Recurrence is surprisingly uncommon after either surgical or nonsurgical treatment.

508. The answer is c. *(Brunicardi, pp 1495–1496.)* This is an inflamed Meckel's diverticulum. This common lesion is often clinically indistinguishable from acute appendicitis. It is the remnant of the vitelline duct. Meckel's diverticula are usually located 60 cm proximal to the ileocecal valve, are antimesenteric, and may contain either gastric and pancreatic or only pancreatic tissue. Hemorrhage or obstruction is a more common presentation than inflammation. ^{99m}Tc pertechnetate has affinity for gastric mucosa, and a scan with this isotope can aid in the diagnosis of this anomaly as a cause of lower gastrointestinal hemorrhage in a child. Angiography is more useful when looking for arteriovenous malformations. Since complications are relatively rare, most authors do not recommend removing asymptomatic diverticula when they are incidentally discovered during abdominal procedures. Those diverticula with a narrow neck, palpable heterotopic tissue, or nodularity are prone to obstruction and should be excised. In addition, patients explored for abdominal pain of unknown etiology should also undergo diverticulectomy, as should those operated on for appendicitis who are to be left with a scar of the right lower quadrant.

509. The answer is c. *(Brunicardi, p 1475.)* The thyroid gland originates embryologically from the foramen cecum at the base of the tongue. Normally, the thyroglossal duct becomes obliterated and resorbed, but portions may remain patent and become filled with serous fluid, which produces a midline cervical mass. Observe that in the scan, the mass is central and appears not to be part of the gland itself.

510. The answer is e. *(Brunicardi, pp 1476–1478.)* This radiograph of a child with a scaphoid abdomen and respiratory disease is characteristic of a congenital diaphragmatic hernia. These defects are posterolateral and occur due to failure of the embryologic diaphragm to fuse between the eighth and twelfth weeks of intrauterine life. The size of the defect does not correlate with the symptoms. Even a large diaphragmatic hernia can be missed on prenatal sonogram if the abdominal contents have slipped back into the abdomen at the time of the study. Hernias of Morgagni are anteromedial and do not present as emergencies at birth. Any abdominal organ—pancreas, kidney, small and large intestine, stomach, liver, or spleen—can herniate into the chest. The abdominal organ acts as a space-occupying lesion and retards growth of the lung, which results in pulmonary hypoplasia. Respiratory problems at birth stem from primary pulmonary hypertension, the consequence of hypoplasia, rather than from compression of the lung by abdominal contents. Most experts recommend stabilizing the pulmonary hypertensive crisis medically or with extracorporeal membrane oxygenation (ECMO) prior to attempting repair.

511. The answer is c. *(Greenfield, pp 1459–1460.)* Coarctation of the aorta is a congenital anomaly that usually causes narrowing of the aorta just distal to the left subclavian artery in the area of the ligamentum arteriosum. Collateral circulation develops around the obstruction by way of intercostal vessels and accounts for the classic x-ray appearance of rib notching. Without surgery, complications in adults arise with eventual death from cardiac failure, rupture of aortic aneurysms or of a cerebral artery, and bacterial endocarditis. Coarctation is often associated with ventricular septal defects (VSDs) and aortic stenosis. Patients who are operated on earlier in life have a better chance of becoming normotensive. Claudication is not a common feature of this disorder.

512. The answer is e. *(Greenfield, pp 1443–1463.)* With the exception of coarctation, in which no shunt (or cyanosis) exists, the anomalies listed cause a shunting of blood between the systemic and lower-pressure pulmonary circulation. Transposition of the great vessels is a right-to-left shunt that leads to cyanosis. Except where there is persistent congenital pulmonary hypertension, patent ductus arteriosus and atrial septal defects cause a shunting of oxygenated blood from the aorta and left atrium, respectively, back into the pulmonary artery and right atrium. These anomalies cause recirculation of oxygenated blood within the cardiopulmonary circuit but not cyanosis. When a ventricular septal defect is combined with pulmonary artery atresia (tetralogy of Fallot), the resulting undercirculation in the pulmonary system joins transposition as a cause of cyanosis. Other, less common congenital lesions in which the pulmonary arterial blood flow is relatively decreased include tricuspid atresia, Ebstein's anomaly, and hypoplastic right ventricle.

513–514. The answers are 513-b, 514-a. (*Greenfield, pp 1443–1463.*) Ventricular septal defect accounts for 20 to 30% of all congenital cardiac anomalies. It may lead to cardiac failure and pulmonary hypertension if the defect is larger than 1 cm, or it may be asymptomatic if the defect is small. Surgery is not indicated for the asymptomatic patient with a small defect since a substantial number of these anomalies close spontaneously during the first few years of life. Operation is indicated in infants with congestive heart failure or rising pulmonary vascular resistance (owing to the left-to-right shunt). Additionally, operation is indicated if the VSD has not closed by age 5. Tetralogy of Fallot, transposition, and tricuspid atresia are cyanotic lesions. Congenital cyanosis that persists beyond the age of 2 years is associated, in the vast majority of cases, with tetralogy of Fallot. Patent ductus arteriosus is associated with the characteristic continuous machinery murmur.

Bibliography

Belkin M et al: Intra-arterial fibrinolytic therapy. Efficacy of streptokinase vs urokinase. *Arch Surg* 121:769–773, 1986.

Blumgart LH, Fong Y: *Surgery of the Liver and Biliary Tract,* 3/e. New York: W.B. Saunders, 2000.

Boucher CA et al: Determination of cardiac risk by dipyridamole-thallium imaging before peripheral vascular surgery. *N Engl J Med* 312:389–394, 1985.

Brewster DC et al: Intestinal ischemia complicating abdominal aortic surgery. *Surgery* 109:447–454, 1991.

Brunicardi FC, et al (eds): *Schwartz's Principles of Surgery,* 8/e. New York: McGraw-Hill, 2005.

Bunt TJ et al: Frequency of vascular injury with blunt trauma–induced extremity injury. *Am J Surg* 160:226–228, 1990.

Cass AS: Renovascular injuries from external trauma. Diagnosis, treatment, and outcome. *Urol Clin North Am* 16:213–220, 1989.

Charlson ME et al: The preoperative and intraoperative hemodynamic predictors of postoperative myocardial infarction or ischemia in patients undergoing noncardiac surgery. *Ann Surg* 210:637–648, 1989.

Cosentino CM et al: Choledochal duct cyst: Resection with physiologic reconstruction. *Surgery* 112:740–748, 1992.

Cummings RA et al: Pneumopericardium resulting in cardiac tamponade. *Ann Thorac Surg* 37:511–518, 1984.

Dutky PA et al: Factors affecting rapid fluid resuscitation with large-bore introducer catheters. *J Trauma* 29:856–860, 1989.

Eisbud DE et al: Treatment of acute vascular occlusions with intraarterial urokinase. *Am J Surg* 160:160–165, 1990.

Erwin TJ et al: Multidisciplinary treatment of advanced squamous carcinoma of the head and neck. *Semin Oncol* 12:71–82, 1985.

Executive Committee for the Asymptomatic Carotid Atherosclerosis Study. *JAMA* 273:1421–1428, 1995.

Flint L et al: Definitive control of mortality from severe pelvic fracture. *Ann Surg* 211:703–707, 1990.

Gobbi PG et al: The role of surgery in the multimodal treatment of primary gastric non-Hodgkin's lymphomas. *Cancer* 65(11):2528–2536, 1990.

Goodnough LT, Shuck JM: Risks, options, and informed consent for blood transfusion in elective surgery. *Am J Surg* 159:602–609, 1990.

Greenfield LJ et al (eds): *Surgery: Scientific Principles and Practice,* 3/e. Philadelphia: Lippincott-Raven, 2001.

Heys SD et al: Nutrition and malignant disease: Implications for surgical practice. *Br J Surg* 79:614–623, 1992.

Landercasper J et al: Perioperative stroke risk in 173 consecutive patients with a past history of stroke. *Arch Surg* 125:986–989, 1990.

Mahmoodian S: Appendicitis complicating pregnancy. *South Med J* 85:19–24, 1992.

McQuaid KR, Isenberg JI: Medical therapy of peptic ulcer disease. *Surg Clin North Am* 72:285–316, 1992.

Merrell SW, Schneider PD: Hemobilia: Evolution of current diagnosis and treatment. *West J Med* 155:621–625, 1991.

Moore EE et al (eds): *Trauma,* 5/e. New York: McGraw-Hill, 2004.

O'Hara PJ et al: Surgical management of aortic aneurysm and coexistent horseshoe kidney: Review of a 31-year experience. *J Vasc Surg* 17:940–947, 1993.

Pasternack PF et al: The value of the radionuclide angiogram in the prediction of perioperative myocardial infarction in patients undergoing lower extremity revascularization procedures. *Circulation* 72:13–17, 1985.

Podolosky DK: Inflammatory bowel disease. *N Engl J Med* 325:928–937, 1991; 114:593–597, 1991.

Reilly HF, al-Kawas FH: Dieulafoy's lesion. Diagnosis and management. *Dig Dis Sci* 36:1702–1707, 1991.

Rhame FS: Preventing HIV transmission. Strategies to protect clinicians and patients. *Postgrad Med* 91:141–152, 1992.

Robinson T et al: Body smuggling of illicit drugs: Two cases requiring surgical intervention. *Surgery* 113:709–711, 1993.

Schirmer BD et al: Laparoscopic cholecystectomy in the obese patient. *Ann Surg* 216:146–152, 1992.

Schroeder T et al: Ischemic colitis complicating reconstruction of the abdominal aorta. *Surg Gynecol Obstet* 160:299–303, 1985.

Schwesinger WH: Is *Helicobacter pylori* a myth or the missing link? *Am J Surg* 172:411–416, 1996.

Thoren T, Wattwil M: Effects on gastric emptying of thoracic epidural analgesia with morphine or bupivacaine. *Anesth Analg* 67:687–694, 1988.

Tondini C et al: Combined modality treatment for primary gastrointestinal non-Hodgkin's lymphoma in the Milan Cancer Institute experience. *Ann Oncol* 4:831–837, 1993.

Townsend CM Jr et al (eds): *Sabiston Textbook of Surgery,* 17/e. Philadelphia: Saunders, 2004.

Trunkey DD: Shock-trauma. *Can J Surg* 27:479–486, 1984.

Way LW, Doherty GM: *Current Surgical Diagnosis & Treatment,* 11/e. New York: McGraw-Hill, 2003.

Weissman C: The metabolic response to stress: An overview and update. *Anesthesiology* 73:308–327, 1990.

Willerson JT et al: Role of new antiplatelet agents as adjunctive therapies in thrombolysis. *Am J Cardiol* 67:12A–18A, 1991.

Wilson SE et al: Operating on HIV-positive patients. What are the risks to healthcare workers? To patients? *Postgrad Med* 88:193–194, 199–201, 1990.

Index

Notes

Notes

Notes

Notes

Notes

Notes

Notes

Notes